SEARCHING FOR THE SECRETS OF NATURE

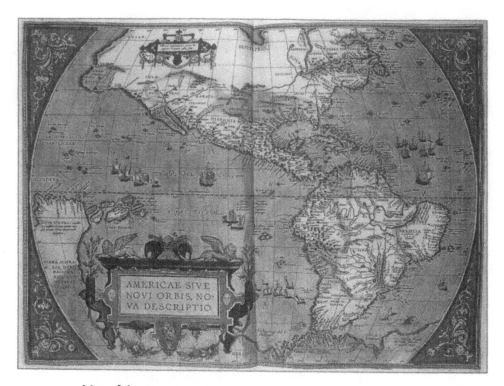

Map of the Americas, drawn in 1587, from Abraham Ortelius,
Theatre of the Whole World, first English edition,
edited and published by John Norton (London, 1606).
Courtesy of the British Library.

SEARCHING FOR THE SECRETS OF NATURE

THE LIFE AND WORKS OF DR. FRANCISCO HERNÁNDEZ

SIMON VAREY

RAFAEL CHABRÁN

DORA B. WEINER

EDITORS

STANFORD UNIVERSITY PRESS
Stanford, California

Stanford University Press
Stanford, California

© 2000 by the Board of Trustees of the
Leland Stanford Junior University

Printed in the United States of America

Library of Congress Cataloging-in-Publication Data

Searching for the secrets of nature : the life and works of Dr. Francisco Hernández /
edited by Simon Varey, Rafael Chabrán, and Dora B. Weiner.
    p.   cm.
  Includes bibliographical references and index.
  ISBN 0-8047-3964-1 (cloth : alk. paper)
    1. Hernández, Francisco, 1517–1587. 2. Natural history—Mexico. 3. Materia
medica—Mexico. I. Varey, Simon, 1951–   II. Chabrán, Rafael. III. Weiner, Dora B.
  QH31.H37 S42 2000
  508.72—dc21

                                    00-026518

Original printing 2000

Last figure indicates the year of this printing:
08 07 06 05 04 03 02 01 00

Typeset by Princeton Editorial Associates, Inc., Scottsdale, Arizona, in
9.75/16 Berkeley Old Style Medium.

CONTENTS

INTRODUCTION

PART I • THE INTELLECTUAL MILIEU OF HERNÁNDEZ

ILLUSTRATIONS

ACKNOWLEDGMENTS

This book results from several initiatives to commemorate the arrival of Columbus in America. The UCLA Center for Medieval and Renaissance Studies sponsored a proposal from David Hayes-Bautista, now director of the Center for the Study of Latino Health at UCLA, and Rafael Chabrán, chair of Modern Languages and Literatures at Whittier College, to produce an English edition of Francisco Hernández's writings. UCLA's Louise M. Darling Biomedical Library had recently acquired a copy of Hernández's famous book *Rerum medicarum Novae Hispaniae thesaurus* (Rome, 1651), thanks to funding from the Ahmanson Foundation generated by that faithful friend of books and scholarship, UCLA's late chancellor, Franklin D. Murphy.

The UCLA Committee for the Quincentenary endorsed this initiative: two of its members, David Hayes-Bautista and Dora B. Weiner, professor of the medical humanities, School of Medicine, agreed to act as principal investigators for a project carried out within UCLA's Center for Medieval and Renaissance Studies, under directors Michael J. B. Allen, then Patrick J. Geary, with the help of the assistant to the director, Susanne M. Kahle.

Several colloquiums and lecture series furthered our task. We thank the National Library of Medicine and Dr. John Parascandola, then head of the History of Medicine Division, for graciously hosting our first workshop, "The Meeting of Medical Traditions in New Spain," in April 1992. A second workshop took place at UCLA that fall. In November 1993 Elsa Malvido and Elena Morales invited the project's southern California scholars to discuss our progress at the annual conference on the history of Mexican medicine, organized by the Instituto Nacional de Antropología y Historia in Mexico City. In the spring of 1995 the Center for Medieval and Renaissance Studies and the UCLA Programs in Medical Classics cosponsored a lecture series entitled "The World of Dr. Francisco Hernández," which was well attended by audiences from both UCLA and the greater Los Angeles community.

We gratefully acknowledge a generous three-year grant from the National Endowment for the Humanities, whose award covered the bulk of our considerable expenses, including foreign travel and research. The anonymous panelists who critiqued our original proposal improved its structure and enriched its contents. The Ahmanson Foundation has been generous with grants at exactly the right moments. We are grateful to Dr. Boris Catz and Dr. Bruce Larson for their continuing support of the whole project.

Our special thanks are due to Professor José María López Piñero of the University of Valencia for his hospitality and generous assistance to our travelers.

Finally, we thank the director of Stanford University Press, Norris Pope, for his guidance and scholarly input; the Center for the Study of Latino Health for financial support of the final editorial work; Hoechst, Marion, Roussel for underwriting the cost of the illustrations; and, for their wisdom and counsel, Michael R. McVaugh and especially the late Mildred E. Mathias. We conceptualize the rich subject matter of this work as an interchange between two cultures—certainly not the "conquest" of one land by the people of another. Hernández's interest in, and deep respect for, the Nahua medical tradition pervaded his work, to which carefully painted illustrations added scientific precision and charm. We attempt to walk in his footsteps.

Dora B. Weiner
Project Director

ABBREVIATIONS

Naturally, several standard and influential works besides those of Hernández are cited repeatedly by different authors in the essays that follow. To conserve space, we abbreviate references to the most commonly cited works, as listed below.

Bataillon, *Erasmo y España* — Marcel Bataillon, *Erasmo y España: Estudios sobre la historia espiritual del siglo XVI,* 2 vols. (Mexico City: Fondo de Cultura Económica, 1950), the translated and revised edition of *Erasme et l'Espagne* (Paris, 1937).

Ciencia y técnica — José M. López Piñero, *Ciencia y técnica en la sociedad española de los siglos XVI y XVII* (Barcelona: Labor, 1979).

Códice Pomar — José M. López Piñero, *El Códice Pomar [ca. 1590]: El interés de Felipe II por la historia natural y la expedición Hernández a América* (Valencia: Instituto de Estudios Documentales e Históricos sobre la Ciencia, Universitat de València–CSIC, 1991).

M — Francisco Hernández, *Opera,* ed. Casimiro Gómez Ortega, 3 vols. (Madrid: Ibarra, 1790).

Medicinas, drogas — José M. López Piñero, José Luis Fresquet Febrer, María Luz López Terrada, and José Pardo Tomás, *Medicinas, drogas y alimentos vegetales del Nuevo Mundo: Textos e imágenes españolas que los introdujeron en Europa* (Madrid: Ministerio de Sanidad y Consumo [1992]).

Nuevos materiales — José M. López Piñero and José Pardo Tomás, *Nuevos materiales y noticias sobre la "Historia de las plantas de Nueva España" de Francisco Hernández* (Valencia: Instituto de Estudios Documentales e Históricos sobre la Ciencia, Universitat de València–CSIC, 1994).

OC — Francisco Hernández, *Obras completas,* ed. Germán Somolinos d'Ardois et al., 7 vols. (Mexico City: UNAM, 1959–84). The prefatory matter in our text volume lists the contents of this and other editions of Hernández.

QL — [Francisco Hernández], *Quatro libros: De la naturaleza, y virtudes de las plantas, y animales que estan recevidos en el uso de Medicina en la Nueva España . . . ,* ed. Francisco Ximénez (Mexico City: Widow of Diego López Davalos, 1615).

T — Francisco Hernández, *Rerum medicarum Novae Hispaniae thesaurus* (Rome: J. Mascardi, 1651).

Somolinos, "Vida y obra" — Germán Somolinos d'Ardois, "Vida y obra de Francisco Hernández," *Obras completas,* 1:97–459.

EDITORIAL METHODS

From 1571 to 1577 Dr. Francisco Hernández undertook an ambitious, royally sponsored scientific expedition to what is now Mexico: our companion text volume, *The Mexican Treasury: The Writings of Dr. Francisco Hernández,* presents substantial portions of Hernández's writings in English for the first time in the modern era. The present volume offers analysis of his achievements by scholars from six distinct disciplines. It brings together critical and contextual essays in broadly defined, chronologically sequential parts, exploring Hernández's intellectual milieu, the medical knowledge and practices of New Spain, the export of drugs and plants to Europe, the dissemination of Hernández's knowledge, and the continuing relevance of Hernández today. The essays explore a range of aspects of Hernández's experience, from the confrontation of a Spanish Christian humanist with Nahua cosmology to the appearance in paintings by Spanish masters of native Mexican flowers described by Hernández, from his education to his place in Latino Catholic civilization. The introduction highlights a number of controversies and hypotheses that invite further study.

We have not sought in any sense to homogenize or regularize the diverse essays or their contributors' voices, but we have endeavored to simplify references and make them consistent.

REFERENCES TO THE TEXTS OF HERNÁNDEZ

This collection of essays is integrally related to our companion volume of English translations of texts by Francisco Hernández, *The Mexican Treasury.* We have organized those texts historically, in order to show how, when, and where the writings of Hernández were disseminated, predominantly in the seventeenth and eighteenth centuries. Our text volume shows that there has been no shortage of Hernández texts in print since the first extracts began to appear in 1607. Yet the perception has long been that there were "really" only three editions: the *Quatro libros* (Mexico City, 1615); the *Rerum medicarum Novae Hispaniae thesaurus* (Rome, 1651); and the *Opera* (Madrid, 1790), the "Madrid edition." In 1960 a team of scholars led by Germán Somolinos d'Ardois, a Spanish exile who settled in Mexico in the 1930s, produced the first of seven volumes of Hernández under the title *Obras completas,* which is the nearest we have to a standard edition. To make references as uncomplicated and as clear as possible, each text in our text volume has been assigned a simple letter and number code (e.g., *QL* for *Quatro libros,* plus book, section number, and chapter). Throughout the essays in this collection, references to the writings of Hernández that appear in our text volume cite those codes (see Abbreviations).

INTERNET CITATIONS

Citations of reviews or articles in scholarly journals published on the World Wide Web follow the recommendations of Andrew Harnack and Gene Kleppinger in their style sheet, "Beyond the MLA Handbook: Documenting Electronic Sources on the Internet," <http://falcon.eku.edu/honors/beyond-mla/#online>.

TRANSLATIONS

A major purpose of the two volumes that make up this project is to introduce the subject of Hernández and his accomplishments to the English-speaking world, where even his name is barely known. To make Hernández accessible, we have tried to provide existing English sources and quotations, not because they are necessarily better than their equivalents in other languages but because they should help to break down linguistic and cultural barriers. Obviously, many of the sources, especially those contemporary with Hernández, are in Spanish and Latin, and a few of them were translated into English in the sixteenth and seventeenth centuries (for example, José Acosta's *Naturall and Morall Historie of the Indies* [1604]). Even though we usually cite the contemporary translations, all our contributors are aware that the translations often differ significantly from their Spanish or Latin originals. Only the most famous of the Mexican chronicles can be found in English, and many of the sonnets of Góngora or the works of Quevedo, which are occasionally quoted in these pages, have never been translated at all. In most cases like these, we have supplied our own functional translations.

In quoted matter, brackets [ ] indicate additions to the text of fragments that we believe to have been in the source text originally but that are now lost or illegible. Bent brackets ⟨ ⟩ indicate the translators' conjectural additions to a text.

As most of the scholarship previously devoted to Hernández is in Spanish, we have similarly sought out English editions of scholarly books, but otherwise we have translated quotations from books and articles. We have, of course, left titles of published works in their original forms and languages. We have translated the titles of unpublished works of Hernández, and in several cases we have invented English titles for works that Hernández himself left untitled in the surviving manuscripts. The most obvious example is the manuscript collection of writings on the plants, minerals, insects, fish, quadrupeds, and birds of New Spain, which is cited throughout the present volume as the *Natural History of New Spain,* but we should emphasize that this title always refers to the manuscripts, never to the many published selections, redactions, and translations that have appeared since 1607.

CHRONOLOGY

Chronology and geography are the eyes of history.

—Francis Bacon

1515	Francisco Hernández born, perhaps of Jewish descent, in La Puebla de Montalbán, near Toledo.
1516	Thomas More's *Utopia* published.
1519	Charles I of Spain succeeds Maximilian to become Holy Roman Emperor Charles V. Leonardo da Vinci dies in France. Chocolate is introduced into Spain as a drink, followed shortly by corn.
1521	(May) Hernán Cortés begins the siege of Mexico City. Martin Luther excommunicated at Worms.
1527	Birth of Benito Arias Montano, who will become one of Spain's most distinguished intellectuals and one of Hernández's closest friends. Birth of the future Philip II.
c. 1530	Hernández begins studies at the University of Alcalá de Henares, School of Medicine. Encounters Renaissance humanism and Spanish Erasmian thinking.
1535	Execution of Sir Thomas More.
1536	Hernández receives degree of "Bachiller" of Medicine. Returns to Toledo to practice medicine, later to Seville, where he undertakes botanical research. Death of Erasmus.
1543	Publication of Vesalius's *De humani corporis fabrici libri septem.*

1547	Birth of Cervantes. Death of Kings Henry VIII of England and Francis I of France.
1550	Introduction of tobacco smoking in Spain and Portugal.
1553	Accession of Queen Mary I of England.
c. 1555	Hernández marries Juana Díaz de Paniagua.
1556	Charles abdicates in favor of his son, who becomes Philip II of Spain.
c. 1557	Hernández is appointed to a prestigious and lucrative teaching position at the hospital attached to the monastery at Guadalupe, where he studies anatomy and performs dissections. Begins to write commentaries on Galen and Hippocrates and comes into contact with Juan Fragoso.
1559	The Treaty of Cateau-Cambrésis ends wars in France and Spain.
c. 1560	After a brief spell at the Hospital of Santa Cruz in Toledo, Hernández moves to the royal court, where he meets the noted doctors Andrés Laguna and Francisco Valles and the great anatomist Andreas Vesalius.
1561	Madrid becomes the capital of Spain.

1563   End of the Council of Trent, which condemns the principal doctrines of the Protestant Reformation.

1564   Deaths of Vesalius and Michelangelo. Births of Galileo and Shakespeare.

1565   Publication of the first of three parts of the work on Mexican medicine by Nicolás Monardes.

1566   The southern provinces in the Low Countries rebel against Spanish rule. Later, they are put down by the Duke of Alva. Election of Pope Pius V.

1567   Hernández appointed royal doctor to Philip II.

1570   Hernández receives royal instructions to undertake the first official systematic scientific expedition to the Americas. He is to study all facets of the natural history of New Spain, including the history of the region. He is also expected to travel to Peru. Sails (September 1) from Seville, accompanied by his son Juan and Francisco Domínguez, a geographer. They stop at the Canary Islands, Hispaniola, and Cuba, where Hernández carries out three series of botanical studies.

1571   Hernández arrives at Veracruz and soon begins his work. Battle of Lepanto.

1572   Leiden joins William of Orange against the Spanish. Election of Pope Gregory XIII.

1571–75 Hernández studies and writes, rethinks, and rewrites his work on the natural history of New Spain.

1575   University of Leiden founded.

1576   Outbreak of an epidemic in New Spain, locally called *cocoliztli*. After years of evasions and delays, Hernández finally sends some manuscripts of his *Natural History of New Spain* to the king.

1577   Hernández returns to Spain with another copy of his manuscripts, which are not intended for the king. These will become the fortuitous basis for an edition eventually published in 1790.

1578   Hernández is named physician to the king's son, the future Philip III. In failing health, Hernández writes his will.

1579   The northern provinces of the Low Countries declare their independence from Spain and form a republic by the Union of Utrecht two years later.

1580   Philip II appoints Nardo Antonio Recchi to make a selection from the work of Hernández. The author's resentment appears in an unpublished poem to his old friend Benito Arias Montano.

1585   The Treaty of Nonsuch, between England and the independent provinces of the northern Low Countries, precipitates a state of war between England and Spain. Election of Pope Sixtus V.

1587   (January 28) Hernández dies in Madrid. The University of Leiden establishes a botanical garden.

1588   The Spanish Armada is destroyed off the coast of the British Isles.

1590   The second edition of José Acosta's *Historia natural y moral* mentions Hernández's epic project in New Spain.

1592   Fabio Colonna becomes the first scholar to incorporate any material from the Hernández expedition in print, when he describes *Datura stramonium* in his *Phytobasanos*. Election of Pope Clement VIII.

1598   Deaths of Philip II and Benito Arias Montano. The Edict of Nantes declares toleration of Huguenots in France.

1607   First English settlement at Jamestown. Juan Barrios publishes *Verdadera medicina, cirugía y astrología* in Mexico City. This book contains a text of Hernández in Spanish.

1611   (April) In Rome, Galileo Galilei, the latest recruit to Federico Cesi's new Accademia dei Lincei, is shown a set of five hundred illustrations from the Hernández expedition depicting Mexican plants. Cesi is seeking to publish Recchi's selection from Hernández as the publication that will secure the new academy's international recognition.

1615   A Spanish translation of Recchi's selection from the work of Hernández, read and approved by Francisco Valles and obtained by Juan Barrios, is published in Mexico City. Francisco Ximénez is responsible for the *Quatro libros: De la naturaleza de . . . Nueva España*.

1616   Deaths of Cervantes and Shakespeare.

SEARCHING FOR THE SECRETS OF NATURE

INTRODUCTION

THE WORLD OF DR. FRANCISCO HERNÁNDEZ

DORA B. WEINER

During his exploration of Mexico in the 1570s, Dr. Francisco Hernández identified more than 3,000 plants previously unknown in Europe. To appreciate the scale of this work, we may note that Theophrastus had inventoried about 350 plants, Dioscorides and the Islamic botanists between 500 and 600 each. Hernández's treasure was too rich and varied to allow for integration into traditional European taxonomy, too voluminous and baffling to encourage speedy publication, too controversial to fit into the orthodox worldview of Philip II's Spain. But the "Mexican treasury" gradually enriched European botany more than any other work. To evaluate Hernández's achievement, we begin by surveying his world.

In Hernández's lifetime, between 1515 and 1587, Spain partook of the revolutions that transformed Europe during the Renaissance, the Reformation, and the Catholic Reform, but on its own terms. It had fought the "infidel" Moors for eight hundred years, its back turned to the Continent while it faced south and east. With the accession of Charles, the king of Spain, to the dignity of Holy Roman Emperor in 1519, when Hernández was a child, the relationship of Spain to the European continent changed, but not its self-

appointed mission. Emperor Charles V, grandson of the Habsburg emperor Maximilian as well as of King Ferdinand of Aragón and Queen Isabella of Castile, had continental interests to defend. He fought Martin Luther, the French, and the Turks, traveling back and forth from his Austrian empire to his Spanish kingdoms. He used Spanish money and soldiers to defend the pope and the Habsburgs. At the same time he watched Spain funnel its most meaningful national efforts into domestic religious reform and expansion overseas, for as soon as the Spaniards had overcome the Moorish kingdom of Granada in 1492, they turned westward beyond Gibraltar, looking across the Atlantic Ocean, particularly to a region they named New Spain.

Thus the sixteenth century ushered in the birth of a powerful national monarchy in Castile, as it did in France and England. But in contrast to northern Europe, where protests against abuses and luxury in the Catholic Church mushroomed into Protestantism, in Spain the spirit of Christian renewal found expression through Catholic reform. Representative leaders included Cardinal Jiménez de Cisneros, who spearheaded the Inquisition; Ignatius of Loyola, who founded and led the Society of Jesus; and Teresa de

Ávila and Juan de la Cruz, who inspired thousands with the poetic expressions of their deeply felt faith.

A unique amalgam of global power and Catholic orthodoxy emerged in Spain under Philip II: Peter O'Malley Pierson analyzes the imperial obligations of Philip in the following essay. Pierson also presents a Philip interested in science and technology, as portrayed by David C. Goodman in *Power and Penury* (1988).

The intellectual milieu of Francisco Hernández's Spain (the focus of Part I of these essays) developed against the backdrop of global imperial ambitions and religious conformity. In the fifteenth and early sixteenth centuries, the Renaissance did not bring to Spain a flowering of the visual and plastic arts or a joyful burst of intellectual creativity as it did in Italy. Spain's Golden Century came later. Rather, in the cultural life of Spain, the Renaissance fostered the rise of Christian humanism, entailing the search for the early religious texts and their comparative and critical study. The humanists' labors reached into philosophy, science, and medicine, but in Spain the basis was grammar and philology. Such studies were important to Christian humanists throughout western Europe, of course, but rarely was the exact meaning of key theological concepts a crucial matter of personal safety and even survival for every mature intellectual, as it was in Renaissance Spain. These preoccupations deeply affected education, including that of a medical student such as Hernández. Rafael Chabrán analyzes these issues in the first essay on Hernández's intellectual milieu. He shows how Cisneros founded the University of Alcalá de Henares to further these studies and how he nurtured that masterpiece of Spanish Renaissance erudition, the Polyglot Bible, in Greek, Latin, and Hebrew, completed at Alcalá in 1514 by Antonio de Nebrija, Juan de Vergara, and others.

A similar scholarly project was occupying the great northern humanist Desiderius Erasmus at this same time—he published his Polyglot Bible even before the Alcalá project was printed. These shared interests brought Erasmus to the attention of Spanish scholars; and Erasmus's learned editions of fundamental Christian texts, his caricatures of superstitious religious practices, and his disagreements with Luther made *erasmismo* the rallying cry of reformers and a major theme of controversy in Spain. Critical scholarship

and the spirit of free inquiry thus challenged obedience to tradition.[1]

Tradition continued to fashion the teaching of medicine when Hernández came to the University of Alcalá de Henares in late 1529. Everyone still accepted the classical theories of the four humors (blood, phlegm, yellow and black bile) and the temperaments (sanguine, phlegmatic, choleric, and melancholic), as well as the natural, vital, and animal spirits, and their physiology according to Galen. The Hippocratic theory of fevers and their crises prevailed, with attention to the "six non-naturals"—air, diet, sleep, exercise, digestion, and management of the passions—and the regimen of health as propagated at the medical school of Salerno.

However, the new spirit of critical inquiry was also making inroads, moving from grammar and philology into botany and the pharmacopoeia as well as the reinterpretation of ancient and medieval medical texts. This new critical attitude furthered study of the *Canon of Medicine* by Avicenna and the *Chirurgia* of Guy de Chauliac, as well as a humanistic interpretation of Galen, based on his *De anatomicis administrationibus,* in contrast to the traditional, scholastic, and Arabist emphasis on Galen's *De usu partium.* The first Spanish chair of anatomy was established at Valencia, and in the 1540s news of the revolutionary teaching of Vesalius reached Spain; the master himself entered the service of Charles V soon after the publication of *De humani corporis fabrici libri septem* in 1543. Pedro Jiménez, a student of Vesalius's at Padua, came to Alcalá as professor of anatomy in 1550. Hernández met Vesalius at court, before the great anatomist left on his fatal pilgrimage to Jerusalem.[2]

Medical students throughout Europe now eagerly sought a chance to watch and perform "anatomies" like the ones that had made Vesalius famous and to gain firsthand knowledge of medicinal plants as well as acquire the skill to formulate medications. In late medieval Castile, the order of the Hieronymites had built monasteries with hospitals that became famous for their medical care and apothecaries' skills. The brothers had long permitted lay physicians and surgeons to practice in their hospitals: the teaching of surgery, as well as possibly some bedside teaching, was pursued at the hospital at Guadalupe when Hernández served as physician at that hospital in the late 1550s. He botanized in the surrounding countryside, profited from the rich library, and surely shared the humanistic, *erasmista* outlook prevailing at this extraordinary institution.[3] In his commentaries on the *Natural History* of Pliny, Hernández alludes to his own dissections of human cadavers at Guadalupe and also—of particular interest for our purposes—the dissection of a chameleon.[4]

It was through his interest in therapeutics and especially in medicinal plants that Hernández was drawn into Philip II's project of sending a scientific expedition to New Spain, a project that Hernández's great friend Arias Montano may have been the first to suggest to the king. Curiosity about the New World, its peoples, fauna, and flora, had flared instantly all over Europe when Columbus and Magellan changed the common perception of a flat, circumscribed earth into that of an accessible globe. Curiosity about nature had a long history in European learned circles. Furthermore, in Hernández's student days, the printing press was making the classics of natural history more readily available and affordable, books such as Aristotle's *Historia animalium,* Pliny the Elder's *Natural History,* and Dioscorides' *Materia medica.* These texts now invited critical study for two contradictory reasons: scholars wished to learn about the ancients' knowledge of nature, but they also nurtured a growing skepticism toward traditional mythical creatures such as the phoenix, siren, unicorn, harpy, and griffin familiar to the medieval public from hundreds of frescoes, capitals, bas reliefs, and manuscripts. Scholars knew, of course, that exotic creatures with peculiar shapes or habits, or dangerous powers, had actually been observed, such as the ostrich, pelican, elephant, owl, hedgehog, and viper. They knew that occult and mysterious powers were being claimed for plants such as the mandrake or remedies such as theriaca. The new task for Renaissance scholars was to check traditional images against features observed in the field so as to arrive at an objective inventory of natural history.

The exact observation of nature was thus a key to the growth of knowledge in pharmacy and medicine, and Hernández's reports from Mexico reveal the modern scientific approach that he had absorbed at Alcalá and Guadalupe.

In the second essay analyzing Hernández's milieu, Simon Varey depicts a restless man of many talents: a physician with some clinical and perhaps even experimental experience, an active botanizer, and by the 1560s already an expert on Pliny's *Natural History,* which he finished translating and annotating while in New Spain in the 1570s. In New Spain, Hernández not only described and depicted plants and animals in every detail but sometimes tested their medicinal properties on himself; he learned and analyzed Nahua traditions and practices and included geography, climate, and anthropological considerations in his writings. He tested his findings in a self-critical manner and added lavish visual representations to his written descriptions. Varey calls Hernández a "Renaissance man," which, in Philip II's Spain and New Spain, meant a scholar and scientist as many sided, inquisitive, secular, and practical as his controlling environment permitted. In Varey's words, Hernández intended to "seek out and describe *everything.*"

To complete Part I, Carmen Benito-Vessels notes the disturbing intolerance in Hernández's intellectual milieu and argues that Philip kept his *protomédico* in exile and censored publication of the *Natural History* in Hernández's lifetime. The reasons are intriguing: Benito believes that Spanish theologians perceived Hernández's naming of animals and plants as a heretical activity, because only God has the power to name and thus create living beings. Hernández presumed to write "the literary equivalent of the book of Genesis in Philip's empire." Besides, Hernández's association with Alcalá and especially with the hospital at Guadalupe meant that he was perceived as the friend of Judaizers—perhaps even being of Jewish descent himself.[5] According to this thesis, Philip therefore decided to silence his protomédico: Benito argues that the king kept Hernández in Mexico much longer than the distinguished naturalist wished to stay and that the king effectively prevented the publication of the doctor's book. Benito's argument parallels that of Georges Baudot, as we shall see later.

When Philip chose a physician to study and collect the animals, plants, herbs, and seeds of New Spain and New Castile, he made a logical choice. The connection of medicine with zoology and botany had traditionally been close, as evinced by the widespread medicinal use of "simples," that is, parts or products of animals and plants, directly applied for therapeutic purposes. In fact, all the outstanding zoologists and many of the botanists among Europe's sixteenth-century naturalists were physicians, but none of them traveled to the New World. Nor did Hernández's famous countryman the physician and botanist Nicolás Monardes (1493–1588), whose three-part *Historia medicinal de las cosas que se traen de nuestras Indias Occidentales* was published in Seville between 1565 and 1574. Only two Spanish nonmedical naturalist authors preceded Hernández as travelers: Gonzalo Fernández de Oviedo y Valdés (1478–1557), official historiographer of the Indies, who journeyed six times to America and wrote the *General y natural historia de las Indias,* partly published in 1526 and 1535, in its entirety only in 1851; and José Acosta (1539–1600), a Jesuit missionary who spent twenty years in Peru and wrote the *Historia natural y moral de las Indias* (1589), which quickly went into numerous editions in all the modern languages. They and Hernández were the pioneer travelers in the Western Hemisphere.

None of the English, French, Dutch, or Portuguese explorers and seafarers of the era was inspired by a grand design such as King Philip's to advance the practice of medicine and the preservation of health in the mother country by importing knowledge and remedies from overseas. Thus one can imagine that Spanish youths, and even older men such as Hernández, believed that it was their destiny, and no one else's, to unlock the secrets of the New World.

Once appointed "general protomédico of all the Indies, islands, and mainland of the Ocean Sea," Hernández outfitted himself and departed, in September 1570, with his son Juan as his personal aide.[6] That a man in his fifties should undertake so hazardous a journey proves enthusiastic dedication. Hernández wished personally to see, feel, taste, measure, test, describe every plant and animal of the New World that might be of use to Spain and to have them pictured in color by able artists. Philip, he repeatedly wrote to the king, would be the new Alexander—meaning, of course, that Hernández's work should be compared to Aristotle's. A proposed expedition of two years took seven, even though Hernández never reached Peru, which the king had initially included in the itinerary.

"Medical Knowledge and Practices in New Spain," Part II of this collection of essays, focuses on the professional context of Hernández's overseas explorations. It opens with John Jay TePaske's discussion of the regulation of medical practice in New Spain. In Hernández's day, colonial city councils regulated their own practitioners; the formal machinery of the *protomedicato* was not instituted until 1646. Hernández had little power as protomédico and seems rapidly to have come to terms with this situation and concentrated on botany.

In "Shelter and Care for Natives and Colonists: Hospitals in Sixteenth-Century New Spain," Guenter B. Risse reconstructs the probable hospital experience of two patients whose names we know—one a native victim of the dreaded *cocoliztli,* the other a Spaniard suffering from syphilis. The varied examples of contemporary hospital establishments give a realistic idea of the institutions, personnel, medications, practices, and obstacles Francisco Hernández encountered in his travels through Mexico. He practiced extensively in these hospitals, and Risse's essay permits us to share Hernández's experience.

Elsa Malvido and David A. Boruchoff, on the other hand, allow us to identify with native thought: Malvido pens an impassioned accusation against the conquerors of her country, especially because they imported deadly diseases. Even though the ensuing near extinction of native populations was unintentional, she finds the white Catholic Spaniards guilty of genocide. Boruchoff explores Hernández's perception of native health practices in the context of Nahua cosmology: to this end he analyzes the *Antiquities of New Spain.* Boruchoff recognizes Hernández's open-minded and objective appreciation of native health rituals and medicinal usage. He finds Hernández well aware that New World natural history as perceived by a Renaissance man was certain to conflict with Catholic moral philosophy. A sixteenth-century Spanish author such as Hernández had deftly to orchestrate two dissonant themes: mindful of censorship, he had to show respect toward medieval medicine's own mixture of mythical creatures, magical powers, miraculous events, and mysterious sympathies. At the same time he had to fulfill his professional mission and record his personal evaluation of native health practices. Part II is followed by a brief descriptive account by Rafael Chabrán and Simon Varey of what Hernández actually did in New Spain: what he studied and how.

Part III, "The Dissemination of Hernández's Knowledge," opens up a wide horizon. In "The Reception of American Drugs in Europe, 1500–1650," by J. Worth Estes, there are few surprises, as we read about guaiacum, balsams, jalap, and sassafras, followed by special attention to tobacco and cacao (which we shall encounter again later, in England). Bezoar stones and coca leaves from Peru are mentioned here, but they remained beyond Hernández's firsthand observation. Estes finds that, every time a new American medicinal plant appeared on the European market, it flourished temporarily as a panacea. What surprises is the author's conclusion that by 1800 the old Galenic remedies again dominated in European medical practice.

Next we read a masterful overview by the doyen of Hernández scholars, José María López Piñero and his colleague José Pardo Tomás. They assess Hernández's contribution to all of European botany and materia medica. They single out vanilla, tomato, and corn but also *Datura stramonium* and peyote. This essay surveys the keen interest of sixteenth- and seventeenth-century European naturalists in Hernández's new American information. It traces the use and mention of Hernández's botanical discoveries all the way to Linnaeus, the nineteenth century, and beyond, viewing later Spanish botanical expeditions to the Americas, especially to New Spain, as a "continuation of Hernández's work."

While this work remains central to the argument, the scene then shifts to the Netherlands and England. Rafael Chabrán and Simon Varey visit botanical gardens and personal libraries, catalogs, and correspondence and follow leads as diverse as personal contacts, the politics of the printing press, the circulation of books, translations, and plagiarism. Chocolate ranks high among prized American imports.

María José López Terrada then offers a strikingly different and magnificently illustrated piece in which she tracks eleven foods, decorative and useful plants described by Hernández and possibly brought to Spain by him. She finds the plants in the paintings of Spanish seventeenth-century masters and in the diet and homes of their contemporaries. The author also traces related issues, such as the religious symbolism associated with the passionflower or the established myths that surrounded the sunflower, and compares Mexican and European contexts. She indicates how gardening skills guided the spread of seeds and flowers toward northern Europe.

Jaime Vilchis follows with an analysis of the reception, absorption, and emulation of Hernández's writings, a process he calls "globalization." Vilchis sees the Accademia dei Lincei, the force behind the publication of Hernández's *Thesaurus* in 1651, as an "invisible college," seeking to propagate its own cosmology, believing that the author was equally keen on harmonizing Nahua and Christian philosophies and religions. A brief analysis of a Jesuit "enlightened countercurrent" closes the essay.

The section's concluding essay by Leoncio López-Ocón evaluates nineteenth- and twentieth-century Spanish scholarship in the history of the natural sciences. Spain needed to redefine its relationship to its former American colonies, lost as a consequence of the Napoleonic invasion and the interdiction to interfere in the Americas, contained in the Monroe Doctrine of 1823. Spain's own reevaluation focused on its cultural mission, particularly on the exploration of nature in Latin America, where Hernández's monumental achievement was accorded pride of place. López-Ocón places the publications of Hernández's works in the historical context of Spanish scientific polemics: the *Thesaurus*, the Madrid edition of 1790, and the *Obras completas* led by Somolinos in the 1960s. These editions, and many other texts that include writings by Hernández, are amply discussed in our text volume.

Two postscripts, one by David Hayes-Bautista, the other by Simon Varey and Rafael Chabrán, record the continuation of a popular tradition of Mexican medicine in Mexico and parts of the United States today.

————

The proof of Hernández's astounding labors was contained in the twenty-two books in Latin that he brought back from New Spain in 1577 and that he had at least begun to translate into Spanish, and probably Náhuatl. He had already transmitted sixteen volumes to the king, who had them sumptuously bound in blue leather embellished with gold and silver.[7] Arriving in Madrid, Hernández realized with a shock that priorities and the climate of opinion had changed at court. In the international sphere, the victory of Don John over the Turks at Lepanto in 1571 was now overshadowed by the Revolt of the Netherlands. Neither troops, money, nor the Inquisition could quell the Calvinists' rebellion. Worse, Queen Elizabeth of England supported them. Therefore Philip II was beginning to nurture his project of a giant naval expedition against England.

International affairs, however, by no means claimed Philip's whole attention. He was now building the Escorial, where he established research facilities, distilleries, even laboratories: Paracelsian influence had by then reached Spain, and even if the "distillers to His Majesty" mixed a little alchemy with research, there is no reason to question their experimental skill and scientific apparatus. Our Spanish contributors argue that Juan de Herrera, the Escorial's architect and adviser to the king, assembled a group of mathematicians, cosmographers, and nautical experts who formed a mathematical academy that began work at the Escorial in 1582, antedating the Lincei by twenty years. And in Spain's botanical gardens, particularly at Aranjuez, Hernández's seeds and plants found fertile soil.

The Spanish scholars contributing to this volume emphasize Philip II's passionate interest in modern science.[8] Their view contrasts sharply with the traditional image of Philip as solitary and morose, dressed in black and absorbed by religious rite and administrative detail and by the fight for a world dominated by Catholic orthodoxy and Spanish power. These clashing interpretations of the personality and psychology of Philip II are perhaps the most startling difference of opinion expressed in these essays. Richard L. Kagan has recently proposed a suggestive explanation: he traces the Anglo-Saxon portrayal of Philip to the early-nineteenth-century American historian William H. Prescott, author of classic histories of the conquests of Mexico (1843) and Peru (1847). Kagan argues that Prescott, wishing to glorify the democratic, enterprising, successful young United States of America, contrasted his perception of his own country with that of an autocratic, stagnant, orthodox nineteenth-century Spain and found in Philip the perfect embodiment of the traits he wished to stigmatize. And that image has been perpetuated in Protestant Western scholarship. Not surprisingly, Spanish scholars decry it as biased.[9]

Another major scholarly controversy apparent in the present essays concerns the eighty-year struggle to publish Hernández's manuscripts. López Piñero and Pardo briefly consider the role of the Neapolitan physician Nardo Antonio Recchi, his selections from Hernández's manuscripts, and the eventual publication in 1651 (matters dealt with in detail in our text volume). They exonerate Philip from any intention to ignore, let alone censor, Hernández. They consider the explorer's poor health to be sufficient explanation for a decision that caused the author ten years of terminal unhappiness.[10] The matter is central to Hernández scholarship.

The king deposited Hernández's manuscripts in his personal treasury in the Escorial, hanging some of the sketches for the illustrations on the walls of his study, where, exposed to too much light, dust, and dirt, they rotted. In 1580 Philip appointed Recchi to make a selection and to "arrange" Hernández's writings. It is not entirely clear if this meant that Recchi was to put the writings on Mexican topics in an order congruent with European medical tradition. Nor is it clear if Recchi's selection was intended to be the basis of an abridged publication. It is possible that choosing an editor rather than Hernández himself might reflect the king's judgment that Hernández had strayed from his original task, that the protomédico with a practical mission had turned into a prolix naturalist and anthropologist. He had, after all, been sent to report on matters useful to medicine in Spain rather than on all aspects of nature in the New World. But there is another, more sinister possibility previously alluded to in Benito's essay: that the king and the orthodox powers around him felt that Hernández had become too friendly with the heathen natives and neglected to instruct and convert them to European Christian ways of ministering to the sick. An analysis of the correspondence between Hernández and the king, argues Benito, shows Philip equally eager to keep his protomédico away and to delay publication as long as possible.

Even stronger arguments in support of prejudice on the part of crown and church can be found in the work of

Georges Baudot, who discriminates between two trends. He confirms a traditional distrust toward the native peoples of New Spain, contempt of their culture, language, and religion. But he also points to genuine alarm among members of the Council of the Indies raised by activities they deemed rebellious. The fears were at first political, stirred by the claims of Hernán Cortés's son Martín in 1566 and those of Moctezuma's grandson in 1576 that there was social unrest on the "silver frontier." But then the members grew more concerned that royal power was being undermined by widespread efforts of Spaniards to understand and educate the Mexican people. The Council of the Indies, the Inquisition, and the king worried about the millenarianism of the Franciscan missionaries who learned Náhuatl and translated Holy Writ in order to convert the native inhabitants; they condemned the ethnographic investigations of Sahagún and the anthropological explorations of Hernández as dangerously sympathetic to native culture and religion. Baudot concludes that, in 1577, when all Sahagún's work was confiscated, Hernández was ostracized.[11]

Tragically, Hernández was ill at the time he might have fought to keep control of his work. He had contracted an undefined, troublesome chronic disease, evidently a urinary condition: New Spain had broken his health. The worst tragedy, however, befell not Hernández but his written work. The sixteen volumes presented to the king perished in the great fire at the Escorial in June 1671. The rest, in Hernández's possession at his death, had vanished from view.

It is at this point that the tragic story yields tantalizing opportunities for the researcher. Several lucky circumstances stand out at the start. Recchi took his manuscript selection to Rome and eventually left it to his nephew. Prince Federico Cesi, the founder of the first modern Italian scientific academy, learned of the manuscript's existence from Fabio Colonna and purchased it, probably in 1609, for an undisclosed high price. A copy of the manuscript mysteriously found its way to Mexico, where it was translated into Spanish and published as *Quatro libros*. Cesi's Accademia dei Lincei then collaborated on and off for another half century until 1651, when *Rerum medicarum Novae Hispaniae thesaurus* finally appeared in print.[12]

There are other lucky aspects. Hernández was a perfectionist, forever revising and polishing his work. Because he was also practical, he left manuscript drafts in Mexico, where they could be put to use. He wrote his original scientific texts in Latin, but, just like Galileo in the younger generation of scientists, he was eager to reach a broad readership. Therefore he translated his work into Spanish (two books of this translation survive among his manuscript drafts) and even into Náhuatl (of which no surviving copy has been identified), thus adding to the number of manuscripts that might be extant. Some of these resurfaced in booksellers' stalls, private collections, and institutional libraries. The most dramatic survival consists of the manuscript index of part of Hernández's work, copied by the librarian of the Escorial, Brother Andrés de los Reyes, for Cassiano dal Pozzo, a Linceo. Cassiano took it to Cesi in 1626. It is now MS H101 in the Montpellier medical archives.[13] Other manuscripts undoubtedly found their way into private hands, for Hernández was widely circulated and parts of his work published in Latin, French, and Dutch, all before the publication of the *Thesaurus* in 1651. The diffusion of Hernández's discoveries is an extraordinary story in its own right, discussed in some detail in *The Mexican Treasury,* our text volume. The originality and breadth of his scholarship will be best appreciated by reading his own words. Francisco Hernández is thus shown to hold an important place in the history of medicine, botany, materia medica, science, exploration, and art.

By the time of Hernández's death in 1587 Spain's rise to supreme world power had been halted, and its intellectual horizon had become somber and narrow. The following year, Spain's wings were clipped by the "Protestant wind" that dispersed the Invincible Armada; English privateers harassed Spain's fleet and Dutch traders took its treasure. The Council of Trent had fortified the Inquisition and imposed the Index expurgatorius, and Philip II prevented most medical students from studying abroad. Spanish medicine and science entered a period of self-imposed isolation. It was fortunate indeed for posterity that King Philip had sent Hernández to New Spain in more optimistic days: eventually, the *Natural History of New Spain* would bear witness to Spanish enterprise and scientific imagination.

NOTES

1. Bataillon, *Erasmo y España,* esp. 1:1–119.

2. José María López Piñero, "La disección y el saber anatómico en la España de la primera mitad del Siglo XVI," *Cuadernos de historia de la medicina española* 13 (1974): 51–110; José Barón, "Vesalio en España," *Cuadernos de historia de la medicina española* 6 (1965): 91–102.

3. Guy Beaujouan, "La Bibliothèque et l'école médicinale du monastère de Guadalupe à l'aube de la Renaissance," in Guy Beaujouan, Yvonne Poulle-Drieux, and Jeanne Marie Dureau-Lapeyssonie, *Médecine humaine et vétérinaire à la fin du Moyen Age* (Paris: Minard, 1966; Geneva: Droz, 1966), 365–457.

4. Idem, "La medicina y la cirugía en el monasterio de Guadalupe," *Asclepio* 17 (1965): 155–70.

5. On "Judaizers," though not specifically on Hernández, cf. Richard H. Popkin, "Jewish Christians and Christian Jews in Spain, 1492 and After," *Judaism* 41 (1992): 248–67.

6. Quotation from *Mexican Treasury,* "Instructions and Letters to the King."

7. There is always confusion about "books" and "volumes." Hernández divided his work into conceptual units that he called books. The six surviving folio volumes of his manuscript drafts, similar to the volumes he presented to the king, contain twenty-four books. The reason that he presented sixteen volumes to the king is that ten of them contained illustrations.

8. Cf. José María López Piñero, "Química y medicina en la España de los siglos XVI y XVII: La influencia de Paracelso," *Cuadernos de historia de medicina* 11 (1972): 17–54, and *Códice Pomar.*

9. Richard L. Kagan, "Prescott's Paradigm: American Historical Scholarship and the Decline of Spain," *American Historical Review* 101 (1996): 423–46.

10. Hernández's will, drawn up in 1578, sheds some light on his feelings toward the end of his life. See *Mexican Treasury.*

11. Georges Baudot, *Utopia and History in Mexico: The First Chroniclers of Mexican Civilization (1520–1569),* trans. by Bernard R. Ortiz de Montellano and Thelma Ortiz de Montellano (Denver: University Press of Colorado, 1995), esp. chap. 9.

12. The secondary literature about the Accademia dei Lincei's "Mexican treasury" is huge. For this introduction the most helpful articles were the three conference papers, by Francisco Guerra, Giovanni Battista Marini-Bettolo, and Carmen María Sánchez Téllez, in *Atti dei convegni Lincei* 78 (1986): 307–42.

13. About one hundred books and manuscripts, taken to France as loot during the Directory's second Italian campaign in 1798, were bought by the librarian of the Montpellier School of Medicine. For a detailed analysis, cf. Ada Alessandrini, *Cimeli Lincei a Montpellier* (Rome: Accademia Nazionale dei Lincei, 1978).

PHILIP II
IMPERIAL OBLIGATIONS AND SCIENTIFIC VISION

PETER O'MALLEY PIERSON

When Philip II of Spain appointed Francisco Hernández to be his chief medical officer of the Indies in 1570, he had recently become the first sovereign in world history to rule an empire on which the sun never set.[1] In 1565 Spanish conquistadores sailing from Mexico had begun to colonize the Philippines, named for their king, which they added to his already extensive dominions in Europe, North Africa, and the Americas. No prince of his time was better prepared for the task of ruling a world empire than Philip. Had it not been for his emphasis on religion and consequent religious intolerance, he might have proved the most enlightened of enlightened despots, fulfilling the expectations of an eighteenth-century philosophe. It is the watershed in thought and sensibility marked by that century and inherited by us that makes Philip in crucial respects seem foreign to us. In Philip's own century there was no separation of church and state, and the spiritual welfare and safety of subjects were as much a concern of government as their material welfare and safety.

The treatment of Philip II by historians from his own time into the eighteenth century reflected religious and national differences, as historians took sides for or against him. During the Enlightenment new prejudices emerged, and the judgments of Philip's enemies were enshrined by thinkers who regarded the Church of Rome as an infamous thing and Spain, where the Inquisition was not finally abolished until 1834, the benighted citadel of bigotry. As ruler of Spain at the peak of its world power, Philip represented tyranny, obscurantism, and intolerance in action and seemed opposed to all that was regarded as enlightened, liberal, and modern. More balanced studies of the man and his reign began to appear only in the twentieth century, as earlier passions subsided. Historians now strive for an objective understanding of the intensity of religious feeling and immediacy of the supernatural in that era; they admit its different standards, values, and priorities and consider its harsher material conditions. More objective treatment of Philip's statecraft has been followed by studies of his art patronage, his interest in architecture and urban planning, in book collecting and printing, in science, mathematics, medicine, public health, and technology.[2]

The Counter-Reformation and Philip's Education

Philip II was born in 1527 in Valladolid. His father, Holy Roman Emperor Charles V (Charles I of Spain), whose own education had been uneven, though Erasmus indirectly had a hand in it, provided that his son would have an education fit for a Christian prince, as propounded by Renaissance humanist educators. Humanist learning had flourished in Spain since the time of Queen Isabella and extolled Plato's model of the philosopher-king, enhanced by Christian precepts. In what has become a trope in Hernández studies, the king's physician would later liken Philip's support of his expedition to New Spain to Alexander's patronage of Aristotle.[3] In Philip's lifetime, as Dora Weiner points out above, the Counter-Reformation chilled humanist criticism of the church and condemned the perceived humanist tendency to skepticism regarding religious doctrine, but humanism's admiration of the ancient classics and determination to surpass the ancients survived.[4]

Philip's tutors introduced him to languages, including Latin, Italian and French, logic, rhetoric, history, ethics, mathematics, science, and religion. But he proved an indifferent student who found other aspects of life at court more agreeable. Some complained that his tutors did not work him hard enough. Yet at his chief task, government, he worked hard indeed, and his long days and nights at his desk became legendary. However lax he seemed in his formal education, he acquired genuine interests in a wide range of subjects and became what might be called an enlightened amateur. While still prince, he began to collect books of every kind and pictures.

At the court of Spain even a lax student could hardly be unaware of the New World across the ocean sea: its discovery, exploration, conquest, and colonization were attended from the start by a powerful fascination with all that was new—the native peoples, the flora, the fauna, and the lay of the land itself. The Renaissance desire to excel antiquity in every way goaded scholars and scientists to new achievements, for which the opening of the New World provided a unique opportunity. Prince Philip knew Gonzalo Fernández de Oviedo y Valdés, author of the *Historia general y natural de las Indias,* who curried royal favor with a courtly

manual, *Libro de la Cámara Real del Principe don Juan.*[5] Philip served as regent of Spain for his absent father during some of the climactic debates about justice and the New World's native populations, between Bartolomé de las Casas, a fiery and passionate advocate of the indigenous people's rights, and Juan Ginés de Sepúlveda, an Aristotelian scholar who had been Philip's chief tutor.[6]

Philip's Empire

Heir to Charles V's many dominions (save for the Austrian lands that Charles bestowed in 1522 on his brother, Ferdinand), Philip began to travel abroad in 1548, when he journeyed to Italy, Germany, and the Low Countries. He encountered the excitement of Renaissance pageantry and erudition in Genoa, Mantua, Parma, and Milan. Across the Alps he halted at Augsburg, a major center of printing and learning, and he found in the Low Countries a flourishing high culture. In Antwerp he would later subsidize the great cartographer Abraham Ortelius and the equally eminent printer Christophe Plantin, whose business much later turned out to have a direct connection with the publication of texts by Hernández.[7] Philip returned to Spain in 1551, the year in which his father's government chartered universities in Mexico and Lima. In 1554 Philip sailed from Spain to England in a splendid armada for his second marriage, to Queen Mary Tudor. After a year in England, he crossed the Channel to the Low Countries, where his father had decided to abdicate his crowns. In 1556 Philip became king of Castile and Aragón, together known as Spain. Charles's imperial crown passed to Philip's uncle, Ferdinand, and after him in turn to Philip's cousin Maximilian II and nephew Rudolf II, but Philip would never wear it; his empire would be different from his father's, though their visions of empire remained similar.

The sheer extent of Philip's empire awed his contemporaries, who called it simply the Spanish Monarchy, but what fascinated most of all was the Americas, opened in 1492 by Columbus and claimed at once by Spain, though the westward move of the 1493 Papal Line of Demarcation between Spain and Portugal by the Treaty of Tordesillas in 1494 gave Brazil to Portugal. The proliferation of new maps gave Europeans a broad impression of two continents connected by a slender isthmus and separated from Asia by the vastness of the Pacific. Only the outlines of the extreme north and south remained unclear; and the Strait of Magellan was still generally believed to be the only certain passage from Atlantic to Pacific. From urban centers and forts, Spaniards effectively controlled the larger islands of the Caribbean, coastal Florida, Mexico, much of Central America, the coastal regions of Venezuela, Colombia, and Ecuador, Peru, coastal Chile, the south bank of the Plate River, and much of Paraguay. All were legally subject to the Crown of Castile. The principal treasure came from the fabled mountain of silver, Potosí, in Upper Peru, today's Bolivia.

When Philip succeeded Charles, the populations of all his European realms stood in the region of 16 million. The Spanish population of the New World may have exceeded 100,000. The Indian population under Philip's scepter declined, largely from diseases against which they lacked immunities, and much more in some areas than others.[8] In many parts of the Caribbean the native population had almost disappeared altogether. The native population in Mexico had declined from perhaps 15 million at the time of the conquest to only 2.5 million and would continue to fall until about 1600.[9] In Peru, the native population seems to have fallen from 2 million to 1.5 million by 1570. Despite the moral qualms of some Spaniards, including Philip, black Africans were imported in growing numbers to replace losses and provide manual labor, especially in the tropics.

To govern so vast an empire in Europe and overseas, Philip posted viceroys to the kingdoms and governors to the other provinces (in theory, if not in practice, for three-year terms) to represent him and preside over local government. In Spain local government rested on municipalities, some directly under the Crown, others under ecclesiastical or noble lords. To those municipalities in the Crown's domain, which included all the larger ones, the Crown appointed corregidores, usually men trained in the law. To supervise the justice meted out by municipal and seigneurial courts, the Crown established chancelleries and courts of appeal. The king, advised by his Royal Council, remained the ultimate source of justice.

In the New World from the start, the Crown frustrated the aspirations of the conquistadores who wanted to create a seigneurial system such as they knew in Spain. The system of encomiendas, the assignment of Indian labor to conquistadores, a system hardly unknown to preconquest Indians, was a compromise. With encomiendas the Crown conceded no juridical powers, which it reserved to itself through municipal courts, regional audiencias, and ultimately the king, advised by the Council of the Indies. During Philip's reign, the council, whose obligations included supervision of defense, was most often headed by a jurist.

In a monarchy, providing justice is only one of the king's powers. The king is also lawgiver, chief executive, and head of the armed might of the kingdom. There is in theory no division of powers. Although by tradition Philip dealt with Spanish representative parliaments known as cortes, only in certain matters of taxation was their consent necessary for him to act. It was, however, politic for Philip to consult them, and he did. The cortes of the Spanish kingdoms were based on the three estates: clergy, nobles, and townsmen. The most important, the Cortes of Castile, met frequently during Philip's reign, made its views known, even when such views did not please the king, and demanded redress of grievances, about which Philip was largely fair. The cortes of the Crown of Aragón (Aragón, Valencia, and Catalonia) met on the few occasions Philip visited his eastern dominions, which were economically depressed and provided few revenues. There was talk in Philip's reign and after of extending the right of representation to American towns or of each American kingdom having its own cortes, but nothing came of it.

Philip, born and by choice a resident in Castile, concentrated on Castile, the richest and most populous of his realms. Contemporaries estimated its population at 6 million. What Philip needed from the Castilian cortes was money, subsidies above and beyond the Crown's normal rights. Despite steady increases in treasure from the Indies and generous grants from the church for his "crusades," the costs of war outpaced Philip's income. Three times driven to bankruptcy during his reign, he dunned cortes to increase tax rates. Responsible for collecting the taxes, Castile's municipalities favored rentiers over producers, which tended to stifle enterprise and, in the long run, impaired the economy of Spain. Philip's American treasure derived chiefly from the "royal fifth" of mineral rights, rooted in Roman law; it provided about 20 percent of Philip's Castilian revenues. Other American income came from tariffs and dues. The colonials enjoyed many exemptions from ordinary taxes and resisted attempts to impose them, even for regional defense.

Philip's Wars

Philip believed that his costly wars were wholly just, in defense of religion and his patrimony, which he thought were inextricably bound. A peaceful man by nature, Philip once described kingship as a form of slavery that brought with it a crown, and he sighed for the simple life of a country gentleman. The peace achieved between Spain, France, and England at Cateau-Cambrésis in 1559 remained fragile, with conflict between Counter-Reformation Catholicism and militant Calvinism the chief destabilizing element. By the standards of the era, religion and politics, church and state, remained just about united: one king, one law, one faith. Holy Scripture validated the political order in Saint Paul's Epistle to the Romans, chapter 13, augmented by the Old Testament. Saint Augustine defined just war, and Aristotle, emended by theologians from Thomas Aquinas to Philip's contemporary Francisco de Vitoria, gave politics its logic.[10] Roman law provided legal language, and Renaissance humanists accorded Christian blessing to Cicero's essays on political duty. Machiavelli's name appeared seldom, and then only to be condemned for daring to secularize politics. Organized religion provided the early modern state with its most efficient instrument of administration and communication.

Religion was a chief dimension of Philip's first major conflict after 1559, war with the Muslim Ottoman Empire. It began in 1560 with a failed expedition against Tripoli. The Turks responded in 1565 with the siege of Malta, which Philip's armada relieved. In 1568 Moriscos, Spanish Muslims supposedly converted to Christianity, rebelled in Granada; it took more than two years to subdue them. In 1570 the Turks turned on Venice and invaded Cyprus. Pope Pius V forged a Holy League of Spaniards and Italians and in 1571 the league's armada destroyed the Turkish fleet in the last great clash of oared galleys at Lepanto.

In 1572, however, the revolt of the Low Countries that had erupted in 1566 and seemed crushed flared anew. The issues were militant Calvinism versus Counter-Reformation Catholicism, dynastic interests and local politics. Because Philip regarded the Low Countries as his by inheritance, he gave priority to suppression of the revolt. By 1575, the costs of war on two fronts drove Philip to bankruptcy. In 1578 he made a truce with the Turks, who emerged from the war with control of Cyprus and most of North Africa. He renegotiated his debts and dunned the Cortes of Castile to more than double basic tax rates. In 1580 he acquired Portugal and its empire, and as his finances improved, he aspired to end the Dutch Revolt. England intervened on the side of the Dutch, which led to the disastrous Armada campaign of 1588. For the rest of his reign, costly war raged through much of western Europe and adjacent waters. In 1597 he declared another bankruptcy. On his death he left his heir, Philip III, a legacy of war, rebellion, and debt, all incurred in the name of God and dynastic right.

With these events dominant, with the routine business of government and church forcing Philip to long hours, it seems remarkable that he found any time for family life, let alone the pursuit of his many other interests. All his interests, he believed, were related to his obligations as king; they were just less pressing. The patterns of Philip II's private life follow both the aging process and his growing despair in the face of events. When young, he participated in state occasions, festivities, and hunting parties. As he aged, the hunting and festivals fell off; he began to dress in black, and little more than religious ceremonies continued—and even those became increasingly private. This has become the dominant image of Philip II: a gray man clad in black, save for the emblem of the Golden Fleece hung by a simple ribbon round his neck as he pores over state papers and annotates them or bows his head and prays at Mass. The state occasion with which he is most often associated is the auto-da-fé, the public spectacle of penance by heretics, Judaizers, and others convicted by the Holy Inquisition, that looming presence that will figure from time to time in the various accounts of Francisco Hernández that follow in this volume. The Inquisition features prominently among several elements in the mix that, according to received opinion, stifled intellectual development in Spain and explained why Spain played no appreciable part in the seventeenth-century scientific revolution.

The Inquisition

Has any institution in all history been so completely connected with thought control and the suppression of the freedom of inquiry as the Inquisition? The Inquisition focused its activities on religious beliefs and behavior. What was forbidden seemed clear: those doctrines on which Protestants differed with Rome, as defined by the Council of Trent, and Jewish, Muslim, and pagan beliefs; and forms of behavior, such as blasphemy (the most widespread offense), that violated God's commandments or church law. The Inquisition touched the fringes of science when it condemned judicial astrology, but it tolerated forms that acknowledged the power of God and the role of free will. It had little interest in alchemy unless "black magic" was involved, nor was it concerned with the Copernican system, which, however, remained an alternative in the curriculum of the University of Salamanca. The Roman Inquisition, not the Spanish, burned Giordano Bruno and condemned Galileo. The Spanish Inquisition's business was the maintenance of Roman Catholic orthodoxy, and in Spain it enjoyed the overwhelming support of the greater part of the population. The people's peace and security, Philip believed, depended on religious unity, and religious difference led inexorably to rebellion and civil war, even as the loss of true faith led just as surely to hell.

Only Christians were subject to the Inquisition, and, in Philip's time, all Spaniards were at least nominally Christian. The Spanish monarchs Ferdinand and Isabella had expelled all practicing Jews and Muslims between 1492 and 1501, so those who had chosen to remain had had to convert and thus became known as "New Christians," in contrast to the majority, the "Old Christians." Persons of Jewish descent were known as *conversos* (in Philip's time, more often *confesos*); those descended from Muslims, Moriscos. The former tended to be urban and given to professions, business, and crafts; the latter were largely agrarian, with some artisans and a smattering of professionals.

The relations between New and Old Christians provide a second and arguably more ominous element in Spain's perceived arrested scientific development. This argument tends to extol the achievements of Islamic Spain, led by Muslims and Jews such as Averroes and Moses Maimonides, and finds its glories blighted by the Christian reconquest and the religious intolerance generated by the Reformation.[11] The threat posed by the Ottoman Empire during the sixteenth century reinforced (with some reason) the bigotry of Old Christians, who suspected New Christians of forming an Ottoman fifth column and saw Protestants as traitors to Christendom. On a more mundane level, conversos competed directly with Old Christians in urban life. Conversos were often disparaged and made the butt of jokes, but much more serious, many corporate bodies, from orders of nobility and city councils to cathedral chapters and university faculties, passed statutes of purity of blood to exclude persons of Jewish or Muslim ancestry.[12] Fears that New Christian physicians who remained secretly Jewish or Muslim would poison their Old Christian patients led to repeated, if not entirely successful, prohibitions against their study or practice of medicine.[13] Though often challenged by lawsuits, the statutes led to public humiliation and a cottage industry in falsified genealogies. Simply to enter a medical or scientific career exposed one to charges of Muslim or Jewish ancestry. As Francisco Hernández knew, accusations of tainted blood spawned by rivalries and envy flew thick and fast. Philip II, determined to find the best talents for his tasks, often ignored the accusations, since few were spared them. But among more anxious sorts, it seemed safest to steer clear of the likelihood of being challenged and to pursue endeavors not historically associated with Muslims and Jews.

A further element in the mix is Philip II's 1558 prohibition, with few exceptions, of Spanish students studying outside the Spanish kingdoms. None of the excepted universities—Rome, Bologna, Coimbra, and Naples—was renowned for science or medicine, and no Spanish university at the time was exactly a magnet for scientific or medical studies in the sense that Padua and Montpellier were. Between 1510 and 1559, 248 Spanish students matriculated at Montpellier; between 1559 and 1599, only 12 did so.[14] Though Philip hoped to strengthen Spain's universities, cutting them off officially from larger European developments encouraged their innate conservatism to stifle them over the long term, even more than was typical of universities everywhere else in Europe in the era.

Both the Inquisition and a large, active church establishment made censorship, hardly unique to Spain, relatively thorough; and although science was not a particular target, any more than philosophy, for example, the process of getting the nihil obstat and imprimatur could prove a time-consuming nuisance and, arguably, discouraged scientific publication.

Science and "Backwardness"

Yet another element in Spain's perceived backwardness is what can be called cultural: what a culture regards as praiseworthy, acceptable, suspect, or unacceptable. Given the longevity and immediacy of the Crusades in Spanish history, the warrior seemed the most laudable of callings to Spaniards, with the missionary a close second. Serving God in his clergy, and serving king and country through the law, were also held in esteem. Lawyers were esteemed more highly and paid better than physicians, who thus hankered to send their sons to law school.[15] Contemporaries repeatedly remarked on Spanish pride, militancy, and zeal, which they found most extreme among Castilians, whose austere and landlocked country seemed to produce in them a closed-minded and tradition-bound character. After 1559 Philip spent all but half a dozen of the thirty-nine years that remained of his life in the Castilian heartland, yet because scientific research interested him far more than it interested most Spaniards, some Spanish scholars even ask if Philip really was the archetypal Spanish king of popular imagination.

Downplaying the received view, David Goodman, in *Power and Penury*, makes a strong case for an economic explanation of Spain's scant contribution to new scientific and technological developments, despite the promising beginnings he finds. Although Philip encouraged scientists, physicians, and technologists, given all the demands on his treasury, he seldom paid them very well. In the royal bureaucracy, lawyers were the best paid, while constant war provided a host of appealing opportunities to those seeking glory: noblemen aspired to be captains general and commanders of regiments and galleons; adventurous youths, to trail a pike in foreign lands and have a crack at booty. A royal physician made half the salary of a galleon commander.[16] Yet Philip repeatedly employed foreigners in technical fields in which few Spaniards were available, and they must have found the wages acceptable. To pursue Goodman's argument would require a comparative analysis of conditions, opportunities, values, and the relative worth of money (Spain's inflation rate led Europe) in those regions—Italy, Germany, Flanders—that provided so many of Philip's technical people.

Of course Philip was not the only employer of scientists and technologists. Wages still had to be competitive, even when the prestige of being "royal" was factored in. How much was Spanish society willing to pay and encourage scientists, physicians, and technologists and promote their endeavors? Goodman finds much public and private interest in the sixteenth century. The Seville physician Nicolás Monardes had a botanical garden famed in his own day for research that attracted interest in Spain and abroad.[17] The city council of Valencia promoted medical studies over theology in its university.[18] Spain pioneered the study of navigation, and inventors flourished.[19] These nascent developments might have been able to thrive and Spain to play a major role in the scientific revolution of the seventeenth century, yet for Spain that century proved disastrous, as available Spanish energies seemed concentrated on the stubborn defense of an overextended empire. Philip II had done what he could to promote science and technology, but he also persisted in the costly course of conflict determined by dynasty, interest, and religion that caused "the Decline of Spain."[20]

Countering the usual view, other essays in this volume show that the scientific and technical achievements of Philip II's Spain, at least in some fields, were impressive and belie the received opinion that Spain from the outset was scientifically backward. Philip II, educated according to the ideal of the philosopher-king, determined to further knowledge and promote the arts and sciences, which he understood in the harmonizing context of religious orthodoxy. To him, a conflict between true religion and true science was unthinkable, and the purpose of science was ultimately practical.

Philip II and the Sciences

The monastery and palace of the Escorial are Philip's enduring monument, an architectural statement of his beliefs. In this royal residence, dynastic mausoleum, and Hieronymite monastery, he also established a college and library, of which he had high expectations, but the Escorial remained remote, its collegians few and chiefly seminarians. The resident Hieronymite monks still regarded theology as the queen of the sciences, although the library embraced all sciences and contained books on every subject. Philip took a great personal interest in the library and its acquisitions, which he often annotated. The works of the fourteenth-century Majorcan Franciscan philosopher Ramón Lull proved a particular favorite with Philip and with his librarian, Hernández's great friend Benito Arias Montano.[21] Lull taught the universal harmony of theology and science, favored mathematical symbolism, and sought the conversion of Muslims (who, according to pious legend, martyred him). Though Rome had condemned some of Lull's propositions, Philip promoted his canonization.

Near the Escorial's royal apartments, a research laboratory took form to seek medicinal remedies through alchemical procedures. When first king and facing bankruptcy, Philip had employed alchemists in the search for a way to transmute base metals into gold, but their repeated failures left him skeptical of metallic alchemy, which he once called a hoax. However, the laboratory was a serious scientific enterprise, as López Piñero has demonstrated.[22]

The principal architect of the Escorial, Juan de Herrera, a Spaniard with service abroad, reflected many of the more promising intellectual interests of the era and might be called Philip's unofficial science adviser. He convinced Philip to establish an academy of mathematics in Madrid in 1582, something Philip urged—though with little success—other Spanish cities to emulate. Opposed by local interests, Herrera and the king also pushed rational city planning in the new and booming capital, Madrid. During Philip's reign,

gunnery, mining, and shipbuilding all flourished. Shipbuilding required knowledge of navigation, which thus encouraged further developments in astronomy, mathematics, oceanography, and geography.[23] It was natural that, when Hernández was commissioned to undertake his expedition to New Spain, Philip should simultaneously appoint a cosmographer—the ill-fated Francisco Domínguez—to conduct a geodetic survey of the new territories.

As other contributors to this volume show, Philip promoted the medical sciences, too, but foreigners still held Spanish medical practice in low regard: "Who hasn't seen it can't believe it," wrote a Tuscan ambassador.[24] The association of medical practice in Spain with Jews and Moors aside, its economic appeal was low. In Spanish universities that taught medicine, the salaries of the chair holders were among the lowest. The salaries of most court physicians remained constant throughout the reign, but inflation caused prices to more than double. Philip's constant shortage of funds prevented him from doing much to alleviate the situation.

Francisco Hernández was fortunate that his mission to Mexico was approved at the beginning of 1570, during a lull in the wars that forever seemed to cut short Philip's promotion of scientific projects. The Revolt of the Granadine Moriscos had been crushed, the Ottoman Empire appeared calm, the Duke of Alva seemed to have pacified the Low Countries, and there was peace with England and France. Philip could at last do something to his liking and launched what Goodman calls "the greatest scientific achievement of his reign."[25] Nine months later, when Hernández sailed in September 1570, serious troubles had developed with England, and Philip had agreed to the Holy League with the pope and Venice against new Ottoman aggression. By the time Hernández returned to Spain in 1577, the crescendo of war had driven Philip to bankruptcy, and Castilian tax rates had been more than doubled to meet the clamor of nervous bankers and mutinous troops. The next summer, the death on a Moroccan battlefield of Dom Sebastian, king of Portugal and Philip's nephew, opened Philip's way to the Portuguese throne, and Spain girded for war once more. Hernández would have to settle for far less than the grandiose publication of his findings that he expected.

NOTES

1. For general studies of Philip II, see Peter Pierson, *Philip II of Spain* (London: Thames & Hudson, 1975); Geoffrey Parker, *Philip II* (Boston: Little, Brown, 1978); Henry Kamen, *Philip of Spain* (New Haven: Yale University Press, 1997); and *Felipe II: Un monarca y su epoca*, Sociedad Estatal para la Conmemoración de los Centenarios de Felipe II y Carlos V (Madrid: Patrimonio Nacional, 1998). To these one might add Antonio Domínguez Ortiz, *The Golden Age of Spain, 1516–1659*, trans. James Casey (New York: Basic Books, 1971).

2. On art patronage, see Jonathan Brown, *The Golden Age of Spanish Painting* (New Haven: Yale University Press, 1991), chap. 2. On architecture and urban planning, see Catherine Wilkinson-Zerner, *Juan de Herrera, Architect to Philip II of Spain* (New Haven: Yale University Press, 1993), and George Kubler, *Building the Escorial* (Princeton: Princeton University Press, 1982). Also of interest is Richard Kagan, ed., *Spanish Cities of the Golden Age* (Berkeley: University of California Press, 1989). On book collecting and printing, see Parker, *Philip II*, esp. chap. 3. On science, mathematics, and the like, for a meticulous, comprehensive treatment, see David C. Goodman, *Power and Penury: Government, Technology, and Science in Philip II's Spain* (Cambridge: Cambridge University Press, 1988).

3. See *Mexican Treasury*, Letter 3 (November/December 1571). For comment, see Goodman, *Power and Penury*, 235.

4. The vast subject of the fate of Erasmian humanism in Spain is the theme of Bataillon, *Erasmo y España*.

5. On Oviedo (1478–1557), who eventually became governor of Cartagena, see José M. López Piñero et al., *Diccionario histórico de la ciencia moderna en España* (Barcelona: Península, 1983), 1:335–37, and E. Alvarez López, "La historia natural de Fernández de Oviedo," *Revista de Indias* 17 (1957): 541–601.

6. On the debates, see Lewis Hanke, *All Mankind Is One: A Study of the Disputations between Bartolomé de las Casas and Juan Ginés de Sepúlveda in 1550 on the Intellectual Capacity of the American Indians* (DeKalb: Northern Illinois University Press, 1974).

7. See *Mexican Treasury*, "The Low Countries, 1630–1648": Juan Eusebio Nieremberg.

8. See Elsa Malvido, "Illness, Epidemics," below.

9. Estimates run as high as 25 million Indians in 1519. The relevant work by Woodrow Borah and Sherburne F. Cook is brought together in their *Essays in Population History: Mexico and the Caribbean*, 3 vols. (Berkeley: University of California Press, 1971–79). Guenter B. Risse, "Shelter and Care," below, and William H. McNeill, *Plagues and Peoples* (Garden City, N.Y.: Anchor/Doubleday, 1976), 204, who records estimates that a population of about 30 million at the time of the conquest was reduced to only 3 million within fifty years and that it fell to about 1.6 million by about 1620.

10. A convenient collection is Francisco de Vitoria's *Political Writings*, ed. Anthony Pagden and Jeremy Lawrence (Cambridge: Cambridge University Press, 1991).

11. See, for example, Américo Castro, *The Structure of Spanish History*, trans. Edmund King (Princeton: Princeton University Press, 1954).

12. See A. A. Sicroff, *Les controverses des statuts de "Pureté de Sang" en Espagne du XVe au XVIIe siècle* (Paris: Didier, 1960). See also Antonio Domínguez Ortiz, *Los Judeoconversos en España y América* (Madrid: ISTMO, 1971), esp. 184 on the dominance of the medical profession by Jews and conversos.

13. See Goodman, *Power and Penury*, 219–21.

14. Ibid., 251–52 n. 26.

15. Domínguez Ortíz, *Golden Age of Spain*, 146.

16. Goodman, *Power and Penury*, 231, treats physicians' salaries. A court physician made about 150 ducats, a galleon captain made 300. [It is worthwhile to note, however, that Hernández's annual salary while in New Spain was 2,000 ducats.—Ed.]

17. See comments on Monardes by J. Worth Estes, "American Drugs," and Guenter B. Risse, "Shelter and Care," below.

18. See José M. López Piñero and José Pardo Tomás, "Contribution of Hernández," below.

19. For example, Michael Florent van Langren, *La verdadera longitud por mar y tierra* (Antwerp, 1644). The author was a Flemish astronomer to the Spanish court.

20. See John H. Elliott, *Spain and Its World, 1500–1700* (New Haven: Yale University Press, 1989), pt. 4.

21. For Philip and Lullism, see Goodman, *Power and Penury*, 9–11, and Wilkinson-Zerner, *Herrera*, 42–45. For Arias Montano and Hernández, see *An Epistle to Arias Montano*, in *Mexican Treasury*, "Spain, 1790."

22. In both *Ciencia y técnica* and "Paracelsus and His Work in Sixteenth- and Seventeenth-Century Spain," *Clio Medica* 8 (1973): 113–41; and see López Piñero and Pardo, "Contribution of Hernández," below.

23. For an account of all of these activities, see *Ciencia y técnica*, 104–6, 168–78, 196–228, 253–70.

24. Quoted by C. D. O'Malley, *Don Carlos of Spain: A Medical Portrait*, UCLA Faculty Research Lecture (Los Angeles: University of California, 1970), 9.

25. Goodman, *Power and Penury*, 234.

PART I ❧ THE INTELLECTUAL MILIEU OF HERNÁNDEZ

THE CLASSICAL TRADITION IN RENAISSANCE SPAIN AND NEW TRENDS IN PHILOLOGY, MEDICINE, AND MATERIA MEDICA

RAFAEL CHABRÁN

That students dedicate themselves to the study of the liberal arts, holy scripture, medicine and the study of languages, grammar, and Greek.

—Constitution of the University of Alcalá de Henares

We must emphasize the usefulness and necessity of letters—what the Greeks call grammar, which nature has linked inseparably with all other sciences; thus all those who dismiss grammar in any discipline are wrong.

—Juan de Brocar

Thanks to the contributions of very diligent and very wise men (many of which have been produced in this century), [the classics] have been returned first to their integrity and original elegance, and later translated into elegant Latin.

—Francisco Valles

Francisco Hernández is still known in some circles today by the nickname he acquired in his own time, "the Third Pliny," and indeed the life and work of Hernández are intimately bound to the work of the elder Pliny (A.D. 23–79), especially to translations, editions, and corrections published during the Renaissance.[1] In the preface to his own translation of Pliny, Hernández referred to the *Natural History* as "the encyclopedia of all the sciences."[2] The works of both Pliny and Hernández can be considered "encyclope-

dias" in the sense that they are "knowledge books" that were written in order to preserve and order knowledge. It could be said that they had a common purpose, at least in the general sense in which Pliny expressed it: "My subject is the natural world, or life—that is life in its most basic aspects."[3] At times, the work of both can seem to be "unwieldy conglutinations" of raw materials. Pliny's work is diffuse and frequently runs squarely upon the problem of presenting encyclopedic knowledge. Both works aim to provide "useful information."[4] Hernández, who spent a large part of his life (at least eleven years, probably many more) translating Pliny's work and composing a long commentary on it, must have been influenced by Pliny's interest in the utilitarian aspects of knowledge derived from natural history. Like the well-known official chroniclers of the Indies, Hernández frequently combined anthropological materials with encyclopedic descriptions of natural phenomena.[5] Natural history fused with moral history. But at times, the new knowledge did not square with the facts of his classic model.

"Between 1550 and 1650," as Anthony Grafton points out, "Western thinkers ceased to believe that they would find all important truths in ancient books."[6] Frequently, the experience of travel and confrontation with a new nature contradicted the views of the ancients, and so "naked experience" began to take the place of written authority.[7] Humanists challenged the scholastics and questioned the authority of the ancients. Following the lead of López Piñero, who underscores the importance of approaching the history of science in terms of "a complex network of interconnections between the disciplines," the present essay explores interconnections between Renaissance developments in philology, anatomy, and botany in Spain during the sixteenth century, within the contexts of tradition and innovation of Spanish medical knowledge at the Universities of Alcalá de Henares and Valencia.[8] We will situate Dr. Francisco Hernández's intellectual development in the context of the history of the University of Alcalá and in an academic environment in which Hernández was introduced to the classic scientific and medical texts of the times. At Alcalá, he was taught the value of studying the classics in the original as well as the usefulness of breaking with tradition by establishing the importance of firsthand experience of observation and research. Of necessity we will have to look at the broad features of Renaissance humanism—a vast subject in itself—and its impact on education and philology as well as its relationship with the sciences, especially medicine, botany, and natural history.[9]

The Dynamic and Dialectic of Tradition and Renovation

In order to examine the intellectual development of Francisco Hernández, we must summarize the principal intellectual currents of tradition and renovation in the areas of philology, medicine, anatomy, and botany in Spain during the sixteenth century.[10] Specifically, we must contextualize these developments within the framework of the confrontation between late medieval "Arabist scholasticism" and Renaissance humanism in Spain.[11] "Arabist scholasticism" is that body of knowledge that resulted from the assimilation of Greek, Hellenic, and Islamic philosophic and scientific knowledge in universities in the late Middle Ages. This body of knowledge and the thought it produced were based on Latin translations of Arabic texts. In Spain during the second half of the twelfth century and the early thirteenth, many translators were engaged in translating Greek science and philosophy, which Arab peoples had preserved, into Latin.[12] As C. H. Haskins has indicated, the circuit of translation was long and complicated, often from "Greek into Syrian or Hebrew, thence into Arabic and thence into Latin and often with Spanish as an intermediary."[13] From Spain came Latin translations of the natural philosophy of Aristotle and the most current versions of Galen and Hippocrates, often accompanied by vast amounts of Arabic commentary. During the thirteenth century, Arabist texts were attacked by scholastic physicians who put together large compilations and commentaries on classic texts. This was the period of "aggregators" and "conciliators."[14]

In medicine, late medieval Arabist scholastic Galenism was a dominant current at Spanish universities during the latter part of the fifteenth century and the beginning of the sixteenth.[15] The basic medical text of this period was the Latin translation of Avicenna's *Canon*.[16] Erwin H. Ackerknecht provides us with a good characterization of this type of medicine and the one medical text that supports it: "The Scholastic medicine of the second half of the Middle Ages was basically a mere repetition of Greek observations, theories, and interpretation. . . . Authority, reasoning, and dialectics were the backbone of this medicine. As a matter of fact, in view of the corruption and contradictions in texts that had undergone so many translations and copyings, dialectial [sic] discussion was necessary if any consistent attitude was to be derived from them."[17] As García Ballester points out, medieval Arab medicine was still practiced by a segment of the Morisco population in the sixteenth century in Spain, and it did not break down as a medical system until the seventeenth century.[18]

Diametrically opposed to Arabist scholasticism was Renaissance humanism, which sought to rescue the knowledge of antiquity through the study of original texts by using critical editions based on philological study. However, throughout the Renaissance there was, as is well known, a continuation of the tradition of classical learning, or what we might call the authority of antiquity. The works of Aristotle were especially revered for the structure and categories of knowledge and the division of the disciplines that he proposed.

Humanism stressed not only the importance of philological accuracy and the need to establish authoritative texts but also the need for a true understanding and interpretation of classical texts. However, new critical editions of scientific works generated a crisis over the lacunae and contradictions they exposed, which in turn brought the whole issue of authority into question. This tendency is evident in all the disciplines but is especially conspicuous in the study of human anatomy, particularly in the humanistic studies of the Galenic corpus that came with the Vesalian reform of anatomy.[19] In this particular reform, anatomical knowledge was based on the dissection of human cadavers, which often produced information that openly contradicted classic Galenic doctrines. The same humanistic current of reform is visible in other disciplines, such as geography, natural history, botany, and materia medica.

Humanism encouraged the "purifying" or "cleaning up" and "refining" of classic texts, but it also emphasized the importance of trying to achieve an authentic understanding of classical thought (a task facilitated by the develop-

ment of printing).[20] After cleansing the texts of the supposed errors and falsifications, the next step was the "Renaissance" task of comparing the contents of the classic texts with observations from nature. This was especially true in anatomy and botany.

The New Renaissance University: Alcalá de Henares

Alcalá de Henares is situated about twenty miles northeast of Madrid along the northern bank of the Henares. The city was built on the ruins of the ancient Roman town of Complutum. Its chief claim to fame, other than being the birthplace of Cervantes, is that it has been a historic college town and intellectual center for more than three centuries. The university was founded in the sixteenth century and as such was Spain's first Renaissance seat of learning. Francisco Hernández attended the University of Alcalá when he was a young teenager and was clearly influenced by the Renaissance humanism that was part of its new curriculum. Alcalá played an important role in the intellectual development of many significant Spanish Renaissance physicians and botanists, prominent among them Nicolás Monardes, Juan Barrios, and Francisco Valles.[21]

Tucked away in an autobiographical reference in his commentary and translation of Pliny's *Natural History,* which is filled with lengthy and diverse digressions by both the author and his translator and commentator, Francisco Hernández mentions that he "lived in Alcalá de Henares during the time of [his] studies."[22] From documents found by Somolinos, we know that on Monday, May 22, 1536, Hernández graduated from the Faculty of Medicine at Alcalá with a degree of "Bachiller en Medicina."[23] In order to receive this degree, he must have already attained the degree of "Bachiller en Artes," which was a prerequisite for entering medical school, and this means that he must have come to Alcalá in 1528, at the age of thirteen. The same documents tell us that present at Hernández's graduation from medical school were the president of his examining tribunal, Dr. Cristóbal de Vega (whom we will discuss later); Professor

Esclarea, rector of the university; and two physicians, Pedro López de Toledo and Gaspar de San Pedro.

During the sixteenth century, the new medical school of the University of Alcalá de Henares became one of the most important centers of learning in Spain.[24] As Risse and others have noted, Alcalá and Valencia were both important centers for the diffusion of the new medical learning.[25] The sixteenth century in particular represents one of the richest periods of growth for Alcalá de Henares, as it evolved into a true "university city" with colleges, student residences, convents, and guest houses all planned within the framework of an urban center. In reality there were two cities: a municipal area and the university city proper, which at its founding had about three thousand students. This pattern of expansion indicates that Alcalá was not just a cultural center but was rather one of the more important Spanish cities of its time.[26]

The creation of the University of Alcalá de Henares was the cornerstone of the religious reform designed by Cardinal Francisco Jiménez de Cisneros (1436–1517).[27] The university was designed to provide the most exhaustive and comprehensive religious training available for those studying for the priesthood in Spain. The central purpose of the university was thus the education of the clergy, as López Rueda makes clear: "Theological study constituted the *raison d'être* of the new university."[28] The latest advances of the new humanistic philology were quickly appropriated to serve biblical studies.[29] Cisneros sought to reform the clergy by establishing a new curriculum of theological and biblical studies and the production of the so-called Polyglot Bible— the first of two, as it happened, that would reverberate in unexpected ways across Europe.[30] Cisneros brought together a brilliant group of Hellenists, Latinists, and Hebraists to work on the bible.[31] The project began in 1502, but the actual printing did not begin until 1514 and was not completed until 1517. According to Otis Green, the publication of this bible was a high-water mark in early scriptural science.[32]

The most common date given for the foundation of the University of Alcalá de Henares is 1508, but the story is much more complicated. In order to carry out his objective of the establishment of the university, Cisneros had to overcome the apparent obstacle of papal approval for the project, but the cardinal seems not to have allowed that problem to worry him. He was already confidently planning his new university in 1492, and he authorized construction to begin in the first months of 1496, three years before official approval was obtained from Pope Alexander VI.[33] Castillo Oreja refers to the early plans for "a true university city," a complex to be made up of various "Colegios," or colleges; the Colegio Mayor de San Ildefonso was the most important of the constructions and the signature building of the university. Pedro Gumiel, a leading architect from Alcalá, was put in charge of the project. Along with the construction of the Colegio Mayor de San Ildefonso and the rest of the university buildings, the entire infrastructure of the city of Alcalá had to be put in place, and for this reason building continued throughout the sixteenth century—and would continue well into the eighteenth century. The construction of the two Alcalás, the city and the university, can be divided into two main periods: 1495–1524 and 1530–91.[34]

The construction of the Colegio Mayor de San Ildefonso was completed during the first period and the principal facade, with its plateresque decoration along with the Patio Trilingüe, during the second. It was in this second period that Hernández attended the university. The Patio Trilingüe, or El Trilingüe, was the building in which Greek, Latin, and Hebrew were taught and so connected the physical structure of the university with Cisneros's pet project—the Polyglot Bible. We should also stress here the expressed purpose of the foundation of the university: "that students dedicate themselves to the study of the liberal arts, holy scripture, medicine and the study of languages, grammar, and Greek." Thus the structure of the university was formally based on the study of Greek and Latin. Students had first to complete a course of study in the lower Faculty of Arts (liberal arts) before going on to the major faculties of theology, law, and medicine.

When Francisco Hernández began his university career at the University of Alcalá, he undoubtedly heard the customary *oratio paraenetica* at the start of the academic year. Each academic year would begin in Spain with a speech known as "the opening of the course," or prolusion. These speeches often formally praised the importance of the liberal arts, and grammar in particular; one of them, Juan de Brocar's *oratio* of 1520, emphasized the value of grammar and its intimate connection with the other disciplines.[35] According to Rico, Brocar's prolusion was greatly influenced by the work and thought of his teacher, Antonio de Nebrija. For Brocar, Nebrija was the prototype of the grammarian who believed that grammar was the key to the other disciplines, such as law, medicine, and—of course—theology or biblical studies.[36] Grammar was the repository of the church's languages: Hebrew, Greek, and Latin. Thus the study of texts was as necessary for theology as it was for other disciplines. Without grammar, there could be no correct interpretation of texts, be they theological, legal, or medical.

Elio Antonio de Nebrija: The New Philology

Probably the most influential figure in the early evolution of Alcalá, Elio Antonio de Nebrija nurtured an important orientation toward humanism at the university that would influence Monardes and Hernández.[37] Nebrija was born in Lebrija in 1444 and died in Alcalá de Henares in 1522.[38] He studied at the University of Salamanca, where he also taught, and his name is always closely associated with that historic university, too. A Latinist and grammarian, he is considered one of Spain's greatest humanists as well as the "father" of Spanish philology, among whose many concerns was the correction of the text of the Vulgate. According to Otis Green, "his position was new in that he proposed to apply all the resources of the new philology of the Italian Renaissance to the understanding of the Scriptures."[39] Nebrija was also known as the "conqueror of barbarism" and the intellectual match of any Italian of the period. For Bataillon, he could be considered the heir to the great Italian humanist Lorenzo Valla (1407–59) with respect to biblical studies.[40] Nebrija's work on Greek pronunciation was just as groundbreaking as his study of the grammar of the vernacular and the vocabulary of law, cosmography, astronomy, and Scripture.[41]

In 1481 Nebrija wrote the first Latin grammar to appear in Spanish, and in the momentous year 1492 he published the first Spanish grammar, actually the first grammar in any modern European language. He wrote and published additional works on mathematics, astronomy, geography, and natural history. Although some research has appeared, far too little emphasis has been placed on Nebrija the scientist, and the connections between Nebrija's humanistic works and his scientific endeavors have been explored inadequately at best.[42] Nebrija's work needs to be seen in terms of the incorporation of Spanish Renaissance science into the humanities, as well a riposte to Arabist scholasticism. Even though his work in the sciences was limited and admittedly small in comparison with the rest of his humanistic production, it was still genuinely significant and had a great deal of influence on many Spanish thinkers and writers.

About 1463, Nebrija went to Italy, where he could taste for himself what has been called the "new learning" and the "new philology" of the Renaissance. With a clear motive in mind, he went to the Spanish college of San Clemente at the University of Bologna to learn Greek, Latin, and Hebrew from classical sources: "So it was that at the age of nineteen I went to Italy, not as others do to obtain a benefice or bring back formulas of civil or canon law, or to return with merchandise: but to restore to the land they had lost the authors of Latin literature."[43]

After ten years in Italy, Nebrija returned to Spain in 1473, bringing with him the new philology of the Italian Renaissance, the basis of which was the belief that the first duty of the interpreter was to go back to the original sources. Although Lorenzo Valla had already died before Nebrija went to Italy, the intellectual climate that Valla had created deeply influenced Nebrija, as it did most people who came into contact with Valla's ideas. Valla's influence lay behind the emergence of historical philological criticism as well as the teaching of Latin, and his *De elegantis linguae latinae* (1471) was demonstrably important to Nebrija.

When Nebrija returned to Salamanca from Italy, he set out to do battle with the "barbarians." At the time the teaching of Latin was in a deplorable state everywhere in Spain, so in Salamanca Nebrija introduced the tradition of the Italians, especially the teachings of Valla. According to this tradition, rhetoric was the key to *studia humanitatis*, whose main goal was to teach students to become interpreters of the classical tradition. To this end one had not only to know the classical languages but also to work with original documents. For Nebrija, the ideal of humanism was the formation of *interpretes* or *gramaticos*—perhaps what we would call philologists today. These *interpretes* would study all types of texts and their specific terms, be they literary, legal, philosophical, or scientific. This task was closely related to Artistole's concept of the art of dialectics, especially with respect to the art of discourse.

Nebrija proposed a new pedagogy, which favored the *studia humanitatis* over medieval scholastic reasoning. Nebrija argued for what has been called the critical philological method as more appropriate to the former than the latter. In this task, Nebrija sided with Francisco Valles and proposed to unite grammar, dialectics, and rhetoric in order to achieve what both men believed would be a true science of discourse. Nebrija's humanistic research inevitably influenced his teaching practices and beliefs. His insistence that teaching be based on direct contact with classical texts led to the creation of a new series of didactic manuals, which replaced texts that had been in use in the Middle Ages with extracts from classical authors.

Spanish humanists like Nebrija were not only cultivators of "humane letters" in the arts faculties of universities: they were also the standard-bearers of a tradition and defenders of a program of learning, the new learning. This program (the *studia humanitatis*), with its critical philological method, sought to renovate all the liberal arts. Humane letters included texts concerning philosophy, mathematics, and medicine. The new learning proposed a new cultural path that was based on a "new" reading, a fresh interpretation of the original classical texts. This implied, of course, direct contact with those original classical texts. This, in turn, also implied the need for new critical editions and commentaries on those texts.

Humanists sought to work from the "exact" or "correct" classical texts, which meant that they wanted to rid themselves of the medieval intermediary and supposedly flawed versions. They used their critical philological method to get as close as possible to the "original" sources and texts. Humanists and scientists collaborated closely in this enter-

prise. In Spain, Nebrija was one of the chief representatives of the incorporation of the humanist endeavor into scientific activity. He was a central figure in the development of "scientific humanism" at the University of Alcalá de Henares, especially with respect to natural history, and he saw to it that the late medieval currents of natural history were replaced with those based on the new learning and the methods of Renaissance humanism. Nebrija may have lectured on Pliny at the University of Alcalá de Henares and may even have carried out some botanical excursions from there.[44] In any case, Nebrija had an enormous influence on subsequent generations of important Spanish physicians, especially those interested in botany. His influence was direct on such physician-botanists as Garcia da Orta and Monardes, more indirect in the cases of Hernández and Andrés Laguna. Nebrija was also instrumental in the development of scientific humanism at the University of Valencia.[45]

Nebrija made a number of important contributions to the field of natural history, especially with respect to lexical items of materia medica.[46] In this area his most significant work was his edition of the Latin version of Jean Ruel's edition of Dioscorides' *Materia medica*, published in Alcalá in 1518.[47] To this edition Nebrija attached an important list of materia medica vocabulary that contained the Greek and Latin common names for various plants, as well as other medicinal cures derived from animals and minerals.[48] The scientific lexicography current of Nebrija's research was continued by several important Spanish humanists, among them Juan Andrés Estrany, Pedro Juan Oliver, and Hernán Núñez de Guzmán.[49]

The most important of these three, the philologist Hernán Núñez de Guzmán (1473–1553) was the first Spaniard to hold the chair of Greek at the University of Alcalá and continue the work of Nebrija. Núñez (also known as "El Pinciano" because he was from Valladolid, the ancient Pincia) studied with Nebrija at the University of Salamanca and with Peter Martyr at the University of Valladolid.[50] Subsequently he followed in the footsteps of Nebrija and others among his countrymen when he went to study in Bologna at the Spanish College of San Clemente. As a professor at the University of Alcalá, Núñez taught Greek and worked on the Polyglot Bible, especially the Greek text.

According to some, he was "the most eminent humanist of his time" and "more of a philologist than any Italian"—high praise, indeed.[51] His most important contributions in the area of philological studies are to be found in his application of textual criticism to the elucidation and emendation of Latin texts, such as his edition and study of Pliny. As José López Rueda pointed out, in the preface to his work on Pliny, Núñez stated that there was "no task more fruitful or more meritorious in the world of letters than the task of cleaning up the errors of copyists in classical texts."[52] In the same preface Nuñez praised scholars who dedicated themselves to the genre of critical studies and editions that contained the following words in their titles: "corrections, annotations, compilations, collected works, obscurities, emendations."[53]

The Medical Faculty of Alcalá de Henares

The medical school at Alcalá began to function during the academic year 1509–10 with two medical chairs, but two more were soon added. The Constitutions of 1510 (chapter 40) stipulated: "Let there be two Chairs of Medicine, held by two physicians of great erudition and tested experience. Each of them must provide two lectures on each working day: one before noon, the other afterwards, in such a way that one lecture or course [shall be] on the Canon of Avicenna, which course he is ordered to elucidate completely in two years."[54] Later, chairs of anatomy (1550) and surgery (1594) were established. Innovations in the teaching of anatomy came about between 1534 and 1559, primarily as a result of the efforts of Pedro Jimeno and Francisco Valles. One of the founders of the new anatomy at the University of Valencia, Jimeno was born in Onda (Castellón) about 1515 and died in Alcalá de Henares about 1555. It is believed that he studied for both his B.A. and his M.D. at the University of Alcalá. From 1540 to 1543, he attended Vesalius's anatomy lessons in Padua, an experience that was to be most influential for the rest of his life. When he returned to Valencia in 1547, he took up the chair of anatomy and simples, which he held for several years. At some time after 1549, Jimeno went to the University of Alcalá, where he became professor of anatomy and was a noted "dissector" who taught with

Valles. Jimeno spent the rest of his years working at the University of Alcalá.

During his time in Valencia, Jimeno converted the university into one of the first places in Europe to teach according to the new anatomy of Vesalius. Jimeno was also important in terms of incorporating Vesalius's ideas about teaching anatomy. In addition, Jimeno was the first to publish an anatomy textbook that incorporated Vesalius's ideas and approach to the teaching and study of anatomy. This book, *Dialogus de re medica,* was published in Valencia in 1549.

Francisco Valles was born in Covarrubia, near Burgos, in 1524 and died in Burgos in 1593. He excelled in medicine and natural philosophy. Like Hernández, Valles studied at the University of Alcalá, receiving his licentiate degree in arts in 1547 and his subsequent degrees in medicine. He was a professor of medicine at that university, and, while Hernández was in New Spain in 1572, Valles was named royal physician by Philip II. At court Valles was known as an "intellectual" as well as a physician. Philip II named him chief medical officer of all the kingdoms and seigneuries of Castile and placed him in charge of standardizing weights and pharmaceutical measures. In addition, Valles was named by the king to form a joint commission with Arias Montano and Ambrosio de Morales to organize the library of the Escorial.

Valles's first work, *Controversiarum medicarum et philosophicarum libri decem* (1556), consists of commentaries on physiological topics. As a Renaissance humanist, Valles always relied directly on the Greek texts and never concealed his disdain for the translations made by the medieval "barbarians." Furthermore, he always based his information and observations on the dissection of human cadavers. It was Jimeno who introduced Valles to Vesalian anatomy, and the "new anatomy" is nowhere clearer than in Valles's second book, *De locis patientibus* (1559). The revealing prologue of this text states that the physician must have "firsthand anatomical knowledge" and not just awareness of philological critical editions. Valles published some eighteen works of very diverse content. In 1587, the year of Hernández's death, he published *De sacra philosophia,* a gloss of biblical texts referring to medical and scientific issues.

Valles was one of the most important figures of European Renaissance humanism, especially with respect to Galenic humanism. That is to say, without questioning Galen's authority or the validity of his system, Valles accommodated Hippocrates to his own medical knowledge and practice. This current of thought has been called Hippocratic Galenism, in recognition of Valles's approach to the Hippocratic corpus from the underpinnings of humanism.[55]

Materia Medica and Renaissance Editions of Pliny and Dioscorides

Side by side with a man such as Valles, producing new books based on Galen were the Spaniards Nebrija, Estrany, Oliver, and Núñez, who followed the intellectual currents of the Italians who had studied Pliny and Dioscorides. The Spanish scholars knew and modeled their work on such Italian humanists as Ermolao Barbaro, Niccolò Leoniceno, and Piero Andrea Mattioli and the French medical humanist Jean Ruel. Niccolò Leoniceno, or Leonicenus (1428–1524), was professor of medicine at Padua, Bologna, and Ferrara. He is also remembered for his translations of Hippocrates and Galen. Perhaps his most important work was his correction of the botanical errors in Pliny: *De Plinii et aliorum in medicina erroribus* (Ferrara, 1492). Barbaro had already corrected some five hundred orthographic and grammatical errors that had been perpetuated by the medieval copyists of Pliny's manuscripts.[56] Indeed, Pliny was a favorite target for the application of the new philological methods of Italian Renaissance humanism from 1492 onward. So too was Dioscorides.

As John M. Riddle argues, it was not a question of humanists rediscovering Dioscorides but rather one of their turning their attention to his work with renewed vigor.[57] Compilations of Dioscorides' *Materia medica* circulated throughout Italy in both Greek and Latin manuscripts. As early as 1478, Peter of Abano lectured and wrote commentaries on these texts. The real flood of textual work and critical editions and translations of Dioscorides began in 1516 and continued throughout the sixteenth century.[58] Editions and commentaries appeared in Greek, Latin, and the European vernacular languages. As we shall see, the Latin, Italian, and Spanish editions are of special interest.

The Italian Piero Andrea Mattioli (1501–77) became obsessed with Dioscorides and set out to become the foremost expert and supreme authority on the *Materia medica*, refusing to take the smallest criticism lightly. In addition to his work on Dioscorides, Mattioli published (in 1530) a work on syphilis and the efficacy of guaiacum in treating it.[59] In 1544 Mattioli's translation of Ruel into Italian was printed by Niccolò de Bascarini in Venice, and in 1554 he published his famous edition of Ruel's work with notes, commentary, and more than five hundred woodcuts. His purpose was to provide Italian physicians and apothecaries with a commentary that would help them to identify medicinal plants and herbs.[60]

Andrés de Laguna and His Edition of Dioscorides

Andrés de Laguna was born in Segovia (c. 1510/1511) and died in Guadalajara in 1559.[61] Like so many of the people who populate the intellectual landscape in which Hernández moved, Laguna was born into a *converso* family. He went on to study arts at the University of Salamanca and later transferred to the University of Paris, where he studied classics and medicine and was a fellow student of Vesalius.[62] Laguna is known for his important contributions in the areas of medicine, anatomy, physiology, and botany. He is usually associated with the University of Alcalá and is believed to have lectured there in 1538.[63] He also traveled and lived in England, the Low Countries, Germany, and Italy. During his relatively short life he published more than thirty works in medicine, history, philosophy, literature, and politics.

Most of Laguna's medical works revolve around his studies and edition of Galen. In the most important of these, *Epitomes omnium Galeni Pergameni operum* (1548), which was republished and reedited many times, he made use of the studies and translations of Erasmus and Leoniceno. In addition, while in Italy, he wrote commentaries on Galen and Hippocrates and annotated Dioscorides.[64] Laguna also published works on the plague and gout, but his most famous medical work was his Spanish translation of and commentary on Dioscorides' *Materia medica*.[65] Throughout his life Laguna was interested in plants, especially medicinal plants, and between 1554 and 1555 he embarked on his new edition of Dioscorides.[66] This work was unique in that Laguna sought not only to correct the errors that had crept into the text but also to verify the descriptions of the plants by doing fieldwork in Europe, particularly around the Mediterranean. According to López Piñero, the clear and precise nature of the translation and its valuable commentary made significant contributions not just to medical botany but to all the scientific and technical terminology of the time.[67]

Laguna's edition of Dioscorides was one of the most popular scientific works of the time. First published in 1555, it was republished some twenty-two times in Spain up to the eighteenth century. Laguna's work was popular in both the scientific community and the world of literature, in which a reference to it even appeared in Cervantes's *Don Quixote,* no less.[68] Popular or not, Laguna's work contained few true innovations. The text was based for the most part on Mattioli, and almost all the illustrations came from the Italian's work.[69] It is interesting to note, as have López Piñero and Fresquet, that Laguna's work was not of the caliber of those works of medical botany produced by Spaniards who studied the flora of the New World.[70] We should remember that Francisco Hernández was well acquainted with the work of Laguna and used it in his own work.

In Hernández's lifetime, though after he had left the university, Alcalá became the principal center of humanistic Galenism in Spain because of the work of such figures as Cristóbal de Vega and Fernando Mena.[71] Cristóbal de Vega was born in Alcalá de Henares in 1510 and died in Madrid in 1573. He studied at the University of Alcalá, earned his M.D. in 1533, and was professor of medicine there from 1549 to 1557. Between 1551 and 1561 he published several important editions of Hippocrates. Fernando Mena was born in Socuéllamos (Ciudad Real) about 1520 and died in Madrid in 1585. He, too, studied medicine at Alcalá, between 1540 and 1545, and became a professor of medicine there. In 1560 he was appointed court physician to Philip II. Mena's works consist primarily of translations of and commentaries on Galenic texts, especially those dealing with the pulse, urine, purges, and bleeding. Mena's ideas with respect to Galen and Hippocrates are similar to those of Francisco Valles and Cristóbal de Vega.

The initial "Arabist" focus at the medical school of Alcalá had been quickly displaced by a Renaissance humanist perspective. Rodrigo de Reinoso, a close friend of Laguna's, was instrumental in the change in focus. Reinoso had studied in Italy, and he came to Alcalá armed with medical humanist approaches to the study of Hippocrates and Galen and a rejection of the importance of the *Canon* of Avicenna, which was central to the "Arabist" Galenism of the late Middle Ages.[72] Reinoso's reforms in the medical curriculum of Alcalá, along with Nebrija's influence after 1513, radically transformed the Faculty of Medicine of Alcalá and made it one of the most important in Spain during the sixteenth century.

Conclusion

After his years of study at the University of Alcalá (that is, after 1536), Hernández went on to practice medicine and continue his postgraduate work. Although this period of Hernández's life is difficult to study because of lack of documents, we do have some information, which has been summarized by Somolinos.[73] It seems certain that Hernández practiced medicine in the province of Toledo and the city of Torrijos. According to Somolinos, he also lived and worked in Seville about 1555, where he did botanical fieldwork with Dr. Juan Fragoso, another physician like himself who came from Toledo and had studied at Alcalá.[74] By the end of the 1550s or the beginning of the 1560s, Hernández was working and studying at the hospitals of the Monastery of Guadalupe, a place whose reputation is explored by Carmen Benito-Vessels in her essay in this volume. As López Piñero has stated, Guadalupe was one of the outstanding centers of anatomical study in Castile.[75] It was also known as a place where a physician could do postgraduate work, especially in anatomy and surgery. During the time that Hernández was at Guadalupe, the techniques of anatomical teaching were undergoing a reform, and the Vesalian approach had already been instituted.

By the time Hernández was named court physician and later *protomédico,* he had already received a solid education in classical languages, philosophy, and medicine at one of Spain's best and most progressive universities. He had also been introduced to the latest currents of Renaissance medicine, anatomy, and materia medica. In terms of both theoretical studies and practice, Hernández was now ready to undertake his study of medicinal plants and native Mexican medical practice in New Spain.

NOTES

1. Hernández was seen as the heir of Gaius Plinius Secundus, or Pliny the Elder: Roman official, scholar, and author. Pliny's most noted work, the *Natural History,* is a comprehensive encyclopedia, which Hernández translated with the addition of his own commentaries. On Pliny, see Roger French, *Ancient Natural History: Histories of Nature* (London: Routledge and Kegan Paul, 1994), 196–255, and Roger French and Frank Green, eds., *Science in the Early Roman Empire: Pliny the Elder, His Sources and Influence* (London: Croom Helm, 1986).

2. Biblioteca Nacional, Madrid, MS 2,862, fol. 4v, pref. to the reader. The full text of Hernández's translation of Pliny is printed in vols. 4 and 5 of the *Obras completas.* Jerónimo de la Huerta published his version of Pliny in 1624 (facsimile ed., Madrid: Instituto Geológico y Minero de España, 1982). It is a shame that a recent Spanish translation of Pliny made no use of either de la Huerta's or Hernández's translation. Cf. Luis Alfredo Baratas Díaz's review of Pliny the Elder, *Historia natural,* bks. 1–2 (Madrid: Gredos, 1995), in *Antilia: Revista española de historia de las ciencias de la naturaleza* 1 (1995), translated into English by Antonio Fontán et al. <http://www.ucm.es/OTROS/antilia/vol 1 -en/rsen1-1.htm>.

3. Pliny, *Natural History,* trans. by H. Rackham, Loeb Classical Library (Cambridge: Harvard University Press, 1967), 1.8, pref. Cf. also John F. Healy's selection and translation, *Natural History: A Selection* (Harmondsworth, England: Penguin Books, 1991), pref., p. 4.

4. Cf. Sarah Myers, review of Mary Beagon, *Roman Nature: The Thought of Pliny the Elder* (Oxford: Clarendon Press, 1992), in *Bryn Mawr Classical Review* 4, no. 3 <http://www.lib.ncsc.edu/stacks/bmcr-v4n3.html>.

5. Pliny served as a model for many of the chroniclers. See Roberto Moreno, "De Plinio y historia natural en Nueva España," in *Ensayos de historia de la ciencia y técnica en México* (Mexico City: UNAM, 1986), 1–22.

6. Anthony Grafton with April Shelford and Nancy Siraisi, *New Worlds, Ancient Texts: The Power of Tradition and the Shock of Discovery* (Cambridge: Harvard University Press, Belknap Press, 1992), 10.

7. Ibid., 1 and 5.

8. *Ciencia y técnica,* 11. For an overview of López Piñero's research and that of his team of scholars, see Rafael Chabrán, "López Piñero y la historia de la historia natural: Las aportaciones de Francisco Hernández," *Arbor* 153, nos. 604–5 (April–May 1996): 161–96. This entire issue of *Arbor* is dedicated to the work of López Piñero. My own work is deeply indebted to the work and thought of José María López Piñero, who has been at every moment generous and forthcoming with materials and encouragement.

9. Two recent articles by Ottavio Di Camillo provide an overview of scholarship on the Renaissance in Spain: "Interpretations of the Renaissance in Spanish Historical Thought," *Renaissance Quarterly* 48 (1995): 352–65, and "Interpretations of the Renaissance in Spanish Historical Thought: The Last Thirty Years," *Renaissance Quarterly* 49 (1996): 360–83.

10. The phrase "tradition and renovation" comes from José M. López Piñero, "Tradición y renovación científica en relación con las grandes corrientes intelectuales," in *Ciencia y técnica,* 149–54; most recently, he and Victor Navarro Brotons have applied these categories to the history of science in Valencia in *Historia de la ciencia al Pais Valencia* (Valencia: Edicions Alfons el Magnanim, 1995).

11. *Ciencia y técnica,* 150.

12. Among these translators was Gerard of Cremona (1114–87), who worked in Toledo and translated Avicenna, Rhazes, and others. See Katharine Park, "Medicine in Society in Medieval Europe," in *Medicine in Society,* ed. Andrew Wear (Cambridge: Cambridge University Press, 1992), 79; M. T. d'Alvery, "Translations and Translators," in *Renaissance and Renewal in the Twelfth Century,* ed. Robert L. Benson and Giles Constable (Cambridge: Harvard University Press, 1982), 422–26, 453.

13. C. H. Haskins, *The Renaissance of the Twelfth Century* (New York: Meridian, 1957), 281.

14. F. H. Garrison, *An Introduction to the History of Medicine* (Philadelphia: W. B. Saunders Co., 1922), 153.

15. As Guenter Risse points out, there is no good account of Spanish medicine in English ("Medicine in New Spain," in *Medicine in the New World,* ed. Ronald Numbers [Knoxville: University of Tennessee Press, 1987], 52 n. 1). Although Nancy Siraisi's *Medieval and Early Renaissance Medicine: An Introduction to Knowledge and Practice* (Chicago: University of Chicago Press, 1990) is useful for a general sense of the period, barely any specific reference to Spain is included. The best sources for this period are still in Spanish: José M. López Piñero, "Los saberes médicos del galenismo arabizado al paracelsismo," in *Ciencia y técnica,* 339–70, and Luís Granjel, *La medicina española renacentista* (Salamanca: University of Salamanca, 1980).

16. On the translations of Avicenna, see L. I. Conrad, "The Arab-Islamic Medical Tradition," in L. I. Conrad et al., *The Western Medical Tradition* (Cambridge: Cambridge University Press, 1995), 115–16; and on the dissemination of Arab-Islamic learning in Spain, 123.

17. Erwin H. Ackerknecht, *A Short History of Medicine* (Baltimore: Johns Hopkins University Press, 1982), 87. See also P. Laín Entralgo on the "arabizing of medical knowledge" in *Historia de la medicina* (Barcelona: Masson-Salvat, 1994), 197–202.

18. Luis García Ballester, "Academicism versus Empiricism in Practical Medicine in Sixteenth-Century Spain with Regard to Morisco Practitioners," in *The Medical Renaissance of the Sixteenth Century,* ed. Andrew Wear, R. K. French, and I. M. Lonie (Cambridge: Cambridge University Press, 1985), 246–70, esp. 246. According to García Ballester, "arabicized" Galenism broke down between the thirteenth and seventeenth centuries.

19. López Piñero outlines this reform in "The Vesalian Movement in Sixteenth-Century Spain," *Journal of the History of Biology* 12, no. 1 (Spring 1979): 45–81.

20. *Ciencia y técnica,* 151.

21. On Monardes, see José M. López Piñero's "Introducción" and "El Autor y su obra," in Nicolás Monardes, *La Historia medicinal de las cosas que se traen de nuestras Indias Occidentales (1565–1574)* (Madrid: Ministerio de Sanidad y Consumo, 1989), 9–22. See also Francisco Rodríguez, *La verdadera biografía del Doctor Nicolás Monardes* (Madrid: Revista de Archivos, 1925), as well as Javier Lasso de la Vega y Cortezo, *Biografía y estudio crítico de las obras del médico Nicolás Monardes* (Seville: Díaz, 1981), and Francisco Guerra, *Nicolás Monardes: Su vida y su obra {ca. 1493–1588}* (Mexico City: Compañía Fundidora de Fierro y Acero de Monterrey, 1961). Barrios is discussed in the text volume and briefly by Guenter B. Risse, "Shelter and Care," and José M. López Piñero

and José Pardo Tomás, "Contribution of Hernández," below. For Valles, see my discussion later in this essay.

22. Book 7, chap. 16, fol. 536.

23. "El Dr. Francisco Hernández y su Graduación Complutense," *La Prensa médica mexicana* 31, nos. 9–10 (September/October 1966): 314–16.

24. *Medicinas, drogas,* 107.

25. Risse, "Medicine in New Spain," 16; José M. López Piñero, "Valencia y la medicina del Renacimiento y del Barroco," in *La Medicina, la ciencia, y la técnica en la historia valenciana* (Madrid: Sociedad Española de la Historia de la Medicina, 1971), 95–108.

26. The seventeenth century, however, was for Alcalá a period of crisis that lasted into the nineteenth century. In 1836 the University of Alcalá de Henares merged with the University of Madrid, and for that reason the University of Madrid is known today as the "Complutense." In 1977 the University of Alcalá became an independent university again in order to ease the overpopulation of the other major universities in the Madrid area.

27. Some of the most useful bibliography on Cisneros and the founding of the University of Alcalá de Henares is still found in Bataillon, *Erasmo y España,* 1:1–44. See also A. de la Torre y del Cerro, "La Universidad de Alcalá: Datos para su estudio," *Revista de archivos, bibliotecas y museos* 20 (1909): 412–23; 21 (1909): 261–85, 405–33; Alberto Jiménez, *Selección y reforma: Ensayo sobre la universidad renacentista española* (Mexico City: El Colegio de México, 1944); and José López Rueda, *Helenistas españoles del Siglo XVI* (Madrid: Instituto Antonio de Nebrija [CSIC], 1973), 17–52.

28. López Rueda, *Helenistas,* 17.

29. Ibid., 18.

30. The other was the *Biblia regia,* produced in Antwerp and printed by Christophe Plantin in 1572–74 under the supervision of Benito Arias Montano, at the behest of Philip II. As a result of this later one, Arias Montano attracted the unwelcome attention of the Inquisition.

31. The Alcalá Bible was made up of six volumes and was divided in the following manner: vols. 1–4, Old Testament in Greek, Latin, Hebrew, and Chaldean; vol. 5, Greek and Latin texts of the New Testament; vol. 6: Hebrew–Chaldean vocabulary.

32. Otis H. Green, *Spain and the Western Tradition: The Castilian Mind in Literature from El Cid to Calderón,* 4 vols. (Madison: University of Wisconsin Press, 1963–66), 3 (1965): 17.

33. Miguel-Angel Castillo Oreja, *Colegio Mayor de San Ildefonso de Alcalá de Henares: Génesis y desarrollo de su construcción, Siglos XV–XVIII* (Alcalá de Henares: Edascal, 1980), 35–36.

34. Ibid. This is how Castillo Oreja organizes his account of the construction (chaps. 2–3).

35. Francisco Rico, *Nebrija frente a los bárbaros* (Salamanca: Universidad de Salamanca, 1978), 120–21.

36. Ibid.

37. *Medicinas, drogas,* 107.

38. Also known as Elio Antonio de Lebrixa or Aelius Antonius Nebrissensis, his last name being a modified version of his birthplace, Lebrija. For more information on his name, see Rico, *Nebrija,* 111–12. See the papers by Francisco Rico, Luis Gil, and Carmen Codoñer in *Nebrija y la introducción del Renacimiento en España,* ed. Víctor García de la Concha (Salamanca: Universidad de Salamanca, 1983).

39. Green, *Spain and the Western Tradition,* 3:12. Cf. David Coles, "Humanism and the Bible in Renaissance Spain and Italy: Antonio de Nebrija (1441–1522)," 4 vols. (Ph.D. diss., Yale University, 1983); Angel Sáenz-Badillos, *La filología bíblica en los primeros helenistas de Alcalá* (Estrella: Verbo Divino, 1990).

40. Bataillon, *Erasmo y España,* 1:30.

41. Much of Nebrija's work on scientific subjects focused on lexicography: see Enrique Montero Cartelle and Avelina Carrera de la Red, "El Diccionario médico de E. A. Nebrija," in *Antonio de Nebrija: Edad Media y Renacimiento,* ed. Carmen Codoñer and Juan Antonio González Iglesias (Salamanca: Universidad de Salamanca, 1994), 399–411. As Sáenz-Badillos states, Nebrija's purpose was focused on correct "naming": on searching for the meanings of so many names of realia (*Filología bíblica,* 116). Carmen Benito-Vessels expands this theme in "Hernández in Mexico," below.

42. A. Cotarelo Valledor, *Nebrija científico* (Madrid: Instituto de España, 1947). Cf. López Piñero, "Nebrija," in *Diccionario histórico de la ciencia moderna en España,* 2 vols. (Barcelona: Labor, 1983).

43. Bologna was long established as one of the great medical centers in Italy as well as a place where the revival of botanical studies took place. On the importance of the medical school of Bologna, see Siraisi, *Medieval and Early Renaissance Medicine,* 55–65. Nebrija is quoted by Green, *Spain and the Western Tradition,* 3:13, who notes that the Latin authors who were to be restored to Spain included the two Senecas, Lucan, Martial, and Quintilian. Apart from Hadrian, Trajan, and Marcus Aurelius, all Roman emperors born in Spain, two other notable writers who lived in Spain or were educated there were Columella and Prudentius.

44. It has been suggested that Nebrija taught botany at Alcalá, but the evidence is not entirely clear. According to Hernándo, Nebrija was well prepared to teach botany, since he had studied Pliny at both Salamanca and Alcalá; as Nebrija himself states in his edition of Jean Ruel, he was well versed in the editions of both Ermolao Barbaro and Ruel. See Teófilo Hernándo, "Vida y labor médica del Dr. Andrés Laguna," in Luis Granjel et al., *Vida y obra del Dr. Andrés Laguna* (Salamanca: Junta de Castilla y León, 1990), 146.

45. Not because he ever taught there himself, but because many of his students went to Valencia.

46. Montero Cartelle and Carrera de la Red, "El Diccionario," 400.

47. Antonio de Nebrija, *P. Dioscoridis Anazarbei de medicinali materia Ioanne Ruellio Suessionensi* (Alcalá de Henares, 1518). Ruel's work was first published in Paris in 1516.

48. For more on Nebrija's edition, cf. Hernándo, "Vida y labor médica," 143–44. It is interesting that the first edition that Laguna used may well have been the one produced under the supervision of Nebrija.

49. López Piñero, "Nebrija," 2:107. Cf. also López Piñero and Navarro Brotons, *Historia de la ciencia al País Valencia,* 74–78.

50. López Rueda, *Helenistas,* 22–23.

51. Green, *Spain and the Western Tradition,* 3:123, and López Rueda, *Helenistas,* 303.

52. José López Rueda, *Observationes Ferdinandi Pintiani . . . in loca obscura, aut deprau[a]ta, historiae naturalis, C. Plinii* (Salamanca, 1544), pref.

53. Ibid., 304.

54. Francisco Guerra, "Medical Education in Iberoamerica," in *The History of Medical Education,* ed. C. D. O'Malley (Berkeley: University of California Press, 1970), 425–26.

55. Among his most important works, Valles also wrote the *Tratado de las aguas deslitadas,* published in 1592, the year of his death.

56. In the 1490s a controversy arose surrounding the corruptions of the Pliny manuscripts and the editions based on them. Among those who engaged in this controversy were Leoniceno, Barbaro, and Pandolfo Collenuccio. Leoniceno in his *De Plinii* pointed out

the confusion of Greek and Latin plant names, while Barbaro's *Castigationes plinianae* (Rome, 1493) blamed the errors in Pliny's work on medieval copyists, and Collenuccio defended Pliny's original work in the face of Leoniceno's attacks in his *Pliniana defensio* (c. 1493). See Karen Meier Reeds, "Renaissance Humanism and Botany," *Annals of Science* 33 (1976): 519–42, esp. 523. Cf. also eadem, *Botany in Medieval and Renaissance Universities* (New York: Garland, 1991).

57. John M. Riddle, *Dioscorides on Pharmacy and Medicine* (Austin: University of Texas Press, 1985), xviii.

58. The first was the edition by Barbaro, *In Dioscoridem* (Venice, 1516).

59. See J. Worth Estes, "American Drugs," below.

60. The first studies of Dioscorides were primarily philological. This changed with the work of Mattioli, who based his approach to Dioscorides not only on philological study but also on botanical fieldwork. See José Luis Fresquet Febrer, "La difusión inicial de la materia médica americana en la terapéutica europea," in *Medicinas, drogas,* 322.

61. The most useful work that we have found on Laguna is that of Hernándo, "Vida y labor médica," 85–204.

62. In Paris he studied with Jean Ruel and other followers of humanistic Galenism. See José M. López Piñero et al., "Laguna," in *Diccionario,* 1:502–6.

63. See Hernándo, "Vida y labor médica," 96–98.

64. Andrés de Laguna, *Annotationes in Dioscoridem Anazarbem* (Lyons, 1554). This was the work in which he first attempted to correct Ruel's errors.

65. Andrés de Laguna, *Pedacio Dioscórides Anazarbo, acerca de la materia medicinal y los venenos mortíferos* (Antwerp, 1555). The most important study and modern edition of this work is by C. E.

Dubler, *La materia medica de Dioscórides: Transmisión medieval y renacentista,* 4 vols. (Barcelona: Emporium, 1953–55). See also Hernándo, "Vida y labor médica," 96–98.

66. Hernándo, "Vida y labor médica," 146.

67. López Piñero, *Diccionario,* 1:505.

68. Part 1, chap. 18.

69. Laguna was influenced, as we have indicated, by Ruel, and he also knew the work of Marcelo Virgilio, Barbaro, and even Leonhard Fuchs. See Hernándo, "Vida y labor médica," 147–52.

70. López Piñero et al., *Diccionario,* 1:505, and Fresquet, in *Medicinas, drogas,* 321–32. References to New World plants in Laguna, as Fresquet has indicated, are confusing and confused, and identification is correspondingly difficult. Among the plants from the Americas mentioned in Laguna's work are: "pimienta de las Indias" (possibly chili, but it is not clear what he means), various balsams, "Indian coconut" (*Cocus nucifera* L., not strictly American but treated as such by Laguna), gladiolus (*Styrax officinalis*), guaiacum, corn, white bean (apparently; *Phaseolus vulgaris* L.), three squashes (Cucurbitae), and *Opuntia* sp. (323–33).

71. López Piñero outlines the evolution of Galenism in Spain in his introduction "Las *Controversiae medicae et philosophicae* (1556) de Francisco Valles y el Galenismo del Siglo XVI," in José M. López Piñero and F. Calero, *Las controversias (1556) de Francisco Valles y la medicina renacentista* (Madrid: CSIC, 1988), 1–67. Cf. also *Ciencia y técnica,* 344.

72. López Piñero, "Las nuevas medicinas americanas en la obra de Nícolas Monardes," *Asclepio* 42 (1990): 6–7.

73. Somolinos, "Vida y obra," 1:116.

74. Ibid., 1:117.

75. López Piñero, "Vesalian Movement," and cf. Somolinos, "Vida y obra," 1:121–27.

FRANCISCO HERNÁNDEZ, RENAISSANCE MAN

SIMON VAREY

In virtually every study of Francisco Hernández, botanist, poet, historian, and author of theological commentary, this polymath is called a doctor or a naturalist. His qualifications and experience made him prominent but hardly unique in the context of Renaissance men, especially when we range him in the galaxy of the great intellects of the Spanish Renaissance. We do well to emphasize that, as Rafael Chabrán has shown in the previous essay, Hernández's education at the University of Alcalá de Henares brought together, crucially, language—in the form of philological and grammatical studies—and medical science. It is unlikely that Antonio de Nebrija, above all a grammarian, sought primarily to train a generation of doctors to write elegantly, or even as persuasively as the *Ad Herennium* would have them do, but eloquence was one consequence of Nebrija's legacy, as the work of Andrés Laguna or Francisco Valles would confirm. The implications of this linguistic influence for Hernández are far-reaching, as Carmen Benito-Vessels argues below.

It is a commonplace in studies of Hernández that he may have been a *converso,* or of converso origins: that is, that he was of Jewish descent. There is no hard evidence to support this view, although circumstantial evidence and propinquity suggest a strong Jewish connection. The Sephardim who survived and attempted to integrate themselves into Spanish society at large after the expulsion of 1492 had to confront violent and mostly successful efforts to displace them.[1] The broad community in which Hernández lived and worked, that of Spanish medicine and science, included plenty of men who were functioning under cover. Later in the sixteenth century nobody would even have to be a converso to be forced underground, because the Inquisition was so unrelenting that it essentially reinforced all the negative and repressive currents of the Counter-Reformation.[2]

Whether or not Hernández was a converso, we know little at first hand about his personality because few contemporaries said much about him, there is not a scrap of evidence about his family or his youth, and he never wrote much about himself, certainly not about his earlier life.[3] Most disappointing of all, there is no substantial collection of his personal correspondence, no extensive series of frequent letters like Arias Montano's to Plantin that might reveal in almost daily detail the workings of his mind. Still, we glimpse Hernández's activities at the isolated monastery of Guadalupe from a couple of fugitive comments in his massive commentary on Pliny, and we can learn more than we might dare to hope from his handful of surprisingly frank and densely packed letters to Philip II written from New Spain. We can also use the scientific writings, as Somolinos did, to draw some conclusions about the kind of intellect Hernández brought to his scientific task in New Spain. Even before this expedition was over and Hernández had brought his monumental work back to Spain, he was quite explicit about what he thought he had accomplished. At the risk of reading Philip II's mind with hindsight, we can project backward from Hernández's achievements to determine what kind of man would have been considered right to undertake the expedition to New Spain. Philip did not need a botanist to do the work, at least not in the specialized sense we would bring to such a term today. Whether or not the king needed a polymath, a Renaissance man is what he got when he appointed Hernández.[4]

The prolific writings of Francisco Hernández reveal an extraordinary range of interests. If he is known today for his epic survey of Mexican plants and animals, it is because that vast and original work catches the eye and because it was his most enduring contribution to the cultures of two continents. And although this volume of essays and our companion volume of texts concentrate, as they should, on the "world" that is spanned by the *Natural History,* no one should ever think that this was all that Hernández wrote or that all his earlier creativity somehow was a preparation for the later fulfillment of his magnum opus. If Hernández had never gone to New Spain, he would still have left behind a sizable and significant oeuvre.[5]

All over Europe, most naturalists among Hernández's contemporaries relied on established networks of correspondents with whom they would exchange seeds and specimens.[6] Hernández must have had such allies and informants while working in New Spain, though their names are not now known, and at different times both before and after his years in New Spain, Hernández was at the very center of a circle of affinity in Europe.[7] Hernández's friends and associates seem not to have been "correspondents" in the sense that members of Clusius's network were: there appears to have been little in the way of exchange of seeds and specimens between Hernández and his circle. Rather, the exchange appears to have been an interchange of ideas, methodologies, and visions.

A list of the names of the men in Hernández's circle of affinity reads like a *Who's Who* of the Spanish Renaissance: Benito Arias Montano, probably his greatest friend and ally; José de Sigüenza and Juan de Herrera; Juan Fragoso; Andrés Laguna (ambiguously); perhaps Ambrosio de Morales, Andreas Vesalius, and Francisco Valles, "the divine, the Hippocrates of Alcalá, the Spanish Galen."[8] These men were not collectors of dried flowers but doctors and thinkers, one of them (Herrera) credited with the design of a new Temple of Solomon but not known for studying peonies.[9] Unlike so many of their counterparts elsewhere in Europe, Spanish medical men were characterized more by their humanism and their promodern experimental philosophy than by any adherence to ancient methods and precepts. If Hernández, who himself certainly had botanized in Spain, ever enjoyed the mundanely practical assistance of a pan-European circle of fellow scientists, there is so little surviving evidence of it that anyone might be forgiven for thinking he must have been almost isolated. The reality, perhaps, is that Hernández was not a botanist in the same mold as Clusius or L'Obel. Designated the "Third Pliny" in his own lifetime, Hernández would be recognized much later as one "who added to his vast medical knowledge no common understanding of natural history, geography, mathematics, and literature."[10] Hernández styled himself "doctor and historian" (in Latin, *medicus atque historicus*), because he was a polymath with the vision of a cultural historian, who saw botany and medicine as two crucially important components in the total history of the world.[11]

When Hernández was appointed to undertake the expedition to New Spain that earned him all his modern renown, he had already established himself as a formidable intellectual force. The ambitious doctor from the small, notoriously Judaizing town of La Puebla de Montalbán rose rapidly to become, probably in the late 1550s, a resident physician at the monastery of Guadalupe, long established as one of Spain's historic pilgrimage sites but also a place with an ambiguous reputation, as Benito shows.[12] After his spell at Guadalupe, Hernández returned, probably in 1566 or 1567, to Toledo, where he had spent many years already, to work at the Hospital of Santa Cruz. As Somolinos puts it, "His experience at Guadalupe, the research and exploration centered in Andalusia, and the vision of the New World emerging from the restless traffic in and out of Seville had made a mature doctor of him" (127). By this time Hernández had certainly been working on his translation of Pliny, as we know because at one point in it he mentions the year in which he is writing, 1566. More tellingly, for an ambitious man such as Hernández there were, again as Somolinos notes, only three choices: the church, the sea, or the court. The court offered the most honor, the most glory. So by taking up residence in Toledo, only two days on horseback from the court at the Alcázar in Madrid, Hernández was perhaps signaling his intention of being noticed, or what Somolinos calls "premeditated proximity to the court" (127–28). Somolinos reminds us that this was El Greco's Toledo, one of Renaissance Spain's exciting cities of intellectual ferment (128), even if the great painter's livid canvases always suggest that the city is about to be struck by lightning.

There might have been an outside chance that Philip II knew who Hernández was when he named him, first in 1567, to be royal doctor and then, in 1570, to be his chief medical officer in the Indies—the two top honors in the Spanish medical profession.[13] Hernández was without question one of the best men available, especially for the second position, which promised to be an extremely demanding task, but no one knows how or why Hernández emerged from the packed throngs of position seekers at Philip's court. Somolinos's guess (139) that Arias Montano may have put in the requisite good word cannot be too far off the mark. When Philip sought someone to carry out a scientific and medical expedition to New Spain, he was looking for a man who could describe and absorb the nature of the medicinal and alimentary riches of the still half-understood territories. The character of Spain's colonial enterprise meant that there were plenty of qualified men to choose from, and, as usual, the job went to the man who happened to be in the right place at the right time, though we have little sense of how anyone else might have viewed this expedition at the time—as an exile, an irresistibly attractive scientific project, an adventure, a dangerous voyage, or what?[14] Scientists, especially those with heterodox views that did not sit too well with the court, could be much more useful to Philip if they were doing their scientific research 5,642 miles away, where they could still glorify (or just explain) aspects of the Spanish empire without spreading dangerous heretical influence in the corridors and anterooms of the royal palace.[15] As it happened, Hernández was a man with the necessary intellectual curiosity, but more than that, he had the driving will—ambition, if that is the right word—to get the job done. Like his equally illustrious contemporaries, Hernández at the age of fifty-five was still spurred by the motivating power of adventure and the need to see new realities for himself. Having taken on Pliny, he now took on a second monumental task: he clearly relished large, complex projects.

The precise nature of the task was set out, most probably by Hernández himself, in the royal instructions:

> It is hereby ordered that you, Doctor Francisco Hernández, our physician, shall hold and occupy the office of our chief medical officer of the Indies, islands, and lands of the Ocean Sea, to which office we have appointed you, and for all other things relevant to the history of the natural things that you shall find in those parts, the following shall apply:
>
> First, that with the first fleet to leave these realms for New Spain you shall embark and shall go first to that land and to no other of the said Indies because we are informed that more plants, herbs, and medicinal seeds are to be found there than elsewhere.
>
> Item, you shall consult, wheresoever you go, all the doctors, medicine men, herbalists, Indians, and other persons with knowledge in such matters, if it seems to you that they have understanding and knowledge and thus you shall gather information generally about herbs, trees, and medicinal plants in whichever province you are at the time.
>
> Further, you are to find out how the abovementioned things are applied, what are their uses in practice, their powers, and in what quantities the said medicines are given, as well as the places in which they grow and their manner of cultivation, and whether their habitat be dry or moist, or if they grow near other trees and plants, and if they occur in different varieties, and you shall write down descriptions thereof.[16]

As the instructions imply, the roles of the *protomédico* and the scientific explorer were intimately linked. Hernández was in New Spain primarily as the investigator of the natural resources of the country, but he was also there as a practicing physician, an official representative of Spanish medical thinking. As matters turned out, Hernández encountered an intractable and hostile bureaucracy that did little to assist his efforts to carry out either of his two related tasks and that cared nothing for the wishes of a monarch who was too distant to have much effect on anyone disregarding his wishes. Besides, in August 1571, about six months after Hernández had landed at Veracruz, he was hauled in to give evidence before the Inquisition in what sounded like a trumped-up case against Dr. Pedro López.[17] Hernández barely cooperated, and the case died, but he had clearly been given an intimidatory warning. Largely because of local difficulties that seemed to him like endless harassment, Hernández was a disaster as protomédico, and in fact he more or less gave up trying to do anything much in that official role, preferring to throw himself energetically into his job as scientific researcher, at least until the outbreak of the epidemic called *cocoliztli* in 1576. His research was finished by then, and instead of returning to Spain as he had planned to do, he suddenly, understandably, and properly resumed his role as a public health officer.[18]

The general idea of the royally sponsored expedition was that the protomédico should undertake a survey of the plants, animals, and minerals native to New Spain and that he should compile a book of "antiquities," an ethnographic history of the region. A geographer was supposed to measure and map the land, and in the declared absence of anyone suitably qualified in Mexico, one Francisco Domínguez was appointed to accompany Hernández from Spain. In the first of a series of fiascoes, Domínguez went on strike and was apparently replaced not once but twice.[19] Hernández was meant to travel as far south as Peru, but in the event he never got past the southern end of the central Valley of Mexico. This is hardly surprising. Anyone unfamiliar with Mexico, especially one arriving from Europe for the first time, must have found that the sheer quantity and variety of natural resources were almost too much for the mind to comprehend. It was quite absurd to expect to cover the natural "reality," as Spanish speakers say, in as little as five years.[20]

The rhetoric employed by Hernández in his descriptions of natural history in New Spain is as revealing of his patterns of thought as his much more personal letters to the king of Spain and his suspicious, embittered verse epistle to Benito Arias Montano, written about 1580, when Hernández was back in Spain. The letters are occasionally used in studies of Hernández, but usually to establish facts, such as the year of his birth (1515, because in a letter dated March 20, 1575, he says he is nearly sixty), or to show glimpses of his changing conception of what he was in New Spain to do.[21] The poem has attracted virtually no attention, although it, too, can be used similarly to determine Hernández's apparent attitude to his situation, to the Mexican artists he employed, to Mexico in general. Together, the poem and the letters convey a number of linguistic and syntactic habits that cast a somewhat different light on the "scientific" work of Hernández. The language of the descriptions is obviously European in conception, revealing little of the traditional Aztec conceptions of illness, life, and death. He seems to keep the native traditions at arm's length, recording them without necessarily embracing them. Yet the way he finally wanted to arrange his material was entirely Mexican, not European.

The format of each chapter is repeated thousands of times. First, Hernández describes the appearance of the tree (herb, shrub, and so on), using a simile to indicate the shape and size of the plant and its leaves, then a description of the fruit, its color, shape, size, smell. Then follow the varieties, the medicinal applications, the climate and terrain in which the plants grow, and sometimes the potential for cultivation in Spain. For example:

The second acacóyotl, also called acoyo or acóyotl, has a fibrous root, thick stems five cubits long, large, almost heart-shaped leaves, and a flower like a large pimento. It is hot and dry in the third degree, very fragrant and pleasant tasting, with a flavor of caucalis and cinnamon, or anise. The tender shoots, which are like fennel, are edible, and are usually prepared with sugar. Although it seems to be entirely like anise in all its virtues, except that it is a little more astringent, the Indians, who recognize some virtue in all their herbs, say only that it binds the stomach and eases stomach inflammation and pain. Perhaps this is a species of the acueyo, of which we shall speak in its place, or possibly it is the same herb, different only because of the conditions in which it grows. It grows in the warm climate of Pahuatlan, next to streams.[22]

When he describes flavors, aromas, and textures, we can almost see him squatting on his haunches, rubbing a leaf between finger and thumb, sniffing a piece of cut fruit, cautiously licking a potentially poisonous berry. This was a man who got his hands dirty, whose sheer curiosity—not to mention the silence of uncooperative natives—got the better of him on occasion, so that he was foolhardy enough to taste the leaves of an oleander and nearly killed himself in the process. Yet personal, anecdotal information of that sort comes not from Hernández but from his editors: he himself stuck to his format. There is nothing eccentric or quirky about Hernández's rhetoric; indeed, his language is entirely consistent with the style of his contemporaries writing in Latin all over Europe, even down to the common exasperating habits of multiplying relative pronouns until a reader has lost any grasp of an antecedent, and continually replacing terminal punctuation with the word *and,* so that whole paragraphs may eventually (at least technically) consist of a single sentence.[23]

Anyone following in the footsteps of Hernández today can witness the incredible exuberance of the natural life of Mexico. Within a few miles of Mexico City, he was confronted with scores of plant species that were entirely new to him, as were virtually all the animals and most of the minerals. Any description of something totally unfamiliar is sure to encourage extravagant use of the simile, so that readers, those "travellers [who] move across lands belonging to someone else, like nomads poaching their way across fields they did not write," may have a point of comparison, an anchor in their own reality.[24] Indeed, the language of the sixteenth-century travel narrative contains copious examples of this simplest of rhetorical figures. Take Peter Martyr, who in 1501 conveyed his sense of the shape of Hispaniola as it would appear on a map by saying "the island in shape resembles a chestnut leaf."[25]

Hernández's language is revealing, even at its most formulaic, because it shows the historian's desire to organize and classify and so to possess. The repeating pattern of the descriptions shows us precisely that the individual quali-

ties of thousands of plants are less important than the taxonomy in which Hernández disposes them. In Hernández's *Natural History* there are exceptions to his use of the formula, especially where he describes plants of such self-evident importance as tobacco, corn, and chili peppers. For example, his description of corn begins:

> How extraordinary it is that, in the origins of the world and the crude beginning of time, all the appropriate things for comfortable living had already been discovered. And lacking wheat, that wonderful find and a gift from mother nature as precious as health itself, people had to resort to acorns and barley, with which today we fatten hogs and the most wretched animals. But let us consider that even in our time some people feed themselves on rice and millet bread . . . others live on tlaolli, which our countrymen call Indian wheat and the Haitians call maize. . . . I do not understand how the Spanish, always diligent imitators of all things foreign, who know so well how to exploit other people's inventions, have still neither adapted for their own use, nor attempted to plant and cultivate this species of grain.[26]

This is the rhetoric of European discovery and the growing awareness that another culture not only predated Europe's but in some respects had already surpassed it before Europe even conceived of glorious things like cathedrals. But Hernández knew that the astonishment he experienced, increasingly, would be barely understood by Spanish readers who had never seen Mexico's vast lagoons, its monstrous fish, and the unearthly forms of its grotesque cacti. His descriptions are quite frequently punctuated with phrases expressing not wonder exactly but a sense that, for readers to understand even the description, it would still be necessary to be there and see with their own eyes:[27]

> What shall I say of the wonderful natural properties of so many plants, animals, and minerals; of such different languages—Mexican, Tezcoquense, Otomi, Tlaxcalteco, Quexteco, Tarascan, Chichimeca, and so many others that can scarcely be listed and which vary within such short distances; of such variety of customs and rituals of the people, of the clothing they wear, the ways in which they decorate and ornament themselves, which human understanding is barely capable of grasping even when we have provided as much help as we can, so that,

somehow, we can present some idea for those who are absent, when the true image can be understood only by those who are here and have the experience of seeing it and representing it for themselves.[28]

For his compilation of antiquities, from which this quotation is extracted, Hernández exploited existing texts, and so he plundered López de Gómara's *Historia general de las Indias* (1552) and fray Bernadino de Sahagún's *Historia general de las cosas de Nueva España*, adding some little material of his own and reorganizing the whole. The two genuinely original chapters promptly reveal more characteristic patterns of linguistic and rhetorical usage. Describing the cold-water baths prescribed by the native doctors known as Titici, Hernández speaks of women giving birth:

> They are obliged to take a steam bath, and to wash themselves and their newborn babies in icy water after first taking a bath known as temaxcalli.
>
>   What can I say? Even people suffering from fever with eruptions and other kinds of outbreaks are given the cold water treatment.[29]

Confronted with a natural abundance that amazes him, as it probably amazed most Spaniards, Hernández resorts to the gesture of the rhetorical question. The wider implications of all this are discussed later in this volume by David A. Boruchoff in his account of Hernández's *Antiquities*.

We now know that Hernández worked on Pliny and rewrote both his *Natural History* and his *Antiquities* during his time in New Spain. We also know that the revisions continued, at least on the *Natural History,* once he got back to Spain. The publication of Hernández's major work on the natural history of New Spain had been deferred, seemingly forever, and in January 1580 Nardo Antonio Recchi had been called in by the king to make a selection from it. In or about 1580, at a time of personal disappointment, discouragement, disillusion, and indisposition, Hernández wrote the poem that Rafael Chabrán and I have called "*An Epistle to Arias Montano.*" This poem, written in stately hexameters, certainly expresses Hernández's unhappy circumstances. It also employs some of his favorite formulas, such as a long sequence of personal questions that function as declarative statements; a seemingly contradictory pairing of self-

effacement and an assertion of the importance of his discoveries and his work; and an almost brooding resentment of unidentified gainsayers who are jealous of all great and new things.

> What do I say? Why did it fall to me to test the medicinal plants on myself?
> And at the same time put my life at great risk?
> Or those diseases, which caused me such excessive fatigue,
> with which I am still afflicted, and which will affect me for the rest of my life—
> how many more years will that be?
> —
> There are those who snap at my heels and spread the poison
> of envy, who try to damn my innocuous labors,
> which they will not see, or—if they read them—even understand:
> they do not deserve to know what the earth conceals, yet the mass of good people
> have to hear the venomous outpourings from their wretched mouths.
> —
> In all important matters, if one takes a great stride
> toward the loftiest heights, the effort
> brings honor to the endeavor—and still curses the ears
> of those detractors by exposing them to a fatal disease that destroys them at the core.[30]

These ordinary rhetorical tactics have precise parallels in Hernández's annual letters to the king, and they speak volumes for the mind behind them:

> Let us suppose that you are Alexander, and name me Aristotle because of what you have commanded me to do in these parts. Your Majesty could multiply Alexander by twelve and that would still not be enough. There are so many things in the new world, with so many wonderful virtues, all of which I see, I touch, I test, I draw, and I describe clearly and precisely in Spanish in a not unpleasing style, and which I am beginning to prepare to transfer to Spain.[31]
> —
> Having done what I have done here, I can leave the rest undone elsewhere; either it is quite like, or very close in form and virtue to what I have already described, or else it is not very important; but because it is Your Majesty's will that what remains must be tracked down, I have laid

such foundations for the project and given them such an order, that the door remains open for those who may follow me to finish that work with ease.[32]

—

But all great and new things always provoke opposition and jealousy, and this work has not escaped either, and thus there is another work, which has robbed me of no little time in the service of Your Majesty, which is my continuing concern.[33]

We can recognize at once that it is not the king's will so much as Hernández's will that "what remains must be tracked down," for this scientific investigator intended to seek out and describe *everything*.[34] Hernández was a perfectionist. In a late memorandum to the king, he affords us a glimpse of just what it was that the protomédico considered he had accomplished:

> Doctor Francisco Hernández declares: that he has resided by order of Your Majesty for nearly eight years in New Spain, during which time he has caused the natural things of this land to be depicted and described better and more accurately than had previously been possible, and caused the land to be surveyed exactly, and he has written the history of the western regions with their states and customs, images of their gods, sacrifices, and other antiquities, and because the natural history of this world is conjoined to that one, he has completed a translation and commentary of the thirty-seven books of the *Natural History* of Pliny, in nine volumes, and furthermore he has described the plants of the islands of Santo Domingo, Cuba, and the Canaries, subject to the little available time he could spend in these places, and the plants of this land that grow in New Spain, distinguishing between those that are native and those that have been transplanted, and how to recognize the plants from here and from there.[35]

His work in New Spain was, in his own judgment, a New World complement to Pliny. And because he had translated Pliny himself, he considered that he had become responsible for the natural history of both worlds. It is little wonder that he was known as the "Third Pliny," but what is more important is that he now realized that he had described the natural history of two continents, or as they were seen then, two worlds. He had omitted nothing. He had covered it all. Yet his manifestly grandiose accomplishments brought him

little solace in his old age. The very plague through which he had worked in 1576 had wiped out so many knowledgeable Mexicans that few, he said, would now know enough of the work he had done to reconstruct or replace it if it should ever be lost (a prescient thought on his part).[36] In ill health, pressured by his monarch and denied publication of his own work, deprived even of control over the fate of his own manuscript, and about to die obscurely, Hernández at the end of his life was like King Henry VII of England in Francis Bacon's words, "sad, serious, and full of thoughts and secret observations. . . . He was indeed full of apprehensions and suspicions."[37] A Renaissance man, indeed.

NOTES

1. As Jane S. Gerber points out, about 175,000 Jews left Spain in 1492, but about another 100,000 stayed and became conversos: the irony is that "Spain had expelled her Jews in order to eliminate their influence on *conversos,* but the expulsion had only succeeded in swelling the ranks of the *conversos* within her borders," and she notes that conversos "could not possibly change their religious identity overnight" (*The Jews of Spain: A History of the Sephardic Experience* [1992; New York: Free Press, 1994], 140, 142, 143). On the thorny question of religious identity, see the controversial thesis proposed by B. Netanyahu, *The Origins of the Inquisition* (New York: Random House, 1995). For a masterly overview of studies of the "secret Jews" of the Iberian Peninsula, Richard H. Popkin, "Notes from Underground," *New Republic,* May 21, 1990, 35–41.

2. See José M. López Piñero, "Paracelsus and His Work in 16th- and 17th-Century Spain," *Clio Medica* 8, no. 2 (1973): 121. Antonio Domínguez Ortiz comments on the dominance of Jews and conversos in the medical profession (*Los Judeoconversos en España y América* [Madrid: ISTMO, 1971], 184).

3. See Somolinos, "Vida y obra," 102.

4. My understanding of the concept of the Renaissance man is, of course, a palimpsest, with Jacob Burckhardt at the bottom of it. Burckhardt's work continues to be assailed—130 years on—for everything from confusions and omissions to not being proletarian enough, yet his name still appears eight times in nine modern essays redefining the concept of the Renaissance man. I have profited from those essays, *Renaissance Characters,* ed. Eugenio Garin, trans. Lydia G. Cochrane (Chicago: University of Chicago Press, 1991). Ágnes Heller, *Renaissance Man,* trans. Richard E. Allen (London: Routledge & Kegan Paul, 1978), is essentially a vast philosophical study in which the Renaissance man is a self-conscious self-fashioner, a category that applies only tangentially to Hernández. If the concept of the Renaissance man is slippery despite its widespread use, we might remind ourselves that "Renaissance" itself does not carry the same implications for the Spain of Hernández or the England of Francis Bacon as it does for the Italy of Michelangelo, Leonardo, and Alberti—or Burckhardt.

5. See Somolinos, "Vida y obra," 142.

6. See, for example, F. W. T. Hunger, *Charles de l'Ecluse (Carolus Clusius): Nederlandsch Kruidkundige, 1526–1609* (The Hague: Martinus Nijhoff, 1927), 117, 145, 349.

7. Hernández certainly had friends and contacts in Mexico whose names are known, but the people who supplied him with botanical

and medical information remain anonymous. See Somolinos, "Vida y obra," on Hernández's circle of helpful acquaintances (169–71).

8. Ibid., 108, 113–15, 117, 132.

9. Herrera was one of the executors of Hernández's will, probably the owner of part of the manuscript of Hernández's translation and commentary on Pliny, and certainly the owner of a wonderful library that may well have been the source of much of the erudition that peppers the pages of Hernández's most learned work (at least according to Somolinos, "Vida y obra," 140, 235, 270–71). For the idea that the Escorial was consciously designed as a new Temple of Solomon, see Sigüenza's commentary and his cautious comparison in his indispensable *Fundación del Monasterio del Escorial,* intro. Federico Carlos Sainz de Robles (Madrid: Aguilar, 1963), 26–27, 431–46. Sigüenza explicitly states that an inscription on the building identifies Philip as Solomon, and it was a commonplace anyway to identify Philip as the "king of Jerusalem." See also René Taylor, "El Padre Villalpando y sus ideas estéticas," *Academia: Anales y boletín de la Real Academia de San Fernando* (1952): 1–65; idem, "Architecture and Magic: Considerations on the Idea of the Escorial," in *Essays in the History of Architecture Presented to Rudolf Wittkower,* ed. Douglas Fraser, Howard Hibbard, and Milton J. Lewine (London: Phaidon, 1967), 81–109. On Herrera more generally, Catherine Wilkinson, "The Escorial and the Invention of the Imperial Staircase," *Art Bulletin* 57 (1975): 80, notes that Herrera, not a professional architect, was barred from holding the office of Escorial architect by members of the profession. See also the same author, now Wilkinson-Zerner, *Juan de Herrera: Architect to Philip II of Spain* (New Haven: Yale University Press, 1993). Agustín Ruiz de Arcaute's study, *Juan de Herrera: Arquitecto de Felipe II* (Madrid: Espasa-Calpe, 1936), is still useful.

10. *Mercurio peruano de historia, literatura, y noticias públicas,* no. 228, March 10, 1793, in vol. 7 (January–April 1793): 169. At least a part of this text was reprinted in *Ocios de españoles emigrados* (1825); see Leoncio López-Ocón, "Circulation of Hernández," below.

11. The headings of many of his manuscripts use the phrase "doctor and historian," for example, "De historia plantarum novæ hispaniæ liber primus, francisco hernando medico atque historico philippi secundi Regis hispaniarum et indiarum, et totius novi orbis medico primario authore" (BN MS 22,436, fol. 1r). When he was nominated royal physician in 1567, Hernández, ever conscious of his titles, signed himself "doctor from Toledo," prior to promoting himself, justifiably, to "doctor to Philip II" (Somolinos, "Vida y obra," 137).

12. La Puebla de Montalbán lies about sixteen miles west of Toledo, about sixty miles from the center of Madrid. For its Jewish population, see Somolinos, "Vida y obra," 98. Idem, 102 n. 30, points out that Guadalupe still enforced the test for purity of blood, which is discussed by Peter O'Malley Pierson, "Philip II," above, and Guenter B. Risse, "Shelter and Care," below. Bataillon (*Erasmo y España,* 1:71) reminds us that there were Jews everywhere, and Somolinos speaks, rightly, of what might have been Hernández's "psychological Jewishness" ("Vida y obra," 103). See also Somolinos, "Vida y obra," 121–31, and Carmen Benito-Vessels, "Hernández in Mexico," below.

13. Somolinos makes the valid point that all over Europe the best doctors of the period were royal physicians in their respective countries ("Vida y obra," 111 and n. 59). On the protomédicos, see John Jay TePaske, "Regulation of Medical Practitioners," below.

14. See Somolinos, "Vida y obra," 111.

15. My view entirely, but based on what seems to be an implication in Somolinos, "Vida y obra," 148. See also Benito-Vessels, "Hernández in Mexico," below.

16. *Mexican Treasury,* "Instructions and Letters to the King."

17. This is an oft-told tale, but still it is hard to make much of it. See Somolinos, "Vida y obra," 178, and Richard E. Greenleaf, *The Mexican Inquisition of the Sixteenth Century* (Albuquerque: University of New Mexico Press, 1969), 106–7.

18. Somolinos speaks of Hernández giving up the struggle over the protomedicato and taking refuge in his research, as scholars usually do (see 143–50, 178, 181, 243). When the plague broke out, Hernández would have been officially obliged to help the sick, but it is in any event hard to imagine him refusing to do so, for any reason. See also Risse, "Shelter and Care," below.

19. See *Mexican Treasury,* Letter 7: March 31, 1573, and Somolinos, "Vida y obra," 111, 154, 253–55.

20. Cf. Somolinos, "Vida y obra," 252. The term that crops up a few more times in this volume is realia, in the philosophical sense of "real things" or the pedagogical sense of actual objects that illustrate daily life and customs.

21. But cf. ibid., 100. For Hernández's changing conceptions, see Jesús Bustamante, "De la naturaleza y los naturales americanos en el siglo XVI: Algunas cuestiones críticas sobre la obra de Francisco Hernández," *Revista de Indias* 52, nos. 195–96 (1992): 297–328.

22. *Mexican Treasury,* M 1.129.

23. In our text volume we have consciously masked this problem in an effort to make Hernández's prose more readily accessible to modern readers. Those of a fanciful disposition might detect a link between the luxuriant growth of wild Mexican plants and the volubility of the author's style.

24. Michel de Certeau, *The Practice of Everyday Life,* trans. by Steven Rendall (Berkeley: University of California Press, 1984), 174.

25. The first Ocean Decade, *Selections from Peter Martyr,* ed. Geoffrey Eatough, Repertorium Columbianum, vol. 5 (Turnhout, Belgium: Brepols, 1998), 60.

26. *Mexican Treasury,* "Five Special Texts."

27. Somolinos, "Vida y obra," 143, notes the fashion for invention, exaggeration, and pure fantasy in contemporary descriptions of the New World written for the benefit of European readers.

28. *Mexican Treasury,* "Antiquities of New Spain," 1.23.

29. Ibid., 2.2.

30. *Mexican Treasury,* "Spain, 1790."

31. *Mexican Treasury,* Letter 3: [November/December 1571].

32. Ibid., Letter 9, March 20, 1575.

33. Ibid., Letter 2, May 15, 1571.

34. A point often made, for example by Somolinos, "Vida y obra," 231.

35. *Mexican Treasury,* "Hernández's Petition to the King, [early? 1577]."

36. Somolinos, "Vida y obra," 245–46.

37. *The Historie of the Reigne of King Henry the Seventh* (London, 1622), in *The Works of Francis Bacon,* ed. James Spedding, Robert Leslie Ellis, and Douglas Denon Heath, 14 vols. (London: Longman, 1857–74), vol. 6 (1861), 243. Also, Somolinos, "Vida y obra," 236. On the almost unnoticed death of Hernández on January 28, 1587, see Somolinos, "Vida y obra," 284. Hernández was buried in the Church of Santa Cruz in the Santiago district of Madrid. The church itself no longer stands, and there remains not a shard that might preserve the tiniest tangible memory of Hernández's residence in the area.

HERNÁNDEZ IN MEXICO
EXILE AND CENSORSHIP?

CARMEN BENITO-VESSELS

The year 1570, when Francisco Hernández's expedition to the New World was about to begin, provided a brief spell of welcome relief from the series of economic and military crises suffered by the government and the people of Philip II's Spain. As Fernand Braudel puts it: "By a happy coincidence, all her problems were temporarily but simultaneously out of the way in these years 1570–1571.... [Even] the anti-Spanish policy skilfully engineered by Cosimo seemed to be in eclipse."[1] It was on March 1, 1571, that Hernández presented his title of *protomédico* at the palace of the viceroy in Veracruz before the High Court of Mexico.[2] In October of the same year the fleet of the Holy League crushed the Ottomans at the Battle of Lepanto, a victory that was surprising in many respects, but, according to Braudel, "if we look beneath the events, beneath that glittering layer on the surface of history, we shall find that the ripples from Lepanto spread silently, inconspicuously, far and wide."[3]

The Spain that Hernández knew suffered from internal conflicts that affected ideologies as much as government and external conflicts that affected the Atlantic as much as the Mediterranean. José Ignacio Fortea Pérez has unearthed a series of documents that help to explain the underlying causes of the deepening crisis during the reign of Philip II. I am concerned here with the factors of that crisis that coincided with Hernández's time in Mexico: "On April 28, 1573 a royal memorandum was read to the provincial deputies, setting out the financial burdens upon the throne, which were a direct consequence of the necessity of having to make fiscal provision—by means of exchanges and contracts, at excessive interest and cost—for ever-increasing costs, charges, and expenses in such matters."[4] One equally interesting fact here is that the corresponding memoranda presented by the ministers omitted any evidence or proof that the "politics of gaining control began with the deputies."[5] A consequence of this situation was the pitiful financial support allotted to Dr. Hernández, and as for the alternative of "gaining control," there was little he could do, despite his impressive new title of protomédico, once he arrived in Veracruz: "The authorities found that the work of the protomédico, when it came to exercising his legal functions and medical duties, could damage their own interests. [Hernández] struggled with the High Court, fought with the viceroy, battled generally with every authority that tried to curb his prerogatives and powers."[6] His precarious economic situation, his near begging for funds, and the frankness with which he addressed Philip II leave a suspicion that it was not just the king but the administration as well that was punishing Hernández by granting him such wretched financial support and by doing nothing at all to help him satisfy his longing to be brought back to Spain.[7]

We should remember, too, that the state bankruptcy under Philip II opened the way for the municipal oligarchies to play a very active role in the distribution of revenues and the approval of ordinary, and extraordinary, services.[8] The expedition of Francisco Hernández could be considered a required service, and as such, there could be no doubt that the Crown did not have sole authority over the project. Hence in the period of Hernández's expedition, "the viewpoints of the Cortes and the municipalities did not always coincide . . . [and] the main resistance to the royal policy statements did not come from the Cortes, but from the individual municipalities affected."[9] Curiously, and perhaps not coincidentally, the agreement based on mutual concessions was signed in 1577, the very year of Hernández's return to Spain.

With this political context in mind, let us explore the ideological circles in which Hernández moved. In most of the studies devoted to him, four facts about his personal life are repeated: his probable Jewish origin; his established connections with the cradle of Iberian Erasmianism, Alcalá de Henares; his well-documented residence at the monastery of Guadalupe, the center of clandestine Judaism; and his steadfast friendship with one of the most prominent humanists or Erasmians of the sixteenth century, Benito Arias Montano, celebrated in the verse epistle that Hernández addressed to him.[10] But naturally the stature of Hernández as a scientist attracts studies of him and his work that tend to neglect such political and ideological factors as irrelevant to his botanical accomplishments.

The purpose of this essay on Hernández is to try to clear the field and to emphasize the consequences that could be caused by his close contact with the most revolutionary ideology of his time, Erasmianism (in the widest-ranging sense of the term), and his connections with the most stigmatized creed in Counter-Reformation Spain: Judaism. Germán Somolinos noted years ago the need to follow this line of inquiry and remarked on the disappointing lack of documentary evidence that might have cast light on some of these issues.[11]

In my view, there is no doubt that Hernández himself felt that his extended sojourn in Mexico was an exile, as suggested by the evidence of his letters to Philip II, as we shall see. It is worthwhile to remember, as Rafael Chabrán has described above, that Hernández was educated at Alcalá, which supported two chairs of medicine, and that as far as humanism was concerned at Alcalá, "there seems to have been a profound correspondence between the welcome reception accorded to nominalism and that other novelty that characterized the theological school at Alcalá, the direct study of the Bible with the aid of the original languages of the Old and New Testaments."[12] In the enterprise of the Polyglot Bible, the leading philologist, Antonio de Nebrija, was thought more appropriate than a theologian to "cast light on the names of the plants and animals that appear in the Bible." As Bataillon puts it, "Almost all of the terms upon which Nebrija shone his philological light belong to what could be called the field of biblical *realia*."[13] The effects of such a milieu on Hernández will be my focus from here on in as I develop my hypothesis that Hernández was possibly exiled and his work probably censored. These are my four points of departure: (1) parallels between the undertaking of the controversial Polyglot Bibles by Nebrija and Arias Montano and Hernández's enterprise in New Spain; (2) the implications of Hernández's spell at Guadalupe; (3) how the expurgation of the work of one who was considered a luminary in his own lifetime could be justified; (4) what could have caused Hernández's desire for repatriation to be refused.

Parallels between the Textual Projects of Nebrija, Arias Montano, and Hernández

Hernández went to New Spain with an exceptional scientific assignment: to name an unknown botanical reality. To all normal appearances there was nothing extraordinary about it, but the very act of naming is, in the Judaeo-Christian tradition, an act of creation, as Hernández would have been continually reminded at Alcalá. Given the intellectual affinities of Hernández, the result of his identification and naming of the *realia* of the New World was likely to be a heterodox version of Spain's overseas imperial ambitions.

The nominalist theory to which Hernández had been exposed at Alcalá supposed that abstract ideas are nothing without rational beings; general ideas do not exist without general signs. This theory is opposed to linguistic realism, which maintained that abstract ideas do have a real existence, hence that universals do exist independent of the things in which they are made manifest. Partisan adherence to one or the other of these ideologies was no trivial question and had already undergone attacks by Erasmus in his *Praise of Folly:*

> And then the most subtle subtleties are rendered even more subtle by the various "ways" or types of scholastic theology, so that you could work your way out of a labyrinth sooner than out of the intricacies of the Realists, Nominalists, Thomists, Albertists, Occamists, and Scotists—and I still haven't mentioned all the sects, but only the main ones.
>
> In all of these there is so much erudition, so much difficulty, that I think the apostles themselves would need to be inspired by a different spirit if they were forced to match wits on such points with this new breed of theologians.[14]

Contemporary with Hernández was the grammarian Francisco Sánchez de las Brozas, who dispensed his wisdom at the University of Salamanca and had to face the Inquisition as a result, in 1584 and 1600.[15] Brozas recognized Nebrija as his predecessor, the difference between them being that "Nebrija's approach consisted of *describing* the phenomena of language by relying on the authority of the classics, while Brozas focused on exploring the *causes* underlying those phenomena."[16] Brozas has been called, with some justification, the precursor of linguistic rationalism and the school of Port-Royal.[17] Hernández was closer to Nebrija's position in the study of "signs," but he allows us to glimpse a rationalist tendency founded in the priority he grants to the "use" of names.[18] So, then, the role of language and the importance that Hernández attached to it arise from a conception of the world that departs from official Counter-Reformation presuppositions. There is therefore a contradiction right away between the spirit of the command given to Hernández

by his monarch, the champion of the Counter-Reformation, and the spirit that guided Hernández as he applied that command to matters of language.

Arias Montano partook of the same theoretical information as Hernández as far as language was concerned, and in the poem addressed to Arias Montano, Hernández confirmed the ideological affinity between the two men. The explicit appeal with which he begins the poem includes four commendatory phrases that I italicize here:

> Montano, do not scorn *your old colleague,* who has
>   already docked at Jerez, who first saw
> you in the land of Romulus and who has come, over the
>   years, to recognize in you
> *a rare miracle of nature, honor of your people,*
> *an ornament of our time.* I have come here now to see
>   you once more,
> long after that retirement in which the nine Sisters
> taught you, Montano, and filled your mind with the
>   causes of things.[19]

Thus Hernández addressed Arias Montano as a dear friend, "old colleague," and defined the uniqueness of Arias Montano as "a rare miracle of nature" and as the "honor of your people" and "an ornament of our time"; later in the poem he adds:

> I will not say a word, O Montano,
> concerning our private affairs, so that by my silence
>   you may know
> how indebted to you are these writings of mine, and
>   how much
> gratitude I owe you, and what glory awaits our
>   efforts.[20]

Given that Arias Montano had had to face the Inquisition, this laudatory poem of Hernández as a declaration of an ideological affinity gives us grounds to presume that the court would not have taken kindly to the relationship between these two humanists. Basically, it was the role performed by Arias Montano in the edition of the Polyglot Bible (the *Biblia regia,* 1572–74) that was the reason for his brush with the Inquisition and with Philip II himself. In summary, Arias Montano and Hernández both took part in major projects with enormous linguistic, scientific, moral, and political significance; the Polyglot Bible project was destined to seek the true interpretation of the Christian *book* par excellence, and Hernández's botanical compilation was—in a figurative sense—the literary equivalent of the Book of *Genesis* in Philip's empire.

Granted that it could not have been the scientific spirit of Hernández that was called into question at Philip II's court, it necessarily has to be this humanist's ideology that explains his enforced isolation from his country and the suppression and expurgation to which his work was subjected.[21] As we shall see below, in the correspondence with Philip II, the king waged psychological warfare against the sick and weak Hernández in an effort to take his work away from him; it looks as if the king had lost confidence in his protomédico and wanted to separate the author from his work, that is, separate the creator from his creation.

José M. López Piñero mentions one facet of the era of Philip II that is relevant here:

> The protomedicato succeeded in being converted into a *controlling organization* for the practice of medicine and measures in the interest of public health. . . . It promoted the *institutionalization* of the chemical laboratory and the "pharmacy" of the Escorial, as well as the botanical garden and the menagerie at Aranjuez . . . and the first modern scientific expedition, which researched Mexican natural history from 1571 to 1577 under the direction of Francisco Hernández.[22] (My italics.)

In view of the narrowmindedness of Philip's era, which would want to turn the protomedicato into a "controlling organization," as López Piñero so rightly puts it, the censorship of the work of a protomédico with such close ties to Erasmianism and Judaism certainly falls within the realm of possibility. What is more, since royal intervention was a determinant in the saga of the Polyglot Bible on account of the exploration of its *realia,* it would hardly be strange if the same thing happened with the exploration of the realia of the New World.

Let us remember, furthermore, that the scientific discoveries made by Hernández cannot be separated from his mode of expression, especially at a time when everyone in his circle was attuned to Nebrija's work. As Francisco Rico says, Nebrija declared that " 'a knowledge of language . . . was . . . the foundation of our *religion* and the Christian

republic,' as much as 'law . . . medicine . . . the humanities . . .' or 'the study of *Holy Scripture*' " (my italics).[23] Religion, law, Holy Scripture, and science are, in effect, the four pillars that propped up Philip II's convalescent empire. Francisco Hernández, just like Nebrija, gave precedence to the pragmatic and didactic functions of linguistic expression and would tolerate neither the isolation of science nor its treatment as "pure" science. These two great thinkers shared many interests that arise from the priority they gave to language as an instrument of power.

The immensely ambitious project that Nebrija brought with him from Italy to Spain was "to combat the barbarism of all the sciences with the weapon of grammar."[24] Although, to be sure, Hernández was no linguistic theorist, he did put Nebrija's theories into practice. Fernando Martínez Cortés observed that Hernández noticed shrewdly that "the names of medicinal plants are derived from the principal action for which the plant is known";[25] in other words, the king's botanist did not restrict himself to recording a name without digging into the etymological meaning and the reason for it—as Brozas stipulated in *Minerva.*

Erasmus expressed the need for care in linguistic expression and warned of its social power in *Lingua,* in which he declared that "the flesh has its tongue, but the spirit has a different tongue."[26] And in *Praise of Folly* he developed the theme of linguistic expression as an act of creation, or desecration in the case of sins committed against the word. With Nebrija and Erasmus of Rotterdam, Spanish interest in philology was aroused. According to Sáenz-Badillos: "It cannot be said that Spanish philologists received from Erasmus the impulse necessary to come close to the Bible. Nebrija was already doing this kind of work before the Dutchman felt he had the linguistic competence to undertake such a task. All the same, Erasmus is something of a convergence point, the one to which all our humanists turn."[27] Thus the impact of Nebrija, that of the linguistic theory of Erasmus, and that of friendship with Arias Montano are all aspects of the life of Hernández that we would be very unwise to underestimate in any search for answers to questions about his life. This is especially true considering that the unknown—the recently conquered paradise—was to be shaped by the words of Hernández. He would be the new Adam going in search of curative plants and as such would be charged with the task of naming in credible words a new and incredible reality to present to the king.

At Guadalupe

Alcalá de Henares and Guadalupe were the two cultural nurseries in which Hernández was nurtured, and there was an active cultural interchange between them. Formal evidence of an affinity between the two institutions is a document published on May 3, 1503, that records the "receipt of the work of Homilías de Orígenes by fray Juan de Constantina who lends it to the monastery of Guadalupe to aid in the publication of the polyglot Bible."[28] The textual project of the Polyglot Bible was just one of many points of contact. Rafael Chabrán has explored the importance of Alcalá in our understanding of Hernández, and to understand the parallel importance of Hernández's spell at the monastery of Guadalupe, one should recall that "the internal life of the converted Jew (the *converso*) and his reactions to a hostile environment can be exemplified by what happened at the monastery of Guadalupe, where clandestine judaizing took place, and the prior, on one occasion, called upon the rabbis of Jerusalem to determine if they were following the orthodox rite."[29] Eugenio Sarrablo Aguareles, Antonio Correa, and fray Arturo Alvarez say that documents have survived that refer to "the examination which took place in 1485 within the Monastery of Guadalupe against fray Diego de Marchena, Jew, and fray Diego de Burgos, Judaizer, and several other brothers of the order of Jerome."[30] Luis de la Cuadra, for his part, compiled a total of 1,337 documents that refer to the everyday life and running of this enclave, and he emphasizes its political, social, and cultural importance.

Half a century before the arrival of Francisco Hernández at Guadalupe, one man was exiled: fray Eugenio, "the pharmacist," who was banished for life by Hernando de Talavera, archbishop of Granada, in 1510. The reason was that Eugenio, with the support of the reputable fray Luis de Madrid, took part in the burning of a document issued by the General Chapter of the order of the Hieronymites and declaring that the lay brothers did not have the same privileges as ordained monks, except in matters involving the rites of the priesthood.[31] Neither was fray Luis free of all blemish despite being a member of the royal *protomedicato*. As Sicroff comments: "In curious contrast to the vague depositions . . . were the surprisingly specific recollections by some monks of events which went back many years. Fray Diego de Guadalupe, for example, was able to recall finding fray Diego de Marchena and fray Luis de Madrid talking together about eighteen years ago and hearing the former use the expression 'asi vos vala el criador,' an utterance apparently deemed Jewish."[32]

As early as the fourteenth century, on Christmas Day, 1340, Alfonso XI granted a royal privilege "for the founding of the Church of Santa María in Guadalupe, and explained that he was mandating a much larger construction than the hermitage that was already there because it was virtually in ruins, and thanked Our Lady for the victory at Tarifa against the Moorish kings of Morocco and Fez."[33] This monastery was thus founded as a standard of Christianity and symbol of the belief in the superiority of one creed above others. From the first few years after its foundation, the monastery enjoyed royal and papal protection.[34] Under the reign of the Catholic monarchs, in 1479, a declaration of privilege confirmed by royal decree expressly required that the solemn feast of the Conception be observed in December every year.[35] On May 8, 1559, one year after Hernández had arrived at Guadalupe, Philip II himself issued a decree "ordering those of the Service of the Province of Toledo that this year 1559 they should not charge for service to the monastery of Guadalupe, and if any had been charged they should be reimbursed, and confirms the decree of the emperor Charles, given in Burgos on 2 June, 1542."[36]

Guy Beaujouan, who emphasizes the long-standing importance of the monastery at Guadalupe in materia medica, mentions how the Catholic queen Isabella had a special liking for this monastery, choosing her personal and family physicians from there. The same author points to fray Luis de Madrid and to the renowned doctor Juan de Guadalupe, member of the tribunal of the royal protomedicato of Castile, in addition to Alfonso Fernández de Guadalupe, another examiner for the protomedicato; Dr. Nicolás de Soto, who practiced in Guadalupe from 1478 to 1483 and became physician to the royal family between 1487 and 1504; and

Dr. Juan de la Parra, a native of Guadalupe who practiced there from 1480 to 1488 and became the queen's physician in 1504.[37]

One might emphasize that in the medical sphere Nicholas V, on August 2, 1451, "granted that the lay brothers who had studied medicine before entering the Order were permitted, under the authority of the prior, to practice and to cure the sick in the hospitals, etc., on condition that they did so free of charge."[38] The prestige of medicine at Guadalupe attracted qualified doctors to the monastery and prompted the expansion and improvement of the physical and cultural facilities at the whole site.[39]

Beaujouan states that from the mid-fifteenth century the papacy authorized the monks at Guadalupe to study medicine and surgery, but, he adds, references to the controversial subject of dissections at Guadalupe are inconclusive. Yet some scraps of indisputable evidence do survive, one of which is the testimony of fray Gabriel de Talavera, who spoke in 1597 of "dissections which the surgeons were permitted to carry out by the indulgence of His Holiness."[40] Of the other two pieces of textual evidence cited by the learned Beaujouan, one is the famous account of Hernández and the chameleon he dissected during his time at Guadalupe, and the other is a well-known letter from Eugenio de Salazar, who describes meat-eating sailors "wielding the knife with the same dexterity they would have if they had spent all their lives practicing anatomy at Guadalupe or Valencia" (381). López Piñero states that Hernández "practiced dissections of human cadavers at Guadalupe in accordance with the principles of the movement spearheaded by Vesalius."[41] Arana Amurrio adds information of great interest for the study of Hernández's ideological, cultural, and scientific development during his time at Guadalupe, from 1558 to 1562, noting that "students of medicine and surgery lived together[,] . . . from the foundation of the School of Grammar by the Catholic Kings at the end of the fifteenth century, with students of grammar."[42] And as far as Hernández himself was concerned:

> Of major importance for a possible understanding of the details of anatomical methods in Guadalupe are the references to what was going on at one time in the hospitals. In this context the work of Francisco Hernández makes

an extremely valuable contribution. . . . [He] was "doctor of the monastery and hospital" and "those who attended practicals in medicine, surgery, and dissection" practiced dissections with him. . . . Hernández generally refers to a group of doctors . . . and only rarely does he speak in the first person ("the autopsies or dissections that I performed while in Guadalupe . . .").

The anatomy performed by Hernández and Micó should be seen as inspired by Vesalius. . . . Thus when Hernández speaks of the uterus he says "Its shape (based on the evidence of the one I saw at Guadalupe where we anatomized the cadaver of a pregnant woman) was round but elongated, quite different from those of cows, goats, or sheep, contrary to the appearance in Galen."[43]

Although we are fortunate to have this glimpse of Hernández performing dissections at Guadalupe, the task of tracing the humanistic works that he might have consulted at the school of grammar is unfortunately hampered because, when 8,260 volumes were transferred from the library at Guadalupe to Cáceres, a great number of them were destroyed on the orders of the Commission for the Sale of Church Lands of 1838—actually the result of a decree of October 1, 1820, that suppressed religious communities and mandated the seizure of their goods by the state.[44] Surviving biographical information and studies of the most renowned luminaries with Jewish connections—Arias Montano and Sánchez de las Brozas among them—are thus all the more valuable.[45]

For Arana Amurrio it is still a mystery that "an order that had suffered such monumental scandal [at the hands of the Inquisition] should be . . . the choice of monarchs such as Charles I and, especially, Philip II, to run the monasteries most intimately connected to them personally: Yuste and the Escorial" (196). It is equally paradoxical that, when the Inquisition visited itself upon Guadalupe, doctors and surgeons were conspicuously absent. Arana Amurrio suggests that "a possible reason could be that the doctors, surgeons, and pharmacists of the Monastery of Guadalupe were utterly absorbed in their work, one of the most, if not the most absorbing of which involved the Hieronymites. . . . But even so, it is hard to imagine that they were totally unaware of the large population of crypto-Jews established right inside the monastery. There must be some other factor that could explain this apparent immunity" (201). In sum, by the time Hernández arrived in 1558, Guadalupe must long have been a disturbing hotbed of ferment that, curiously, enjoyed extraordinary protection from the state and the church. This explains why, after his second voyage to the New World, Columbus should have taken "the first Indians for whose baptism there is documentary evidence" to be baptized at the monastery of Guadalupe, and it also explains why Queen Isabella of Portugal, wife of Charles V, had "ordered two of the eight Indians who came from the island of Fernandina to be taken to this sanctuary to be educated."[46]

The last piece of evidence I want to mention connecting Hernández with crypto-Judaism at Guadalupe is that "the Jewish extraction of the Guadalupe doctors explains that, to them, medicine as it was practiced in the hospitals of the Puebla was quite technical and modern within a religious milieu."[47] Sicroff makes it clear that "to the indignation and frustration of the Old Christians of Guadalupe there was more than ample justification for the word that circulated among Conversos to the effect that 'it was prophesied that the church was going to come under the rule or governance of the lineage of the Jews, and that it was already being fulfilled because there were so many prelates and cardinals of that lineage, even within our order of St. Jerome.'"[48]

So, then, in a period in which the hunting of suspects gave carte blanche to Old Christians and suspicion of others turned into a national pastime as well as a national paranoia, any suspect such as Hernández would have had good grounds to write what Somolinos calls "the most extraordinary of all his works," the *Christian Doctrine* in hexameters.[49] Let me add that "the definitive legitimizing of the statutes of pure blood by the Spanish monarchy took place in the reign of Philip II, when the High Church of Spain took the decisive step of proclaiming its own statute of purity," and "Philip ordered his ambassador in Rome to press upon the Pope the importance of these statutes in Spain, and to request him to establish a tribunal to examine the credentials of those who were elected to ecclesiastical prebends in Spain."[50] In 1547, not long before the arrival of Hernández in Guadalupe, the statute of the church of Toledo was proclaimed, in defense of the purity of blood. "It is curious to observe that as late as 1575, and again in 1608, important

works were dedicated exclusively to defense of the statute adopted by the Church of Toledo."[51] Indeed, the *Christian Doctrine* is very much like one of these works, a boldly defensive argument justifying the "discovery" of correspondence that exonerated the Jews and their Spanish *converso* descendants from the charge of deicide. Among the other defenders of this "discovery" were intellectuals of the stature of Juan de Vergara and Arias Montano, who, according to Sicroff, actually had good personal reasons to maintain the myth of a "discovery" that recognized the innocence of "New Christians."[52]

Expurgation of Hernández's Work

Hernández's attitude toward groups of people generally considered inferior or even thought to have no soul was philanthropic. Philip must have found this attitude just as intolerable as Hernández's revolutionary scientific thinking. In Hernández's vast botanical documentation of the New World were "*volumes in Náhuatl,*" a language that Hernández had learned well enough to translate "*for the benefit of the native population.*"[53] The fundamentally human dimension of his project, together with such consideration for the native people, would surely have struck a dissonant chord at Philip's court. What is more, the translation into Náhuatl does not chime with the disdain that Hernández expressed elsewhere for people living in "a savage condition ... insincere, reluctant to reveal any of their secrets.... The Indians are for the most part feeble, timid, mendacious; they live from day to day, they are lazy, given to wine and drunkenness, and only somewhat devout. May God help them!" But at the same time Hernández recognized that "they have a phlegmatic nature and are notable for their patience, which enables them to master even the most demanding of arts, which we do not even attempt, and to make exquisite copies of any work, without any help from their masters."[54] It surely would make little sense to translate three volumes into Náhuatl if they were to be dedicated to Philip, and not much more if those volumes were written for people held in contempt. A third option, perhaps more viable, would be that Hernández wanted to make himself indispensable as an intermediary for making his work comprehensible and useful in New Spain. Interest in Náhuatl in Hernández's time was more economic and religious than scientific, as the works of Arenas and Alonso de Molina demonstrate.[55] In contrast, the interest that Hernández showed was more than scientific: it was political, too. Martínez Cortés shows that when Hernández was looking for information on the *chuprei,* the "king's investigator" said, "The natives consider this plant to be priceless and guard their knowledge of its properties with great secrecy, but with diligence and care I will manage to get it out of them."[56] No doubt the discovery of the secrets of curative properties would help to eradicate the beliefs in natural magic and the superstitions to which Ruiz de Alarcón referred when he said that "the Indians . . . lack this knowledge because of their small reasoning power and total ignorance of medicine" and so "consult some curer-sorceress of the sort called *tiçitl.*"[57]

Hernández, says Martínez Cortés, wrote his *Natural History of New Spain* because he was ordered to do so but also because it was a satisfying task that he was capable of accomplishing;[58] a comparison of this work with commentaries on superstition would also furnish evidence that could justify the censorship of Hernández, a subject that is worth a study to itself. Even though Recchi's abridgment certainly could be justified, at the expense of giving the impression that it was Hernández's complete work,[59] there were other factors in play, particularly the ideological differences that I have noted, that would certainly explain exile and censorship.

The omission of the name of Francisco Hernández is just as significant as his prolonged but reluctant stay in Mexico and the censorship of his work. It was not just his work but his actual name that was sometimes expurgated, in a "tradition" that lasted into the Franco era. For example, his name is surprisingly absent from the list of celebrated doctors given by Luis Alonso Muñoyerro, who extracted them from fray Quintanilla's *Archetypo de virtudes . . . Cisneros* (Palermo, 1653). But if we remember the ideology that Hernández embraced, then Muñoyerro's subsequent statement can perhaps be seen as a case of censorship: "Besides the influence of the college and university milieu, both well disposed to confirm students in the faith and foster piety, certain rules and practices existed precisely to achieve those ends."[60] And even more significant is the final paragraph of

Muñoyerro: "Let us bring this work to an end, then, and liken it to a Christian soul, in praise of the Lord, who is the knowledge and source of all things, who has granted us his favor in the beginning, the middle, and the end of this work" (296). Finally, let us note that Muñoyerro added as an appendix "The dogma of the Immaculate Conception of the most holy Virgin in the University of Alcalá de Henares" (299). This, without a doubt, points to the monastery of Guadalupe, since one of the weapons in the battle for crypto-Judaism practiced in the monastery was questioning of this very dogma. Arana Amurrio, as Sicroff pointed out in 1955, reminds us that in the monastery of Guadalupe, "the virginity of Mary, a dogma fundamental to Catholicism, was doubted on numerous occasions, and almost as often was the object of ironic or comic commentaries."[61]

Muñoyerro, who was bishop of Sigüenza, mentions that Dr. Fernando Mena—licensed in medicine in 1543 at the University of Alcalá—was personal physician to then Prince Philip. He then goes on to eulogize Dr. Juan Ramírez, who succeeded Mena on November 18, 1560, and who, he says, was protomédico to Philip II. There is no mention here of Hernández, even though Dr. Cristóbal de Vega is cited as royal doctor in the mid-sixteenth century. The name of Francisco Fernández, native of La Puebla de Montalbán, figures only once, in the list of bachelors for 1536. Another Francisco Fernández, from Torrejón de Alcolea, is similarly listed for 1554, and someone else with this name, from Agreda, graduated in 1565. With such scant mention the future protomédico would become the most revolutionary of them all, though he is given short shrift in one recent study of the University of Alcalá, a collective and ambitious work with a wide scope that incorporates virtually everything ever written about Alcalá up to the time of its publication. Curiously, and disappointingly, the section on medical studies merely redirects readers: "Everything about the professors, their appointment, salaries, etc. is fully treated in the work of Alonso de Muñoyerro," and continues: "The faculty of medicine enjoyed its own golden age in the sixteenth century; it was reformed several times, before falling into serious decadence in the middle of the seventeenth, when it was dominated by the dead weight of scholasticism, which got rid of its scientific and practical character, the basis of its study.

In this century the number of matriculating students was sparse, and the faculty never recovered the prestige of the sixteenth century, when Dr. Valles—well known as a divine—personal physician to Philip II, was professor at Alcalá."[62] Thus, to cite the work of Muñoyerro as the primary source of information on the faculty of medicine is an indirect way of putting the name of Hernández on the censored list.

Finally, we know from the research of Georges Baudot that the work of Hernández—not the *Natural History* but the *Antiquities*—was to be censored in 1577, though not necessarily for the same reasons that I have outlined here.[63]

Refusal to Repatriate

The letters from Francisco Hernández to King Philip make a very interesting contribution to the theory that the great botanist/physician was exiled. In his letter of September 22, 1572, Hernández thanked Philip "for Your Majesty's memory of my works, that I am granted this favor. I will do what Your Majesty commands by sending whatever I do with great secrecy, leaving a copy in translation here, and thus I will send what I can when Our Lord pleases that the fleet sets sail." It does seem somewhat incongruous that a doctor and botanist of such standing should tell the king that he is suffering from a "a long and serious illness from which at present the Lord as by a miracle has spared me, because my works remain to be finished, and Your Majesty to be served"; perhaps this peculiar phrasing comes from the same motivation that lay behind the *Christian Doctrine*.

Hernández was well aware of the importance of his own work and, betraying his strong philological background, says in his third letter that in the eight months since he began work on this project, he has written descriptions of more than eight hundred new plants, in Latin and Spanish, and "that there will be no need to bring to the Indies medicines from Spain, nor to Spain from Alexandria." This letter affords fleeting glimpses of self-justification: "God knows that I speak true, that I am up all night every night thinking of ways to serve Your Majesty more successfully and speedily and less expensively, and thus I have conceived a thousand designs by which before my death this benefit to the world may be placed in the hands of Your Majesty."[64] The letters of Hernández constitute a cry of despair, as the next sentence in this letter demonstrates: "But all great and new things always provoke opposition and jealousy, and this work has not escaped either, and thus there is another work, which has robbed me of no little time in the service of Your Majesty, which is my continuing concern; for which reason, if it pleases Your Majesty that this project continues with the same felicity with which it began, it is vital that I be favored with your royal inspiration and encouragement." One might say that these letters are dominated by four repeated themes: complaints and requests for more money; a desperate plea to return to Spain, most explicit after 1575; praise of his own work as a valuable text; and his intent to handle delivery of the work himself, in exchange for safe conduct on his way back to Spain.

There is no deception in these letters, since the third letter informs the king of the progress of the *Natural History* and how Hernández is following the king's instructions conscientiously, but there surely is a strain of tension in them, prompting the suspicion that Hernández thought his sojourn in Mexico was a punishment and that now he had served his time.

On the other side of the Atlantic, in the comfortable ambience of the royal palace, King Philip felt entirely safe (but, one may ask, safe from what?) keeping Hernández so far away and officially barred from returning. Philip II wanted the work of Hernández but did not want Hernández, as we can learn from a note written on the cover of the next letter: "I have read this and written to the Viceroy telling him that this doctor has frequently promised to send these books, but he never does send them; he is to pack them up and send them on the first ship for safe keeping."[65] We should note here the running feud between Hernández and the viceroy, which gives us a better taste of the implicit sentence passed by the king.

Conclusions

The throne did not act alone in the provision of funding. The power of the citizen oligarchies and the control to which I alluded earlier could be ranged for or against any given project. The dissident ideology of Hernández was, as we know, enough to cause any citizen to be declared persona non grata, and Judaism was, as we also know, the worst stigma in Philip's reign, so it is easy to draw the conclusion that Hernández had two black marks against him when one alone would have been enough to guarantee exile.

Francisco Hernández was a humanist who drank in the philological theories advanced by Nebrija and Erasmus. He was aware of the act of naming and its implications and thus of the intrinsic relationship between things and their names. Like Arias Montano, Hernández undertook a textual project that Philip II sponsored without wanting to take responsibility for the consequences. The time Hernández spent in Guadalupe added to his prestige as a doctor and perhaps also intensified suspicion that he was a "Judaizer," a suspicion that hung on even into the Franco era in the work of Muñoyerro, the bishop of Sigüenza. His ethnographic work became subject to censorship, less spectacularly than that of Sahagún, which was confiscated, and anyway it was damaging in 1577 even to be associated with Sahagún. Lastly, the letters of Hernández to Philip II contain so many desperate pleas that alert the reader to a tension, a conflict between the botanist and his king that could not be openly expressed but must forever remain between the lines.

Consequently, if we can still not produce absolute proof that would place Hernández on the inquisitorial scaffold, I am certain that if any zealous inquisitor had wanted to, he could have gone so far as to bring together the arguments presented here to disgrace Hernández. The doctor's only hope of protection would have been the official state interest in medicine and recognition of his major contribution to the subject. The king's botanist/physician was more useful alive and far away from the court than he was sitting next to the king, and his work could be rendered as harmless as his royal patron desired—all the king had to do was give it to an obedient and innocuous subject such as Recchi.

NOTES

1. Fernand Braudel, *The Mediterranean and the Mediterranean World in the Age of Philip II,* 2 vols. (New York: Harper & Row, 1973), 2:1105.

2. Somolinos, "Vida y obra," 1:161.

3. Braudel, *Mediterranean,* 2:1089. For some implications of Lepanto as the epitome of "all that was most glorious in the crusade against Islam [and] . . . a divine deliverance of Christendom from the power of the oppressor," see J. H. Elliott, *Imperial Spain, 1469–1716* (1963; reprint, Harmondsworth, England: Penguin, 1990), 241.

4. José Ignacio Fortea Pérez, *Monarquía y Cortes en la Corona de Castilla: Las ciudades ante la política fiscal de Felipe II* ([Valladolid]: Cortes de Castilla y León, 1990), 44.

5. Ibid., 45.

6. Germán Somolinos D'Ardois, *El doctor Francisco Hernández y la primera expedición científica en América* (Mexico City: SEP, 1971), 29–30. On Hernández's problems in detail, see Somolinos, "Vida y obra," 160–93.

7. Hernández's salary of two thousand ducats may seem a large sum for a doctor (see Peter O'Malley Pierson, "Philip II," above), but it was inadequate for his task.

8. Philip sought to levy new sales taxes to pay for maintaining the regime of *encabezamientos,* which meant negotiating with the *cortes* and the municipalities. The latter, more accurately, were oligarchies that controlled the *regimientos* and were seen as threatening on too many fronts to accept passively what had to be demanded from others. They boycotted the *encabezamiento* of 1575, and, mobilizing the constitution—the mandatory concession of powers for the approval of ordinary and extraordinary services—they forced the Crown to review all the projects. In 1577 an agreement was drawn up based on mutual concessions. Admitting his own contradictions, Philip reduced his demands, and the municipalities prepared to agree to some taxes, which, despite all this, were considerably increased. See Fortea Pérez, *Monarquía y Cortes,* 509–10.

9. Ibid., 512.

10. On Alcalá, see Somolinos, "Vida y obra," 108, and the comments in the essays by Rafael Chabrán, "Classical Tradition," and Simon Varey, "Renaissance Man," above. On the Guadalupe monastery, see Albert A. Sicroff, "Clandestine Judaism in the Hieronymite Monastery of Nuestra Señora de Guadalupe," in *Studies in Honor of M. J. Bernadette* (New York: Las Américas, 1955), 81–115. *An Epistle to Arias Montano,* in *Mexican Treasury,* "Spain, 1790."

11. Somolinos, "Vida y obra," 98, 102, and n. 30.

12. Bataillon, *Erasmo y España,* 1:21–22.

13. Ibid., 1:39.

14. Erasmus, *The Praise of Folly,* trans. Clarence H. Miller (New Haven: Yale University Press, 1979), 90.

15. See Antonio de Tovar and Miguel de la Pinta Llorente, *Procesos inquisitoriales contra Francisco Sánchez de las Brozas* (Madrid: CSIC, 1941).

16. Francisco Sánchez de las Brozas, "El Brocense," in *Minerva,* ed. Fernando Riveras Cárdenas (Madrid: Cátedra, 1976), 6. A preliminary text of *Minerva* appeared in Lyon in 1562, but what is usually taken as the first edition is the expanded version, Salamanca, 1587.

17. For a convenient text, see Antoine Arnauld, *The Art of Thinking: Port-Royal Logic,* trans. James Dickoff and Patricia James (Indianapolis: Bobbs-Merrill, 1964). Arnauld's hugely influential treatise, *La logique, ou l'art de penser,* was first published in 1662.

18. We should note that for Brozas "use arises from reason [and] authority from use. . . . These levels coincide completely. Anything that does not admit reason cannot be in use" ("Brocense," 18).

19. *Mexican Treasury,* "Spain, 1790."

20. Ibid.

21. Philip II and his successors alike recognized the intellectual distinction of Hernández. The founding of the Botanical Garden in Madrid in 1755 and the corresponding politics of research lasted far beyond the end of the sixteenth century. Jacqueline Durand-Forest states that eighteenth-century interest in Linnaeus was a direct consequence of the "discovery" of Hernández's work ("Hernández y la botánica mexicana," *Caravelle: Cahiers du monde hispanique et luso-brésilien* 55 [1990]: 53–64). See Jaime Vilchis, "Globalizing the *Natural History*," below.

22. *Códice Pomar*, 13.

23. Francisco Rico, *Nebrija frente a los bárbaros: El canón de gramáticos nefastos en las polémicas del humanismo* (Salamanca: Universidad de Salamanca, 1978), 49–50.

24. Ibid., 55.

25. Ibid., 287.

26. There is no English translation of *Lingua*. This quotation is translated from Erasmus, *Opera omnia*, vol. 4, pt. 1A (Amsterdam: North-Holland, 1989).

27. Angel Sáenz-Badillos, *La filología bíblica en los primeros helenistas de Alcalá* (Estrella: Verbo Divino, 1990), 31.

28. Luis de la Cuadra, *Catálogo-inventario de los documentos del monasterio de Guadalupe* (Madrid: Dirección General de Archivos y Bibliotecas, 1973), 162.

29. Angelina Muñiz-Huberman, *La lengua florida: Antología sefardí* (Mexico City: FCE, 1989), 262.

30. Ibid., 85.

31. Cuadra, *Catálogo-inventario*, 202.

32. Sicroff, "Clandestine Judaism," 95.

33. Cuadra, *Catálogo-inventario*, 7.

34. On October 10, 1475, Sixtus IV excommunicated "those who did any harm to the churches and monasteries, their goods and persons, reserving the right of absolution in those cases" (ibid., 130), and on November 14, 1547, an "apostolic letter" declared that "Jacobo Unteo, apostolic auditor . . . prohibits the bishop and chapter of Avila from intervening in matters of tithing concerning the monastery of Guadalupe" (ibid., 197).

35. Ibid., 136.

36. Ibid., 207.

37. Guy Beaujouan, "La Bibliothèque et l'école médicale du monastère de Guadalupe à l'aube de la Renaissance," in Guy Beaujouan, Yvonne Poulle-Drieux, and Jeanne Marie Dureau-Lapeyssonie, *Médecine humaine et vétérinaire à la fin du Moyen Age* (Paris: Minard, 1966; Geneva: Droz, 1966), 379.

38. Cuadra, *Catálogo-inventario*, 320.

39. In 1520 a plan was conceived for "reform of new and old infirmaries; detailed description by Juan Torello, master of works at the convent, dated January 1520," and in 1516 the "College of humanities and grammar at Guadalupe" was designed. Plans for "the rectangular cloister for the infirmary" were drawn up perhaps about 1528, while similar plans for the infirmary's outbuildings date from 1532. "Plans for the new and old infirmary, by Antón Egas and Alonso Covarrubias," date from February 6, 1525. See Cuadra, *Catálogo-inventario*, 374–76.

40. Beaujouan, "Bibliothèque," 381 n. 46, citing Talavera's *Historia de Nuestra Señora de Guadalupe* (Toledo, 1597).

41. *Códice Pomar*, 19. Somolinos, "Vida y obra," 105, points out that surgery at Alcalá was a serious academic enterprise, and López Piñero states that dissections were regulated and commonly performed all over sixteenth-century Spain.

42. José Ignacio de Arana Amurrio, *Medicina en Guadalupe* (Badajoz: Diputación Provincial de Badajoz, 1990), 158. On the subject of dissections Arana Amurrio comments: "As far as Iberian centers are concerned, the first to be granted a privilege of this type was the University of Lerida, which King John I authorized to perform one autopsy every three years on someone condemned to death. That was followed in September 1402 by Martin I granting Barcelona the right to perform two autopsies a year on human cadavers. Years later, in the second half of the fifteenth century, John II granted a privilege to the Guild of Surgeons and Barbers of Valencia to dissect cadavers (1447), and Ferdinand the Catholic in 1488 granted a similar one to the brotherhood of doctors and surgeons of Zaragoza for their activities at the Hospital of Our Gracious Lady" (165).

43. Ibid., 168.

44. Eugenio Sarrablo Aguareles et al., *Inventario del Archivo del Real Monasterio de Guadalupe (Cáceres)* (Madrid: Dirección General de Archivos y Bibliotecas, 1958), 14.

45. Other surviving biographies are those of Benito Montero, Calderón y Aguinaco, Carvajal, Donoso Cortés, Martínez Silíceo, Monroy, Moreno Nieto, Muñoz, Diego Sánchez, Sánchez de Badajoz. See "Legajo 15," in ibid., 89.

46. Arturo Alvarez, *Relaciones entre el Emperador Carlos V y el Real Monasterio de Guadalupe* (Madrid: Instituto de Cultura Hispánica, Ciudad Universitaria, 1958), 1, 4.

47. Arana Amurrio, *Medicina en Guadalupe*, 213.

48. Sicroff, "Clandestine Judaism," 125.

49. Somolinos, "Vida y obra," 427, and see *Mexican Treasury*, "Mexico, 1571–1615." For the distinction between "Old" and "New" Christians, see Américo Castro, *The Structure of Spanish History*, trans. Edmund L. King (Princeton: Princeton University Press, 1954); Peter O'Malley Pierson, "Philip II," above; and Somolinos, who notes that most petitions to the king seeking royal favor or reward conspicuously paraded a phrase to the effect that the petitioner was an Old Christian, thus of pure blood, free of all taint of Jewish, Moorish, or *converso* blood. But, Somolinos adds, nothing like this appears in any surviving document by Hernández ("Vida y obra," 102).

50. Sicroff, *Los estatutos de Limpieza de Sangre: Controversias entre los siglos XVI y XVII*, trans. Mauro Armiño (Madrid: Taurus, 1985), 124, 176.

51. Ibid., 191.

52. Sicroff, *Estatutos*, 215.

53. *Mexican Treasury*, Letter 9: March 20, 1575 (my italics).

54. *Mexican Treasury*, "Antiquities of New Spain," 1.23, and see David A. Boruchoff, "Anthropology, Reason," below.

55. The *Vocabulario* (1616) of Arenas enjoyed great popularity and went through five printings in the eighteenth century. It is interesting for two reasons: its awareness of the politico-economic power inherent in the command of a language and the possible existence of a public interested in learning Amerindian languages. The second edition added to the conversation guide a summary of grammar. This text was also translated into French. On the other hand, fray Alonso de Molina, as befitted his calling, compiled two Náhuatl/Spanish dictionaries for doctrinal purposes in 1569.

56. "La historia de las plantas de Nueva España: Aspectos médicos," *OC* 7:287.

57. Michael D. Coe and Gordon Whittaker, *Aztec Sorcerers in Seventeenth Century Mexico: The Treatise on Superstitions by Hernando Ruiz de Alarcón* (Albany: Institute for Mesoamerican Studies, State University of New York, 1982), 223.

58. "La Historia," *OC* 7:268.

59. *Códice Pomar*, 21.

60. Luis Alonso Muñoyerro, *La facultad de medicina en la Universidad de Alcalá de Henares* (Madrid: Instituto Jerónimo Zurita, CSIC, 1945), 131.

61. Arana Amurrio, *Medicina en Guadalupe*, 192.

62. *La universidad de Alcalá de Henares*, ed. Carlos Bustos Moreno, 2 vols. (Madrid: Graficinco, 1973), 2:38 n. 59 and 2:39.

63. Georges Baudot, *Utopia and History in Mexico*, trans. Bernard R. Ortiz de Montellano and Thelma Ortiz de Montellano (Denver: University of Colorado Press, 1995), esp. chap. 9.

64. *Mexican Treasury*, Letter 3: [November/December 1571].

65. Ibid., Letter 9: March 20, 1575, note.

PART II ❧ MEDICAL KNOWLEDGE AND PRACTICES IN NEW SPAIN

REGULATION OF MEDICAL PRACTITIONERS IN THE AGE OF FRANCISCO HERNÁNDEZ

JOHN JAY TEPASKE

Early in 1974, having been diagnosed with bone cancer and with an inkling that his death was imminent, my mentor, colleague, and friend, John Tate Lanning, called me in to ask if I would complete his manuscript on the royal *protomedicato* in the Spanish Indies, a project to which he had devoted almost thirty years. I agreed with the proviso that I had other projects of my own to finish first. When Lanning died in 1976, he left me with a mass of notes and two thousand pieces of manuscript—semifinished drafts of some chapters, bits and pieces of others, and an outline and only notes for still others. In 1983 I finally completed the manuscript, which was published in 1985 by the Duke University Press as *The Royal Protomedicato: The Regulation of the Medical Professions in the Spanish Empire*. Like that book, this piece bears Lanning's imprint, and I wish to pay tribute at the outset to his monumental contribution. Lanning insisted that the *protomedicato* book focus on regulation, not the practice of medicine; thus the emphasis in this essay, too, is on regulation of practitioners in early colonial Mexico. Working as I did with his notes and manuscripts, however, I was unable to check all the references in this essay, particularly the archival citations, yet I am confident most are correct.

In 1570, when Philip II appointed Francisco Hernández "chief medical officer of all the Indies [the Spanish empire in America]," the king was presumably taking a major new step to regulate medical practice and medical practitioners in Spain's overseas possessions.[1] In Spain itself royal medical officers, the *protomédicos,* and the *protomedicato,* an examining board made up of these protomédicos, were already well-established institutions. Evolving in the late fifteenth century, the royal protomedicato became responsible for the examination and licensing of physicians, surgeons, and other medical practitioners, for inspecting pharmacies, and for punishing practitioners guilty of malpractice and those practicing medicine without proper licenses. Moreover, the protomedicato in Spain was responsible for directing and regulating the training of physicians, surgeons, and pharmacists. Protomédicos serving on the protomedicato were supported by fees collected from those examined, initially one mark of silver or five *doblas* or *castellanos* of gold for physicians and surgeons, three doblas for pharmacists, and one dobla for dealers in aromatic herbs and spices. By the end of the reign of Ferdinand and Isabella, the protomedicato had become the state regulatory body to ensure the health and well-being of the populace by licensing medical practitioners and ferreting out and punishing illicit charlatans.[2]

Regulation of Medical Practitioners in Mexico: The Municipal Phase

The appointment of Hernández as *protomédico general* in 1570 did not, however, signal the arrival of the protomedicato in the Spanish Indies. In fact, it took 150 years after Spain's discovery of the New World for the protomedicato to make its appearance. Protomédicos, though, emerged in Hispaniola within two decades after discovery when the royal protomedicato in Castile appointed two physicians—Licentiates Pedro López and Fulano Barreda—to examine and license physicians and surgeons and to ensure proper dispensation of drugs on the island.[3] In 1519, however, Charles V nullified these appointments both because the protomedicato, not the newly crowned king, had vested them with office and because the city council of Santo Domingo had complained that if the protomédicos began challenging unlicensed practitioners who had been ministering to the populace, it would seriously disrupt the island.[4]

Not surprisingly, the two rejected protomédicos moved on to newly conquered Mexico. Here in Mexico City in 1525 the city council first designated Barreda as protomédico; then in 1527 it replaced him with López, who was given the power to fine illicit practitioners "twenty pesos for the first offense, a mark of gold for the second, and banishment from New Spain for the third."[5] John Tate Lanning believes that López probably used the commission he received as protomédico in Hispaniola to convince the municipal authorities to appoint him.[6] Barreda, meanwhile, had returned to Hispaniola in 1526 at a salary of three hundred thousand maravedís annually, an enormous stipend by the standards of the day.[7] The island, it turned out, was without a single

licensed physician when López and Barreda departed for greener pastures in Mexico.[8]

The appointment of Barreda and then López as protomédicos began the municipal phase of the regulation of medical practice in Mexico. Since Charles V did not see fit either to appoint a royal protomédico for New Spain or to establish a more formal Spanish-style protomedicato during the immediate postconquest epoch, the city council of Mexico City filled the vacuum by appointing its own municipal protomédicos to regulate the practice of medicine. In this tumultuous epoch the severe shortage of doctors had stimulated the appearance of a rash of unlicensed physicians and practitioners, who preyed on those in need of medical assistance: for dealing with epidemics of *matlazahuatl*, smallpox, measles, and other diseases that ravaged the city; widespread venereal disease; broken bones; urinary problems; cataracts; childbirth; respiratory infections and viruses; and a host of other ailments.[9]

The town council's desire to root out quacks and charlatans became evident in 1530 when the council received a multitude of complaints that a certain Bartolomé Catalán was going around treating buboes without a license. When the council demanded to see his license, he could not produce one. The council thus fined Catalán one hundred pesos and condemned him to perpetual exile. This case is particularly revealing because of the outcry against Catalán, who must have been totally incompetent. In most cases such as these, the patient who had been aided or cured by a quack staunchly defended the latter's right to practice, even if he or she was unlicensed. The empirical evidence of a return to good health was an obvious reminder of the curer's legitimacy and right to practice. Catalán, however, could find no such defenders.[10] The next year, however, when Alonso Guisado was ordered not to practice, he rounded up a number of witnesses who testified to his effectiveness as a healer. In this case the alderman agreed to let him continue to treat sores, ulcers, and the private parts, but "nothing else."[11] Guisado was obviously an expert on venereal disease.

Normally during this epoch, those audacious or daring enough to put up a sign and assume the title "doctor" claimed to have a bona fide degree in medicine, usually from a foreign university such as Paris, Montpellier, or Leiden. Conveniently, though, they somehow lost their medical diploma or proof of certification on the voyage to the New World. (These illicit physicians were careful not to claim a degree from a Spanish university whose authenticity was more easily ascertained.) Pedro de la Torre, who claimed a medical degree from the University of Bologna, was one of these bogus physicians. Charged and convicted by the city council in 1545 of practicing without a license, he was sentenced to sequestration of half his property and permanent exile. Death was the penalty if he remained in New Spain. Pedro de la Torre, meanwhile, defied the authorities by tarrying. Instead of being executed, he paid five hundred pesos to stay on in the viceroyalty. Moreover, distinguished residents of Mexico City, including the ecclesiastical council and Bishop Juan de Zumárraga, appealed to the Crown to let him continue his practice. In the interim, the municipal council suggested that protomédicos in Mexico City subject de la Torre to a rigorous examination and, if he passed, let him practice until the king decided on the appeal. Not surprisingly, de la Torre continued to practice. The need for experienced physicians in Mexico City was desperate, especially in view of the impending departure for Spain of a Doctor Juan de Alcázar, which would have left the urban populace with only three licensed doctors, including de la Torre. Quite clearly, de la Torre had had either enough good luck or enough expertise to cure his patients and to acquire defenders, distinguished ones at that.[12]

Price gouging by apothecaries and physicians was another object of the council's watchful eye during the post-conquest era. When, in 1537, a rash of complaints over the high price of drugs reached the council, it lowered and fixed prices for drugs and set firm regulations for the compounding of prescriptions. Meanwhile, the apothecaries in the city appealed the new regulations. When a commission appointed by the council got an admission from the pharmacists that they had charged too much, they agreed to a more moderate price list drawn up by the commission.[13] Ten years later, however, in the face of a raging epidemic, prices again shot up in the city, indicating that the problem of outrageous charges for drugs had not been resolved.[14] At the same time, with a severe shortage of doctors, a rising white population, and increasing wages, doctors also began

charging excessive fees. As a result in 1535, the city council ruled that no physician could charge more than half a peso for a visit on pain of a fifty-peso fine and a two-month suspension from practice. If a patient called a physician, however, the doctor could charge what he wished, and he did.[15]

Thus, the council of Mexico City gradually emerged as the principal regulator of medical practitioners and apothecaries to ensure the health of the urban populace. What became apparent also is the increasing concern among the aldermen for providing medical services to those who could not pay for medical care or had in some way become wards of the state. To fill these needs, the council began the practice of appointing what might be termed "city doctors" and other practitioners in the service of the municipality. Between 1607 and 1643 the council named six licensed physicians, eight apothecaries, six surgeons, three bone-setters, one oculist, and three phlebotomists.[16] Paid substantial salaries by the city, these practitioners served the needs of those in jail and those in local hospitals or charitable institutions too indigent to pay for medical care. In the century after the conquest, the council did more than simply license doctors and surgeons, inspect drug stores, and ferret out quacks. The aldermen also believed it essential to assist the dispossessed in obtaining medical treatment.

The appointment of Francisco Hernández as proto-médico general of all the Indies might have inaugurated a new direction in the regulation of medical practice in New Spain, perhaps even a new royal protomedicato for New Spain. In his instructions to Hernández, Philip II laid out two major tasks for the distinguished doctor. Most important, given Hernández's expertise as a botanist and the keen interest then sweeping Europe concerning New World curatives, was the injunction to collect information on "herbs, trees, and medicinal plants." He was to disembark first in New Spain because of the prevalence of such diverse flora in that viceroyalty and then move on to Peru. He was to consult with the appropriate doctors, surgeons, and herbalists on their experience with New World medicants and to send back to Spain herbs, plants, and seeds unknown in the Iberian Peninsula. In short, the Crown expected Hernández to organize a botanical expedition in New Spain to survey New

World plants and herbs and to determine their curative properties.[17]

Another part of his instructions as protomédico general, however, outlined a second set of regulatory responsibilities. From the seat of the royal *audiencia,* presumably Mexico City, he was to examine and license all physicians and surgeons and to inspect apothecary shops within a five-league radius of the city. Those practitioners and apothecaries outside the five-league limit could ask to be examined and licensed if they wished, but this was not required.[18]

This second set of instructions clearly challenged the power that the city council and its appointed protomédicos had appropriated by default to regulate medical affairs. Whether the aldermen felt threatened by Hernández is not clear, but they were well aware of his presence in Mexico. One indication is that during his sojourn in New Spain council members no longer referred to their municipal medical officers as protomédicos but called them *visitadores médicos* instead. Significantly, though, they returned to using the term *protomédico* once Hernández left New Spain.[19]

In the end Hernández constituted no threat at all to the council's authority because he ignored the second part of his instructions. In fact, there is no evidence that he examined or licensed a single physician or inspected a single pharmacy in Mexico. He devoted himself instead to his botanical pursuits. The council and its protomédicos continued as before in their regulation and discipline of medical practitioners, protecting the urban populace from quacks and charlatans. In fact, it was not until 1646 that a royal protomedicato finally came to New Spain.[20]

Physicians and Surgeons: Training and Control

If Francisco Hernández had taken up his medical responsibilities as protomédico instead of pursuing his botanical and scientific interests, what kinds of medical practitioners in New Spain would he have examined and licensed? What kind of medicine did they practice? Highest ranking among these various practitioners was the licensed physi-

cian, whose requirements for the practice of medicine were essentially the same throughout the colonial epoch. To get a medical diploma and a physician's license, the candidate had to know Latin, be of pure blood, and spend eight years at the university, four getting the bachelor of arts degree and four studying medicine. After an internship of two years with an established physician, the candidate presented himself to the protomedicato or protomédico for examination and certification. If he passed the exam, he became a licensed physician. Since the four years spent studying arts corresponded to high school years in the United States, a would-be physician began his medical training at approximately the same time a contemporary American student enters college. Thus, with the two-year internship, he might become a fully fledged physician by age twenty-two or twenty-three.[21]

Two additional medical degrees were also available— the licentiate and the doctorate. In Spain and the Indies the licentiate demanded a bit of additional reading from the established authorities such as Galen, Hippocrates, and Avicenna, but those aspiring to the licentiate neither had to take more classes nor had to engage in more laboratory or practical training. The doctorate in medicine was totally honorific and required no additional study, only a well-filled pocketbook to pay the required fees and to provide a sumptuous feast and entertainment for those certifying the degree. On occasion, the doctorate was awarded only three or four days after the licentiate.[22]

Those seeking to become physicians could not be trained adequately in Mexico until the seventeenth century. By a Spanish law of 1617 the university needed three chairs of medicine to train would-be physicians and to award medical degrees. At the Royal and Pontifical University of Mexico, the first chair of medicine was established in 1578, a second of "vespers" in 1599, and a third in surgical methods and anatomy in 1621.[23] Appointment of this third chair thus gave the Royal and Pontifical University of Mexico the minimum number of faculty members to award medical degrees. After 1578 a student could take courses in medicine and receive a degree, but he did not meet the standards set later in 1617 for getting a medical diploma. That was only possible after 1621.

The standing of the medical faculty at the university was very low. Salaries reflected this lowly status, particularly when compared with others on the faculty. At the outset, chairs in medicine at the university in Mexico City received little more than three hundred pesos annually, whereas colleagues in theology, law, and sacred canons got more than thirteen hundred pesos a year, although over time stipends of the medical faculty increased somewhat. Significantly, when the third chair of surgery and anatomy was established in the 1620s, the appointee agreed to serve gratis.[24] The medical faculty could not carry swords and marched last in university processions. No professor of medicine or surgery could serve as rector of the university. Although a medical doctor's usual mode of dress was black with silver accessories, in Chile physicians seemed to make up for their lack of status by wearing green gloves and powdering their beards with gold dust and also by wearing ostentatious gold chains around their necks.[25]

Once legally certified, physicians had to subscribe to certain rules and regulations. They were obliged to serve the poor without payment of fees, to make house calls, and to perform in such a way as to provide for the patient's spiritual well-being as prescribed by canon law. Moreover, a doctor was required to respond to requests from municipal authorities to make night calls. Then as now, Saturday-night and festival-eve carousals often required a doctor's presence to care for someone whose head had been bashed in during a drunken brawl. Physicians were specifically prohibited from leaving town when an epidemic struck. If they did, they were subject to criminal prosecution and loss of their license.[26]

For the most part, though, a legally licensed physician serving the white inhabitants of Mexico enjoyed both high status and a good living. The extreme shortage of qualified medical men in the large cities of colonial Spanish America ensured a plenitude of patients. If a young doctor achieved early success in his cures, he could quickly build up a practice among the urban white elite and be assured of being paid well by those calling on his services. Moreover, those who practiced in Mexico City or similar urban areas in the Indies generally ignored the duty imposed on them to serve the poor without payment of fees or to go out on Saturday nights when called by the authorities to attend to those hurt in brawls. Such duties fell to municipal physicians appointed and paid by the town council. At the same time, regular and secular clergy often practiced as surrogate physicians in their parishes or hospitals to fill the vacuum left by the lack of licensed physicians, who ministered primarily to rich clients.[27]

The licensed physician was not the only practitioner available to the urban populace. Although the rich and the powerful, the *gente decente,* generally used legally certified doctors, surgeons also practiced in Mexico. Surgeons were of two types: the Latin surgeon and the romance surgeon (*romancista*). The more qualified of the two, the Latin surgeon, labeled as such because he had to know Latin, was required to have a certificate of blood purity, take three advanced courses in surgery beyond the bachelor's degree, and undergo a two-year apprenticeship with a licensed surgeon. If he saw fit to seek a license, he could then go before the examiners and certifiers, either the protomédicos or, in Mexico after 1646, the protomedicato.[28]

The romance surgeon most likely never darkened the door of the university. In fact, he could be illiterate. To qualify as a *romancista,* he only had to assure the authorities of his purity of blood and undergo a four- to five-year apprenticeship with a licensed surgeon. If he chose to be examined, he could then put up his sign, which he usually did even if he was not examined and licensed.[29] Most surgeons of this sort, even Latin surgeons, did not seek licenses. In fact, in the last fifty years of the seventeenth century in Mexico, only one surgeon of either type was ever examined and certified.[30]

Fees collected by surgeons for their services were so minuscule that they found it hard to accumulate enough to pay licensing fees. A surgeon's fee for setting a bone, for example, was the same as for shaving a man's head.[31] Any simple surgical procedure such as removing a cyst cost one peso, more complex operations two. To amputate one leg a surgeon charged one peso, for two legs four pesos. For the most part, without anesthesia and unable to control infection, they were the last recourse for those who sought out their services and seldom achieved much success in major operations. In fact, the satiric Limeño poet Juan de Caviedes compared surgeons to executioners.[32]

Phlebotomists, Apothecaries, and Midwives

Still another class of practitioner was the phlebotomist, the bloodletter. Most were not licensed at all until the beginning of the nineteenth century, but if they were, they had to serve two to three years of apprenticeship in a hospital, somewhat like a modern-day orderly, and four years with an experienced phlebotomist. If they chose to practice legally and get their license, they could be examined orally if they did not know how to read or write. The phlebotomist had to know about veins and arteries, how to bleed properly with cupping glasses and leeches, how to extract teeth, and how to lance ulcers and boils. Some were under contract to hospitals, to which they were called in to practice their art when needed.[33] Pregnant women also used phlebotomists. It was thought that by the third month, since the parturient had lost her menstrual flow, with no natural outlet, the blood was retained in the blood vessels that loaded the membranes of the uterus, made the nerves more irritable, and caused the vomiting associated with morning sickness. Bleeding would relieve this state.[34] Following the dictates of Galen, bleeding was also prescribed for a host of other ailments and illnesses.

Closely associated with all medical practitioners were apothecaries, who dispensed the necessary medicines prescribed by licensed doctors and surgeons. Unlike a physician, who could be younger, the apothecary had to be at least twenty-five years old, establish his blood purity, know Latin and the pharmacopoeia, and undergo a four-year apprenticeship. To become licensed, he had to undergo an examination by protomédicos, assisted by a licensed pharmacist.[35]

Once the apothecary began dispensing drugs, a number of regulations governed his conduct. No woman could become an apothecary; no physician or surgeon could own an apothecary shop; and no physician or surgeon could have his prescriptions filled by a relative or in-law in the same town or fill them himself. No apothecary could close his shop without special permission. To prevent a monopoly over drug dispensation, no apothecary could operate a shop in two different towns.[36] Each apothecary shop was subject to inspection every two years by protomédicos and after 1646 by the protomedicato. As in the qualifying examination, a licensed pharmacist assisted in the inspection. The inspection team ascertained that only licensed pharmacists dispensed drugs, that the shop contained the proper stock of drugs, and that drug prices were fair. The inspection team also determined if the apothecary was related to any physicians or surgeons in the city, and if so, whether he was filling prescriptions for them. The inspectors could close the shop if they found the apothecary violating any of the regulations he was obliged to follow.[37]

What the pharmacist dispensed in Mexico City provides a useful index to the state of medical practice, which may seem appalling by modern-day standards. On the other hand, the shelves of an apothecary shop in Mexico during the colonial period were not much different from those in Spain or the rest of Europe, particularly since medical training in the New World in the sixteenth and seventeenth centuries emulated that provided in Europe. Interestingly, given Philip II's firm desire to establish increasing state control over Spanish and imperial society, in the world of Francisco Hernández there was no official pharmacopoeia. Although in 1594 the king finally ordered one drawn up for all apothecary shops in both Spain and the empire, it was not until 145 years later, in 1739, that the well-known *Pharmacopoeia matritensis* finally appeared.[38] This pharmacopoeia included many of the medicines commonly prescribed over the previous three centuries in both Europe and America and was beholden in many ways to the pharmacopoeia drawn up by Félix Palacios in 1706.[39]

The stock of a pharmacy in Mexico City contained a variety of exotic animal and avian powders and liquids as remedies for a variety of ills. Among them was the tusk of the narwhal, good for treating smallpox, pest, and measles. Cochineals, crawfish, tumblebugs, toads, and frogs were prescribed as diuretics and blood purifiers. Crawfish, vipers, serpents, deer antlers, human cranium, hoof of the tapir, and blood of a she-mule cured palsy and apoplexy and served as antidotes to poison and as coagulants. Powdered crawfish eyes alleviated problems with kidney stones, bladder contusions, hemorrhoids, and side aches. Dried frog intestines were said to dissolve kidney stones. Dried wolf's liver and also its intestines were good for windy colic. Pulverized swallow wings with blood on them combined with

REGULATION OF MEDICAL PRACTITIONERS ❧ 61

salt and certain powders helped with bladder infections. Epilepsy, paralysis, apoplexy, and other such ailments could be relieved by taking a powder made from a pulverized human cranium of one who had died by violence. Dried fox lungs helped with asthma and chest ailments. Nervous disorders could be relieved by tapir hooves. Urine and excrement of animals including the goose, ass, peccary, ox, cow, goat, stork, serpent, horse, chicken, human being, sheep, sparrow, turkey, dog, buzzard, squab pigeon, and fox could all bring out the humors through the skin by stimulating perspiration and helped to eliminate those that caused epilepsy, apoplexy, paralysis, and palsy. How the patient fared after taking such drugs can be left to the modern observer to decide, but these were the kinds of cures recommended by licensed physicians in Mexico City.[40]

Perhaps the largest group of medical practitioners in Mexico, except for the omnipresent native healers (the *curanderos*) who pervaded the land, was midwives (*parteras*), who assisted women through their pregnancies and at childbirth. Since midwives plied their trade so widely in Mexico, state regulation by protomédicos or the protomedicato was virtually impossible. Moreover, in the sixteenth and seventeenth centuries, there were no licensing standards for midwives. In fact, it was not until the mid-eighteenth century that concerned physicians in Spain sought to establish qualifications for midwives, seek their licensing, and provide professional advice for them.

How a woman became a midwife in Mexico is not clear, but many were the daughters of midwives who assisted their mothers in what constituted an apprenticeship. Others were women who gained experience early helping an established midwife at childbirths. After gaining such experience, they went out on their own to offer their services to those who needed them. If they proved helpful and built up a record of births that went well under their supervision, they became much sought after by pregnant women who needed their services.

The Spanish ideal for a midwife was reflected in the eighteenth-century handbook by the Spanish protomédico Antonio Medina, published in 1759, nine years after it was decided in Madrid that midwives needed licensing.[41] Medina believed that local doctors should train midwives in

their communities. Midwives, he insisted, should not preside over difficult cases. In these situations she must call on the services of a "good surgeon." He stipulated that a midwife was to be a mature adult, not a youngish women, be literate, and undergo an apprenticeship under a seasoned practitioner. The ideal midwife also had to be healthy, with good hands and no bent fingers. She was to aid the poor when asked and be "patient, cheerful, and modest" and temperate—she was to shy away from imbibing too much wine. Discretion was also an essential quality. She must keep silent in cases in which the honor of the parturient was at stake.[42]

Medina hoped that, in her training, a midwife would learn about female anatomy, particularly that of the pelvic area—sacrum, coccyx, uterus, mons veneris, frenulum clitoridis, vulva clitoris, urethra, nymphae, and hymen. In cases of rape and in determining virginity, such knowledge was crucial. If situations arose in which a midwife was required to give a deposition in a legal case, she was to consult first with a bona fide physician. She was prohibited emphatically from providing a parturient with information on abortion techniques. In her advice to a pregnant women, she was to suggest that the parturient not have frequent intercourse, not exercise vigorously, not wear restrictive corsets, avoid stress, and report any unusual physical changes during the pregnancy to the midwife.[43] Based on evidence from Spanish hospitals in the sixteenth century, fees paid to these midwives ranged from two reales to one peso.[44]

This was the eighteenth-century ideal, but reports circulating in Mexico throughout the colonial period indicate that midwives plying their trade might well have profited greatly from Dr. Medina's sensible advice. Some midwives prescribed a host of strange remedies to reduce the parturient's labor time and to ensure a more rapid delivery—clysters, a chicken cut open down the back and put on the parturient's stomach, a mule's sweat pad cooked in urine, and infusions of feather grass or senna. One Mexican doctor serving in the countryside—not a midwife but a highly regarded physician—prescribed a concoction made up of horse manure and wine to do the same.[45] Another recommended remedy to ease a parturient's difficult labor was simply to enter the birthing room with a turkey heart.[46] As already pointed out, bleeding during the third month was also recommended as a standard procedure for those who went to a bona fide physician or surgeon.[47]

Conclusion

Implicitly or explicitly this brief discussion of the regulation of medical practice and practitioners in Mexico has emphasized a number of factors. First, in the age of Francisco Hernández, regulation was confined to large cities where fully licensed doctors served the populace. Self-interest gave them a special reason for rooting out illicit practitioners posing as doctors and for eliminating quacks and charlatans. They wanted the medical arena exclusively for themselves so that they might build a large and lucrative practice, unchallenged by other would-be physicians. Outside the large cities, however, the inhabitants were left to their own devices to rely on native healers, midwives, romance surgeons, phlebotomists, priests, or illicit foreign doctors who put up a sign. These practitioners posed no challenge to licensed physicians in rural areas or small towns because there were simply no trained doctors in the countryside. These rural and small-town practitioners also provided a modicum of advice and cures to those who sought them out and in other ways filled the vacuum caused by the dearth of licensed doctors in the community. On balance, though, the countryside may have been as well served as the large cities with licensed practitioners, who, in the sixteenth and seventeenth centuries often, like Pedro de la Torre, practiced with false credentials. They served only the rich and powerful and used drugs and bleeding practices that did far more harm than good. As in Europe, physicians in the Spanish Indies attached themselves to the dictates of Galen and Hippocrates, which oftentimes did little to relieve the sick and the injured.

A second, more positive factor to emphasize for Mexico City is that in the pre-protomedicato period the city council assumed responsibility for regulating medical affairs—ascertaining that physicians had proper credentials, challenging those who did not, inspecting drug stores, and exposing quacks. Moreover, the appointment of a host of city doctors and other medical practitioners during this epoch demonstrated the rising social concern of Mexico City aldermen, who felt an obligation to meet some of the medical needs of the poor. City doctors and municipal practitioners of one sort or another served those who fell ill in jail and visited local hospitals, orphanages, and poorhouses to minister to the impoverished who could not pay an established practitioner. In the early days after the conquest, the council also attempted to prevent price gouging in the city's pharmacies during critical periods when epidemics were sweeping the city and to regulate the fees licensed doctors could charge their patients. As the first bona fide royal protomédico to arrive in Mexico in 1570, Francisco Hernández posed no challenge to the city council's authority to regulate medical practice. Although the aldermen were clearly aware of his presence, Hernández chose to ignore the medical side of his instructions and to pursue his botanical interests instead, which he did with great distinction. Thus, the municipal phase in the regulation of medical practice and practitioners continued until 1646 when the royal protomedicato finally took root in Mexico.

Still a third tendency during the century after the conquest was the freedom of the unlicensed practitioner to ply his or her trade, unfettered and unregulated. Romance surgeons, phlebotomists, and midwives were neither licensed nor rigidly controlled, except when their behavior became a matter of public complaint. Moreover, they were simply too poorly paid to accumulate the fees for an examination and certification, which might have given them additional prestige and more legitimacy in the community. For licensing midwives, there was no interest in Spain until the middle of the eighteenth century, while in Mexico the first licensing of *parteras* did not occur until 1816 and 1818, when two women presented themselves to medical authorities for examination.[48] In their own way native healers, surgeons, phlebotomists, and midwives seemed to have performed a useful service in their communities. Many successfully built up a clientele, who, by luck or by good advice, were cured of their maladies by a native healer's remedy. Others went under a surgeon's knife and sometimes recovered, as did those being bled by phlebotomists or assisted by the midwife at childbirth. Many of those who sought out these practitioners staunchly defended their right to practice. They were cheaper than established physicians and were readily available when no other doctor was about to minister to them. Only in cases in which a rash of complaints against a practitioner flooded the desks of municipal authorities, such as occurred in 1530 with Bartolomé Catalán, did the aldermen take decisive action. But sometimes, as with Pedro de la Torre, vigorous and powerful defenders of the illicit practitioner forced the city council to back down.

Finally, the regulation of medical practice in Mexico during the sixteenth and early seventeenth centuries, prior to establishment of the protomedicato, demonstrated the concern of the state for the welfare of the populace and indicated that municipal authorities saw a real need to protect the citizenry from the quack and the charlatan and a responsibility to look after the health and welfare of the inhabitants, even the most needy.

NOTES

1. For quotation, see *Mexican Treasury,* "Instructions and Letters to the King."

2. For the early history of the protomedicato in Spain, see Pascual Iborra, "Memoria sobre la institución del real protomedicato," *Anales de la Real Academia de Medicina* 6 (1885): 183–207, and Tate Lanning's summary dismissal of it in *The Royal Protomedicato: The Regulation of the Medical Professions in the Spanish Empire* (Durham, N.C.: Duke University Press, 1985), 7.

3. Archivo General de Indias (hereafter cited as AGI), Indiferente General, 419, authorizing salary of 50,000 maravedís [about 135 ducats—Ed.] to Barreda (Madrid, July 22, 1517).

4. AGI, Indiferente General, 420, royal patent to Rodrigo Figueroa barring protomédicos and apothecaries from practicing (Barcelona, July 16, 1519).

5. *Actas de Cabildo de México* 1.115 (January 11, 1527).

6. Lanning, *Royal Protomedicato,* 25.

7. AGI, Indiferente General, 421, Barreda's appointment (Granada, September 14, 1525).

8. AGI, Santo Domingo, 1123, royal patent to the appellate court of Santo Domingo (Valladolid, June 1, 1527).

9. [*Matlazahuatl:* Possibly typhus, according to Francisco J. Santamaría, *Diccionario de Mejicanismos,* 4th ed. (Mexico City: Porrua, 1983)—Ed.]

10. *Actas de Cabildo de México,* 2.30–31 (January 24, 1530).

11. Ibid., 2.145–46 (November 17, 1531).

12. AGI, Justicia, 199 (Mexico City, March 28, 1545).

13. *Actas de Cabildo de México,* 4.95 (September 14, 1537) and 4.202 (June 18, 1540).

14. Ibid., 5.191 (October 10, 1547).

15. Ibid., 4.43 (October 13, 1536).

16. See Lanning, *Royal Protomedicato,* 33.

17. Archivo General de la Nación, México (hereafter cited as AGNM), Reales cédulas (Dup.) 47.262, art. 1–6. See *Mexican Treasury,* "Instructions and Letters to the King."

18. AGNM, Reales cédulas (Dup.) 47.262, fols. 157v–58r, arts. 6–12, and *Mexican Treasury,* "Instructions and Letters to the King."

19. *Actas de Cabildo de México,* 8.282 (April 15 and 19, 1577).

20. For the establishment, organization, and operation of the protomedicato in Mexico, see Lanning, *Royal Protomedicato,* 62–134.

21. Ibid., 332.

22. Ibid., 333.

23. Francisco Fernández del Castillo, *La Facultad de Medicina según el Archivo de la Real y Pontificia Universidad de México* (Mexico City: Consejo de Humanidades, 1953), 86–138. [Following the example of the medieval University of Salamanca, the chair of vespers indicated the evening—the time of day when teaching took place. See the Alcalá constitution quoted by Rafael Chabrán, "Classical Tradition," above—Ed.]

24. Fernández del Castillo, *Facultad de Medicina,* 136–37.

25. Ricardo Palma, *Tradiciones peruanas,* 6 vols. (Madrid, n.d.), 1:170. Palma describes the dress of a typical Lima physician in the seventeenth century.

26. Miguel Eugenio Muñoz, *Recopilación de las leyes, pragmáticas, reales decretos, y acuerdos del Real Proto-Medicato* (Valencia, 1751), chap. 13, art. 1, p. 158. See also Lanning, *Royal Protomedicato,* 200–216, for other charitable obligations of the medical profession.

27. Despite this requirement, physicians usually avoided these obligations (and for their methods of evasion, see Lanning, *Royal Protomedicato,* 201–8). In Mexico the city doctors or the clergy usually ministered to the poor and needy; licensed physicians served the white population who could afford them. As indicated above, although there were limits to what a licensed physician could charge, because of the desperate shortage of doctors, their services were much sought after and their fees were often very high.

28. *Nueva recopilación (Recopilación de las leyes de estos reynos . . .),* 3 vols. (Madrid, 1640), bk. 3, title 16, law 9, par. 9, and bk. 1, title 7, law 13.

29. Ibid., 1.7.13.

30. J. M. Reyes, "Historia de la medicina: Estudios históricos sobre el ejercicio de la medicina," *Gaceta médica de México* 1 (1865): 256.

31. Hospital de Nuestra Señora Santa María de Esquiva, Valladolid, n.d., Libros de Despensas 35, fol. 58.

32. Caviedes, *Obras de don Juan del Valle y Caviedes,* introduction and notes by Rubén Vargas Ugarte, S.J. (Lima: n.p., 1947), 213. In one passage Caviedes refers to medical practitioners as "idiots" (140).

33. Archivo Colonial, Bogotá, Médicos y Abogados, 3, fols. 576v–578v. Miguel de la Isla to the viceroy, Bogotá, May 1, 1805; AGI, Indiferente General, 473, royal patent to the governor of the island of Cuba, Valladolid, June 19, 1615.

34. Joseph Erasistrato Suadel, "Carta segunda," *Mercurio peruano* 3 (June 5, 1791): 89–95.

35. *Nueva recopilación* 1.16.13; Muñoz, *Recopilación,* chap. 2, arts. 1, 2; chap. 14, art. 9.

36. Muñoz, *Recopilación,* 14.2.170; 15.8.198. Royal provision, Aranjuez, June 23, 1743; 14.8.180; 14.14.181; 15.8.106.

37. *Nueva recopilación* 8.3.3–4. Muñoz, *Recopilación* 15.8.195 (Aranjuez, June 23, 1743). P. D. Rodríguez Rivero, *Historia médica de Venezuela hasta 1900* (Caracas: Parra León, 1931), 133.

38. *Pharmacopoeia matritensis regii, ac supremi hispaniarum pro-tomedicatus auctoritate, jussu atque auspiciis elaborata* (Madrid, 1739; reprint, Madrid, 1762).

39. Félix Palacios, *Palestra farmacéutica, chimica-galénica* (Madrid, 1706, 1723, 1730, 1737, 1753, 1763, 1778, 1792, and 1797).

40. Ibid.

41. Antonio Medina, *Cartilla nueva, útil, y necesaria para instruirse las matronas que vulgarmente se llaman comadres, en el oficio de partear* (Madrid, 1759).

42. Ibid., prefatory chapter.

43. Ibid., chaps. 2, 3, 4.

44. Hospital de Tavera, Toledo, Despensas, July 5, 1588, and January 10, 1596.

45. *Compendio de la medicina: O medicina práctica* (Mexico City, 1788), 157.

46. AGNM, Inquisición, 986.17, fol. 193v.

47. An inveterate researcher, John Tate Lanning uncovered a host of sensational cases of quacks, charlatans, and incompetents practicing midwifery in the Spanish Indies. As a result, in chapter 13 of his *Royal Protomedicato,* he leaves the strong impression that the midwife was more of a charlatan than a helpmate. Probably, though, the cases he describes are more atypical than typical, and experienced midwives, of whom there is no record, most likely served pregnant women very well in most Spanish colonial communities.

48. Archivo Histórico de la Facultad de Medicina de la Universidad de México, Protomedicato, 10, fols. 1–2 (1816). (The file is incomplete.) Protomedicato 12.15, fols. 1–2 (1818), examination of María Francisca Ignacia Sánchez.

SHELTER AND CARE FOR NATIVES AND COLONISTS

HOSPITALS IN SIXTEENTH-CENTURY NEW SPAIN

GUENTER B. RISSE

When an unidentified pestilential fever erupted mostly among the surviving native inhabitants of New Spain in April 1576, the government, headed by Viceroy Martín Enríquez and the church's highest official, archbishop Pedro Moya de Contreras, called on members of the colonial elite to offer assistance to those affected by this scourge. The epidemic, termed *huey cocoliztli*, or "great pestilence," began to spread from east to west, overwhelming all assistance services, including a network of hundreds of hospitals scattered in all regions of the colony.[1] Among them in Mexico City was the Hospital Real de los Naturales, founded by a royal decree dated May 18, 1553, in response to a suggestion from the *audiencia* a year earlier to the emperor Charles V citing the lack of housing and care for poor Indians and travelers coming to the capital city. Its immediate predecessor is said to have been the Hospital Real de San José de los Naturales, a shelter open to all native people residing in New Spain that was established on royal orders around the year 1531 with the assistance of the Franciscans.[2] Placed under royal patronage and functioning primarily as a hostel, the hospital was expanded several times beginning in 1568 until it had eight wards with a capacity of about fifty patients,

including one ward devoted solely to contagious cases. Its main function during the epidemic was to retrieve the dying for the provision of last rites.[3]

At the height of the epidemic, the Hospital Real de los Naturales was visited by none other than Francisco Hernández, the famous *protomédico* who had already spent five years studying the value of native medicinal plants throughout New Spain.[4] Hernández was no stranger to hospital life, having worked in the infirmary belonging to the monastery of Guadalupe and served a stint as medical consultant to the Hospital de Santa Cruz in Toledo before his appointment as court physician in 1567. Later, following his arrival in the New World, he held a similar position at the Hospital de Santa Cruz in Huaxtepec, where Hernández is said to have studied and clinically experimented with native remedies around the year 1574.[5] Anxious to discover a useful remedy against the dreaded *cocoliztli*, Hernández briefly took residence at the Hospital Real de los Naturales, where he treated patients and had some of those who perished dissected, presumably by Alonso López de Hinojosos, a Spanish barber-surgeon and author of a surgical treatise published in 1578.[6] As a result of his institutional experiences, Hernández himself wrote a brief treatise concerning the clinical and pathological manifestations of this most lethal epidemic disease.

Conventional histories of the European-American transfer of institutions often describe early colonial hospitals as charitable foundations established by enlightened rulers or local town councils to ensure the provision of medical care for both Spaniards and native inhabitants in the face of widespread disease. However, given their small size and limited resources, these hospitals actually played a minor role in the service of the sick.[7] Indeed, while millions of New World inhabitants perished, only a few thousand found shelter and care in such establishments. Nevertheless, although their importance as centers of medicine was negligible, hospitals constituted early contact points between two distinct cultures and unique instruments of assimilation as the native populations were exposed to the institutions of colonial society. One side was represented by religious personnel, apprenticed surgeons, and a mere handful of university-trained European physicians whose activities were all guided by the Galenic humoral system. The Americas, meanwhile, featured a variety of tribal folk healers with equally comprehensive explanatory schemes coupled with the command of an impressive variety of local medicinal plants.[8]

Events surrounding the celebration of America's quincentennial have forced historians on both sides of the Atlantic to reexamine the ideological foundations of earlier interpretations regarding the "discovery" of the "New World."[9] It is perhaps useful to adopt the recent perspective articulated by Mexico's renowned scholar Miguel León-Portilla. To characterize the first contact and subsequent colonial process, León-Portilla employed the Spanish word *encuentro* (encounter) to convey simultaneously the meanings of collision, conflict, and opposition but also approach, convergence, and connection between cultures representing the Old and New Worlds.[10] This view demands a new conceptual framework capable of including all participants in the colonial enterprise along a broad spectrum of activities, from violent confrontation to peaceful fusion.[11]

To illustrate this approach, a pair of plausible clinical histories has been constructed, based on available documentation.[12] These cases are presented here to symbolize the scope of hospital trajectories in early colonial times. The first features a Christianized Tarascan native to be known by his baptismal name, Juan Manuel, who was presumed to suffer from an infectious disease called *cocoliztli*. This young man in his early twenties lived in Mexico's central highlands, where he was admitted to the Hospital Real de la Purisima Concepción in Uruapan at the height of an epidemic during the fall of 1545.[13] The second case deals with a middle-aged Spanish colonist and former soldier of fortune identified as Xavier Vázquez residing in Mexico City. During the summer of 1585, Vázquez was referred to the local Hospital de Cosme y Damián, better known as Amor de Dios, for treatment of his syphilitic symptoms.[14] The deliberate juxtaposition of the likely institutional experiences of Juan Manuel and Xavier Vázquez is meant solely to convey a clearer understanding of the various roles played by hospitals in New Spain during the sixteenth century.

Hospital Ideology and Patronage

How was the colonial hospital's mission constructed? Based on scriptural injunctions to assist the poor and visit the sick, hospitals had traditionally been incorporated into the network of Christian symbols and institutions. In Europe, setting up shelter-hospitals and providing assistance to the needy were time-honored responses already in place for more than a millennium.[15] Since hospitalization was designed to renew Christian faith and values through the redemptive quality of human suffering, it quickly became another effective instrument in the conversion of native Americans to Christianity after the institution was established in Spain's new colonies.[16]

The hospital's evangelical agenda was part of a broad policy confirmed by a bull of Pope Alexander VI dated May 4, 1493, conceding to the Spanish Crown the right to Christianize the inhabitants of the New World.[17] As early as 1493, Franciscans began arriving in the colonies with Columbus to start the conversion of more than three thousand natives on the island of Hispaniola.[18] In a letter dated March 20, 1503, King Ferdinand and Queen Isabella of Castile ordered Ovando, governor of the island of Hispaniola, "to build hospitals where the poor can be housed and cured, whether

Christians or Indians."[19] This official request reflected not only a medieval Christian tradition of charity and good works deeply embedded in Spanish culture but also a willingness to use a well-known European institution such as the hospital to enhance the process of Christian conversion and Europeanization among the native inhabitants of the New World.[20]

After the conquest of the Aztec empire, further missionary efforts targeted New Spain. Soon, hospital foundations linked to new churches, monasteries, and schools began to dot the countryside outside Mexico City, reaching the Pacific through Michoacán and expanding south to Guatemala, Honduras, and Panama. The area of greatest concentration was the more densely populated region of central Mexico, with an estimated preconquest population between 10 million and 25 million people.[21] It was here in Michoacán and the Valley of Mexico that hospitals, which had no distinct pre-Columbian analog, were integrated into existing Tarascan and Nahua ethnic population centers called the *altepetl*.[22]

Sixteenth-century Spaniards characterized hospitals as *templos de piedad* (temples of pity and compassion).[23] Their charitable services played an important role in restoring some measure of social cohesion to the native population in the face of serious upheavals caused by the wars of conquest.[24] Moreover, in the view of Christian colonists, to die without assistance on the streets or in the fields like beasts was to forfeit eternal life. By contrast, hospitals could not only offer welcome shelter to the homeless and sick but also provide the last sacraments that ensured salvation. In larger urban areas such as Mexico City during the sixteenth century, hospital personnel in fact are said to have regularly searched the city's barrios for sick and dying paupers, who were brought to the institution and suitably prepared there to meet their new Christian maker.

One of the most important elements of the missionary effort, especially after the 1550s, was the recruitment of local native people such as our Juan Manuel to establish lay brotherhoods (*cofradías*) in established villages and new settlements.[25] As the ranks of the indigenous nobility became reduced during the wars of conquest and the ensuing epidemics, preconquest networks of social organization

and dependence broke down, blurring traditional distinctions of social class and hierarchy. Rudderless, often deprived of family through massacres and disease, young men such as Juan Manuel scattered, fleeing from forced labor in the *encomiendas,* only to congregate again around the European newcomers in reorganized colonial pueblos, where they could resume their traditional services as *macehuallis,* or commoners.

Laboring within a new Christian service industry created by the presence of churches, monasteries, and hospitals, many native inhabitants established new social relationships and bonds. This widespread community-building effort spearheaded by the mendicant friars was critical to both the Spanish evangelizing and assimilation processes.[26] Following Spanish prototypes, most lay brotherhoods focused on the humanity of Christ and the mercy of the Virgin Mary, their members identifying with the sufferings of the Holy Family, thus drawing moral support for themselves while performing a series of charitable acts, including care of the sick. Lay brotherhoods were, in the words of one member, "a safe refuge for those who sail upon this sea of furious pains."[27]

A royal political agenda contributed to the creation of hospitals. As expressed in a royal decree issued by Charles V to all colonial viceroys on October 7, 1541, hospitals were to be founded in all Spanish and Indian towns.[28] At this point, the Spanish government had already become painfully aware of the problems caused by the dramatic postconquest mortality and dispersal of the native population. Thus, in their view, it was imperative that this ever dwindling native population be channeled into productive endeavors, especially agricultural tasks and the exercise of various crafts. Able-bodied individuals, organized around the institution of the hospital as well as churches and monasteries, would ultimately produce economic benefits. Therefore, while serving the well-advertised evangelizing function, new hospitals also became, in the 1550s, important mechanisms of a royal policy to aggregate dispersed native inhabitants and achieve a measure of political, economic, and social control over them.[29] At the same time, hospitals rapidly became community symbols, cultural centers in which native and European beliefs and ideas blended.

In their quest to create hospitals, religious and lay Spanish leaders were also influenced by new ideas derived from Renaissance humanism that attempted to recast the traditional religious role of the hospital. Here the works of Erasmus and Thomas More were quite persuasive. More, for example, argued in 1516 for the care of the sick in hospitals in *Utopia*. Such institutional attention was to be a rational and routine activity of the community. Just as important, More's utopian hospitals were no longer conceived as shelters for the poor but designed to be medicalized institutions for the care and isolation of sick citizens.[30]

This humanistic model was partially adopted by Vasco de Quiroga, one of the judges of New Spain's *audiencia,* or governing body under the viceroy.[31] Shrewdly combining religious, humanistic, and economic motives, Quiroga proposed in 1531 that vacant lands be made available to establish new pueblos, or "hospital-republics" arranged around the activities of an infirmary. These centers would be populated by young, Christianized native people of both sexes many of whom had been orphaned by the wars of conquest. Participating Indians were to be baptized, sent to schools to become literate and learn a trade, get married, and have families.[32]

The effects of epidemic disease in the form of a demographic catastrophe profoundly influenced all subsequent political and economic policies of the Crown and the colonial government.[33] By the 1580s, following the demise of another half million native inhabitants from the dreaded cocoliztli, a deliberate royal policy of *congregación* encouraged all villages with the rank of head town to build hospitals with the labor, money, and alms of the native people themselves. Indians were now deliberately herded from rural areas and small population centers to larger, more manageable urban units under the direct jurisdiction of the Crown and the official church. Even native chiefs were pressured to assist in this resettlement. City living was now seen as an essential part of the effort to Christianize and civilize the remaining native people. Since labor shortages caused by the steep decline of the native population were especially acute in urban areas, rounding up Indians became an economic necessity.[34]

Clearly, then, instead of simply medical motives, political and economic agendas meshed with religious and humanistic concerns to establish hospitals in the New World.[35] Public health arguments, such as the prevalence of devastating epidemics, were additionally advanced to justify the establishment of such institutions. Yet hospitals, in removing the sick to their premises, played only a minor role in protecting the healthy. Institutional isolation of a handful of individuals and the provision of reassurance, food, and shelter to a very limited group of wretched survivors were actually insignificant when compared with the detrimental effects of congregating the native people in towns and cities and thus fostering further contagion.[36] The Spanish policy of urban colonization worked in tandem with economic dislocation and cultural disintegration, thus magnifying the impact of epidemic disease. In the meantime, a revolution in colonial transportation brought about by wheeled carts with draft and pack animals only helped to spread further sickness from one part of New Spain to the other.[37]

The Franciscans were the first among the mendicant orders to arrive in New Spain. Prominent clerics such as Juan de San Miguel traveled through the populated Mexican highlands of Michoacán, trying to reorganize previous Tarascan villages into what the Spanish broadly described as "pueblos," ranging from small settlements to larger-sized towns. Hospital foundations such as the Hospital Real de la Purísima Concepción, erected in Uruapan about 1538 and where the Christianized Juan Manuel later sought refuge, occurred as part of the construction of monasteries and schools that were dedicated to the Virgin Mary and her Immaculate Conception.[38] Franciscans were followed by the Augustinians, who often also imitated Quiroga by founding new towns, complete with *cabildo,* school, convent, and hospital around the town's central plaza.[39] By the late 1540s, the entire region belonging to the ancient Tarascan kingdom around Lake Patzcuaro had been more or less pacified and reorganized under ecclesiastical jurisdiction.[40]

In addition to the mendicant orders, the Crown, local governments, and a few private individuals attempted to implement similar agendas. One example was the foundation of the Hospital de Cosme y Damián (Amor de Dios) through a personal initiative of the local bishop, Juan de Zumárraga. This institution was designed to care exclusively for Spaniards suffering from venereal diseases or other contagious ailments, such as our second featured patient, Xavier Vázquez. Local residents or transients, many individuals—sometimes even regardless of social class—who were afflicted with venereal diseases were already shunned by other charitable establishments on account of their grotesque disfigurements and visibly infected sores.

However, throughout the sixteenth century, the official participation of the Spanish state remained limited, often merely ensuring the financial viability of existing establishments through the donation of land, small construction grants, and tax exemptions. Indeed, the Crown was reluctant to intervene in charitable activities traditionally regarded as being in the purview of the local church and civil authorities. Its perceived role was that of patron to institutions devoted to the care of native people. In addition to the Hospital Real de los Naturales in Mexico City serving the indigenous population of the valley, examples of royal sponsorship for specific hospitals abounded. In 1535, the bishop of Tlaxcala founded the Hospital de Nuestra Señora de Belén at a sheep ranch on the plains of Perote. The institution cared exclusively for sick Spanish travelers and pilgrims arriving at the nearby port of Veracruz.

Wealthy individuals such as the conquistador Hernán Cortés, the New Spain physician Pedro López, the judge Vasco de Quiroga, and a Spanish soldier of fortune, Bernardino Alvarez, took advantage of a law that permitted private persons to use their own money in founding monasteries, churches, hermitages, and hospitals, as well as placing them under their patronage.[41] Worried about the physical decay and depopulation of the former Aztec capital, Cortés tried to rebuild streets, aqueducts, bridges, and buildings with the help of native labor. In exchange, returning workers were to be exempted from royal tributes. Included in this building program was the Hospital Jesús Nazareno o de la Concepción de Nuestra Señora founded by Cortés in 1521 to care for sick Spaniards. Some private donors such as Cortés and Alvarez officially expressed the hope that their charitable gesture would, in the eyes of God, serve as atonement for their previous sins of greed and exploitation.

Mirroring developments in Europe during the 1550s, local colonial authorities in New Spain also began to take over the responsibility for charity from the church.[42] Unfortunately, the reluctance of wealthy Spanish landowners to make sizable contributions fostered a chronic lack of local resources, thus hampering numerous plans to build and maintain hospitals. In Puebla, the local council with papal patronage eventually created the Hospital San Juan de Letrán, supported by a number of local confraternities. Some hospitals in Spanish America were exclusively devoted to the care of specific occupational groups: soldiers, sailors, and even priests.

From the very beginning, both ecclesiastical and civil authorities sought the participation of the local population in the establishment of hospitals. Traditional Nahua labor and tribute mechanisms were preserved and placed at the disposal of the colonists for hospital construction and staffing. Indeed, surviving local noblemen became actively involved in many Franciscan foundations, eventually becoming administrators of such institutions. As time went on, many used their new positions to recoup some of their former power over the commoners and channel hospital resources for their private gain.[43]

Often the foundation of a hospital was aided or made possible by the establishment of one or more lay confraternities.[44] In Franciscan institutions, native inhabitants belonging to the confraternity not only took turns in rotation in ministering to the sick but also performed agricultural chores and were involved with a number of crafts for the benefit of the hospital. In Quiroga's pueblo-hospitals scheme, Indians willing to move to the newly established "republics" also worked the land and built the houses, helping to make these communities entirely self-supporting. The most successful, such as the Hospital de Santa Fé pueblo with three thousand inhabitants near Mexico City, added vineyards and urban properties to their original endowment and even placed some of the excess revenues in the market for lending purposes.

Both at home and in the colonies, one of the most important themes in Spanish hospital history was the constant jurisdictional disputes created among the various patrons: kings, church, pope, missionaries, and local authorities. As the patrimony of some colonial hospitals increased through successive donations, the labor of confraternities, and their tax-free status, these institutions became targets for takeovers. Searching for ownership titles, challenging bequests, demanding privileges, and claiming further tax exemptions, each party zealously sought to protect its rights to hospital property and income, often engaging in petitions and lawsuits, conducting visits and inspections, taking inventories, and verifying the execution of royal and episcopal decrees. Given the overlapping jurisdictions and complexity of issues involved, these disputes kept a vast Spanish bureaucracy in slow but perpetual motion.[45]

Institutional Organization and Patients

Not surprisingly, Spanish colonization in New Spain took advantage of preconquest sociopolitical organizations based on the existing Nahua *altepetl,* an urban unit that was gradually transformed from the 1530s onward into a Spanish municipality. Following the baptism of the native elders, a sanctuary and patron saint were usually selected and the town's perimeter established.[46] Here hospitals were expected to be part of most newly reorganized population centers, to be located next to the church in the heart of towns and cities. As such they decisively contributed to local community identity, pride, and wealth.

In contrast to some of the newly erected monumental and richly decorated churches, hospitals were mostly spartan constructions. Architecturally designed like other existing Nahua and Spanish residential complexes, these rectangular or square buildings were located on a separate lot of land, usually facing one of the streets of the urban grid. Most hospitals were one- or two-story institutions, composed of adobe or wooden walls with beamed, straw, or shingled roofs, with their various rooms looking inward and organized around a central patio with an altar, chapel, or even a garden. Private largesse and expanding endowments allowed some hospitals to move into brick or even richly sculptured two-storied stone buildings. Kitchens, in turn, were generally located in a separate building, with the usual grain bins and corrals or animal pens for chickens and pigs. Sweat houses were also popular. Such traditional spatial arrangements, also common to the Nahua, bore an uncanny similarity to the rectangular Aztec cosmos with its magical center represented by a green stone, an arrangement that may have reinforced the hospital's religious significance among the native people.

Some hospitals probably planted their central gardens with medicinal plants and vegetables or, depending on size, even possessed their own agricultural plots out of town. In addition, many establishments had separate chapels dedicated to Our Lady of the Immaculate Conception where the ambulatory sick inmates, lay brothers, and other personnel could congregate. These shrines also provided sites for religious festivals as well as wakes and masses for the dead.

Like Europe, Spanish America came to possess a wide spectrum of hospital establishments. They ranged from small one-room infirmaries next to monasteries in rural communities located in the densely populated Mexican highlands, especially Michoacán, to multistoried institutions in larger urban centers such as Mexico City, where they might be composed of several wards, a chapel, even a pharmacy together with administrative quarters. Many of these hospitals were only temporary structures, often erected as isolation huts during epidemics. Some institutions were constructed along major travel routes, such as Bernardino Alvarez's chain of establishments extending westward from Mexico City to Acapulco and eastward to Veracruz.

Once in operation, hospitals could expect some financial aid from one-fifth of the royal colonial income reserved for churches, monasteries, and other charitable organizations. Most of the resources, however, came from the fruits of native labor, especially the sale of grain and livestock. In the case of hospitals exclusively devoted to the Indians, the colonial government was authorized to collect a tax of half a *real* per year from every native person living in New Spain who was not individually exempted. After 1587, one measure of corn for every hundred grown on public lands was also expected from every native community in the colony.

In urban areas, however, private donations became an important source of income. Royal and papal patronage was frequently requested to supplement such private income and to obtain exemptions from taxation. Since the land on which the hospital was erected belonged to the Crown, taxes were usually in order unless requests were made to place the institution directly under the auspices of the pope. If the

Holy Father agreed, a bull was issued, and the institution was thereafter entitled to special privileges and indulgences for its benefactors. Often, this patronage consisted in an affiliation with the Ospedale di Sancto Spiritu in Rome, an establishment that in the sixteenth century had hundreds of affiliates scattered across Europe and the Americas, including the Hospital de la Concepción in Cuitzeo, Guanajuato. In return for an incorporation fee and yearly membership dues, these hospitals were authorized to offer special dispensations to those who served the institution.

In the 1570s, implementation of resolutions passed at the Council of Trent placed all hospitals as religious institutions under episcopal administrative authority. The Spanish Crown retained its supervisory position, but this move weakened the power and financial advantages previously enjoyed by the mendicant orders. In fact, citing financial irregularities or insolvency, regular clergy increasingly replaced founding friars at the helm of colonial hospitals. At the same time, the third Mexican Ecclesiastical Council of 1585 decreed that hospitals could no longer admit paying patients, a valuable source of revenue that violated traditional notions of charity intended solely for the poor.

Individual donors usually deeded their land and city stores to the hospital and then made detailed and often complex financial arrangements enshrined in wills to have all future income from these properties assigned to finance ongoing institutional services. When the donors died, their individual dispositions were often contested by surviving family members. Pleas to local lay and episcopal authorities, petitions to the king and the pope, and costly lawsuits were inextricably woven into the hospitals' perennially precarious and contested finances. At the outset, many missionary institutions seemed to flourish, their physical plants expanding and agricultural lands thriving under the strict administration of frugal friars and indigenous nobles still commanding respect from their former subjects. All too often, however, corruption set in after the founding generation had passed from the scene, also a common occurrence in the history of medieval and Renaissance hospital management in Europe.

About 1600, the Order of St. John of God became involved in the management of several New World hospitals. This brotherhood was brought in by secular authorities for the purpose of taking over the administration of declining Franciscan, Augustinian, and private institutions. The order's appearance marked an important turning point in hospital management away from traditional medieval models. Instead of being solely concerned with preserving the institution's original patrimony, the brotherhood established an aggressive fund-raising program, charged higher rents for properties belonging to its endowment, and systematically collected all income due. Another measure was to wean the hospital budget from an excessive dependence on alms, a notoriously modest and unstable source of funding. Administrative costs were also trimmed. Moreover, attention was given less to the material conditions of the hospital's chapel, its ornaments and precious stones, than to the physical plant of the hospital itself, with patient services improving as more servants were hired.[47]

Following contemporary Spanish models, colonial hospitals could be complex organizations. Some were governed by an administrator, frequently the founding friar, or a native deputy, who often was obliged to hire a steward to manage the institutional funds and report to the patrons. In the early period this post was often given to a local native of social prominence. Given the frequency of donations through wills and the numerous legal matters arising out of hospital business, lawyers often needed to be consulted.

Aside from an administrative staff, hospitals usually had in-house monks or priests and assistants able to perform the religious services and dispense the sacraments that were always central to the mission of such institutions.[48] In most Franciscan and Augustinian hospitals, the friars themselves, aided by native practitioners whose languages they spoke, carried out many of the healing and nursing tasks. A contingent of servants and assistants, both male and female, and sometimes slaves, performed the cooking and cleaning chores, brought supplies such as water, firewood, and food, and transported the sick and wounded. They also buried the dead.

Because of the scarcity of religious personnel, a key role was increasingly reserved for the indigenous "church people." Lay confraternities composed of singers, custodians, and servants actively participated in the organization and administration of colonial hospitals. In the more democratic Franciscan model created in Uruapan, each year the native confraternities freely elected the hospital's director, who was responsible for spiritual care in the institution. Also selected or appointed was a steward responsible for the accounts, alms, expenses, and admission of patients.

In Quiroga's infirmaries, the confraternity divided its members in groups of eight or ten for one-week stints of service to the sick. During such rigorous rotations, the native weekly workers lived in the hospital, functioning as nurses and burying the dead, while also participating in religious ceremonies and studies. In Augustinian establishments, barefoot *semaneros* consciously pursued their nursing services as a form of penance, a vehicle for communal cooperation, and renunciation of the material world. Hospital service thus became an essential component of Christian indoctrination and education as well as a pathway toward eternal salvation through the awarding of indulgences. "I do not really use the word penance when speaking of the brotherhood and our activities," recalled one member. "Every Christian is called to penance. We send our gifts, our sacrifices. Our gifts of what some people may call penance are really acts of love."[49]

In a few, more medicalized establishments located in larger urban areas, such as Cortés's Hospital de la Concepción de Nuestra Señora and Zumárraga's Hospital del Amor de Dios, salaried medical practitioners made rounds and ordered diets and medicines.[50] In most rural areas, however, the severe shortage of Spanish physicians and surgeons in the colony prompted the employment of native healers who knew the curative virtues of local medicinal plants. Thus, because of his practical botanical knowledge and effective first aid skills, the Aztec *ticitl* found a temporary, albeit narrowly defined, niche among colonial medical staffs, especially in New Spain's Franciscan institutions. When available, apprenticed Spanish barber-surgeons practiced their craft by providing emergency aid and bloodletting, as well as pulling teeth and changing dressings. In a few instances, a pharmacist or herbalist familiar with Old World drugs was added to the professional staff and directed to compound remedies and fill in-house prescriptions.

Among the traditional recipients of European and colonial hospital care were the frail elderly and chronically disabled, no longer able to work and look after themselves. Other potential patients were transients and travelers, individuals who arrived in New Spain weakened and sick after their extensive transoceanic voyages. In the colonies, the authorities carefully divided inmates by race, creating separate establishments for Spaniards and Indians. For blacks, mestizos, and mulattoes, a private hospital opened its doors in Mexico City in 1582 to house the local homeless and sick. The main goal of the Hospital de Nuestra Señora de los Desamparados, privately founded by Pedro López, was to shelter mestizo children, especially the illegal offspring of Spaniards and native women, persons who at the time were the target of widespread infanticide or subject to abandonment in the streets.

Because of their economic value to the colonial authorities, native people whose poor health was caused by hard work, malnutrition, repeated infections, and cultural disintegration were especially singled out and encouraged to seek hospital care. Among the Crown-sponsored institutions was the Hospital Real de los Naturales, founded in Mexico City in 1553. In contrast to pueblo-hospitals scattered in the countryside, such urban institutions were viewed by the native people with considerable fear and suspicion. Indeed, hospitals were often the very source of the oppression of native inhabitants because these establishments demanded tributes and stints of forced labor. Unwillingness to be separated from their families and limited means of transportation also discouraged native use.

The incipient medicalization of the hospital prompted an admission and segregation of patients based on their diseases. Fevers were commonly seen, especially the more serious ones described by Juan de Barrios, a Spanish physician in Mexico City who attended at the local Hospital de los Naturales. Barrios's *Verdadera medicina, cirugía y astrología* presented a spectrum of febrile illnesses, their clinical manifestations, prognosis, and treatment. The text ranges from trivial, one-day fevers to synochas, the more malignant *tabardete* sometimes identified with the indigenous cocoliztli, tertian and quartan intermittents, and the recently described *mal de bubas,* or syphilis.[51]

Another specialized institution, the Hospital de San Lázaro, was built in 1572 outside Mexico City to house lepers. Privately founded by the physician Pedro López, it replaced an earlier establishment founded by Cortés in 1521. This hospital had four large wards, administrative offices, and an annex with a church and small farm. Lepers from all regions of New Spain and all social classes and races, including foreigners, were to be admitted there.

The mentally ill, in turn, found shelter with the old in Bernardino Alvarez's Hospital de San Hipólito, established in Mexico City after 1567. At that time these individuals were already classified into mentally retarded or so-called innocent mad, the regular demented, and the violently deranged.[52] Only the last were usually isolated in caged cells so that they could not harm others. Most of the attention was devoted to the first category, a group of harmless people who traditionally needed institutional protection because they could not successfully beg for their survival and were frequently attacked and beaten in the streets. At the Hospital de San Hipólito, all inmates including poor teachers and students were also provided with temporary lodging and food, and even school activities were allowed to proceed on the premises. Treated with some dignity, the inmates were placed within an ordered communal life routine of work and play. This institution also sponsored a public soup kitchen in which ambulatory poor and homeless people could congregate for meals.[53]

Hospital Life

As noted earlier, colonial hospitals were designed primarily to provide charity and hospitality, including lodging, rest, and food, to the poor who were allowed to enter. Ambulatory, prospective patients waited patiently at the gate until a staff member periodically checking the entrance confronted them. For those who could not walk, Bernardino Alvarez with members of his brotherhood designed an ambulance service, removing some of the sick from the insalubrious city of Veracruz with the help of carts and mules. Following the usual protocol of the times, the arriving party probably assumed the role of supplicant, bowing and standing before the authorities who made a judgment of

need. The charitable character of these hospitals dictated that as many persons as possible were admitted. In the event of an epidemic, emergency admissions were often placed in temporary huts, as the authorities sought to remove to the institution those deemed contagious and dying without the benefit of spiritual aid.

In 1545, the first "great pestilence," or huey cocoliztli, erupted throughout New Spain, although coastal areas suffered greater mortality. After hitting Tlaxcala and Choluca hard, the disease spread throughout Michoacán and Jalisco, prompting Franciscan friars to convert some monasteries into makeshift infirmaries to isolate and assist the sick poor. Among them may have been our Juan Manuel, perhaps a farmer or weaver living in a Franciscan pueblo located in the well-irrigated and fertile valley of Uruapan, in Michoacán. Like other inhabitants of the region, this commoner must have been Christianized during his teens by the arriving monks and was undoubtedly recruited into a local brotherhood devoted to the cult of the Virgin Mary, the Cofradía de la Concepción.

Although the widespread epidemic primarily affected the old people and the young children of the indigenous population, the twenty-five-year-old Juan Manuel, who as a child had already survived an encounter with smallpox during the first postconquest epidemic wave, became quite sick. His febrile symptoms, including intense headaches, combined with recent nosebleeds, incipient jaundice, and a bloody diarrhea, prompted his family or friends to take him to the local hospital. Located at the banks of the Cupatitzio River, Uruapan with its nine barrios had its very own Hospital Real de la Purísima Concepción, a two-floor, rectangular building—known as Guatapera—with separate wards for men and women, as well as distinct accommodations for contagious cases and a room for ambulatory and convalescent patients. The entire complex also had facilities for caregivers, a central courtyard, and a large chapel. To fulfill its mission of mercy, this hospital had been placed under the jurisdiction of the local government in 1540. Not only did this hospital receive donations of agricultural land and cattle from wealthy locals, including the offspring of former Tarascan chieftains and Spanish settlers, but it had also been placed under royal patronage to be exempt from taxes.[54]

Four decades later, our other patient, the Spanish colonist Xavier Vázquez, entered the Hospital del Amor de Dios in Mexico City, a specialized institution reserved exclusively for Spaniards suffering from syphilis as well as other contagious diseases.[55] Vázquez was in his mid-fifties, a former official responsible for drafting native labor from the surrounding towns in the Valley of Mexico.[56] Caught making illegal assignments in return for substantial bribes, Vázquez had not only lost his job but apparently contracted syphilis from one of the women he attempted to shield from some work assignment in exchange for sexual favors.[57]

Bishop Zumárraga's foundation attested to the growing concern about the spread of syphilis in the colonies. Beginning in the late fifteenth century, similar specialized establishments had appeared throughout Europe, frequently founded by local town councils and self-proclaimed healers of the disease. Their purpose was to treat venereal disease sufferers aggressively with what was then perceived to be a curative regimen.[58] After its completion in the 1550s, this Mexico City hospital had about forty beds with a room exclusively devoted for mercurial inunctions.[59]

Once newcomers were admitted to a hospital, most institutional rules demanded that their names be inscribed in registers and that they be immediately referred to the resident priest for confession. Here again, Christian and native concepts of sin and disease, including supernatural intervention, exhibited a considerable degree of similarity. Confessing one's sins and receiving the sacraments, especially the last rites, were the paramount goals for all Christians. Subsequently placed in a bed, the recent arrivals then underwent a number of ritual cleansing ceremonies such as the washing of feet, clipping of hair, and the cutting of finger- and toenails. Preparation for death, suggested by the severity of Juan Manuel's case, involved the sacrament of anointment and disposition of one's earthly possessions. Ensuring that death took place in a well-orchestrated and dignified Christian manner in blessed surroundings, along with subsequent burial in nearby consecrated ground, was among the most important services a hospital could render.

As recommended by authors such as Barrios, clerics and medical personnel first needed to carry out a careful inspection of the new arrivals, attempting to determine their physical constitution within the traditional Galenic model. Because of their white complexion, Spaniards, including Vázquez, were usually categorized as cold, whereas native people such as Juan Manuel were considered hot, choleric, or melancholic. The patient's relative girth provided the second essential quality, with thin people tending to be cataloged as dry and more robust individuals as humid. Given the prevailing epidemic, Juan Manuel's sudden fever, multiple bleedings, and incipient jaundice clearly suggested a hot and humid constitution reflective of the lethal cocoliztli. Native healers, in turn, postulated a pathological accumulation of phlegm around the heart.

By contrast, Vázquez appeared with severe generalized pains in his bones and joints and significant loss of weight. He exhibited a number of painful, ulcerated swellings on his right temple and forehead lacking the usual inflammatory signs but discharging a foul-smelling fluid. Together with similar inguinal ulcerations, this symptomatology probably posed no diagnostic challenges for the Spanish attending: Vázquez was diagnosed as suffering from *bubas*, or syphilis, a severe illness believed to be neither hot nor cold. As another Mexican author, Juan de Cárdenas, observed, syphilitic Spaniards such as Vázquez usually also displayed a darker facial complexion caused by the wearing of a piece of black velvet over their face to hide the telling and disfiguring signs of their disease.[60]

Operating within such a basic body typology, healers were enjoined to observe the alterations brought about by illness and urged to prescribe foodstuffs and medications endowed with opposite qualities to reestablish a healthy balance. A somewhat similar calculus of bodily humors and their qualities was accepted among the tenets of Nahua healing. Thus interpreted, the presenting symptomatology provided the basis for an individualized interpretation of disability within the frameworks of both European and Nahua humoralism. To restore the balance of the disturbed bodily humors, contemporary hospital regimens thus focused attention on symptomatic control and management of the six non-naturals, including food and drink, sleep, rest, and exercise, as well as the use of drugs.

Following admission, most inmates displaying no signs of acute illness were placed together, often two or three assigned to each bed, and asked what they wanted to eat. Franciscan rules allowed newcomers to express their wishes freely, and efforts were made to comply with such requests within the economic constraints of each institution. Before eating their meals, patients and those nursing them joined in prayer, giving thanks to the hospital's past and present benefactors. In Mexico, well-baked wheat bread was recommended. If the hospital possessed adjacent farms, a European diet of boiled vegetables and eggs, chicken, lamb, pork, and even beef could be offered as a substitute for traditional foodstuffs. Fruits such as grapes, melons, and figs were frequently available. For drinks, patients received atolle, a native gruel made by boiling corn, and chocolate. Diluted wine was a commonly prescribed restorative, obtained from grapes grown at nearby vineyards. For the truly sick, however, dietary restrictions were the rule. Although food seems to have been usually plentiful and nutritious at rural institutions, larger urban hospitals were often frustrated by inadequate or tainted supplies, including adulterated breads and rotting meat. The relative comfort and nourishment provided to the limited number of inmates unquestionably saved lives.

In addition to dietary adjustments, ritual cleansing such as purging and bloodletting played a major role. Nature attempted to free the body of the morbific matter by spontaneously eliminating it through urine, feces, sweat, and pustules, abscesses, ulcers, and other discharges. If this was unsuccessful, healers merely imitated or supplemented the natural discharges through the use of drugs and other physical methods. Bloodletting, practiced extensively in European folk healing and monastic life, retained both its symbolic and medical value in the colonies as a method of unburdening the human body of such potentially harmful substances.[61]

Given the characteristics of New Spain's climate and the presumed humoral makeup of its indigenous people, Barrios recommended venesection in almost all fevers. Prescriptions for withdrawals of four to six ounces of blood at a time to a maximum of twenty to twenty-four ounces in cases such as Juan Manuel's cocolitzli were common. Here the additional decision to bleed may have been influenced by the presenting symptomatology, which suggested that the

patient's body was attempting to rid itself of excessive or tainted blood. Even Xavier Vázquez may not have escaped the lancet. Most often, blood was withdrawn through phlebotomy, cupping, and the application of leeches; the first of these methods prompted bitter debates concerning optimal sites for the incisions. Following classical models, Renaissance physicians argued against medieval practices, which recommended that phlebotomies be performed "by revulsion" far away from the bodily parts presumed to be diseased.

Other purification routines, such as sweating and bathing, common to both native and European cultures, were usually available in colonial hospitals, including native hot vapor baths known as *temascales*. Sufferers from cocolitztli such as Juan Manuel in Uruapan may have received cold head and foot baths to counter delirium and convulsions brought about by the high fever, the head bath made with milk, presumably designed to neutralize the severe headaches. In Mexico City, European barber-surgeons and newly specialized "pox doctors" considered mercury to be the preferred antidote to syphilis. In their view, the disease would not yield to anything else. After entering the body, the foul-smelling venereal poison had to be detoured away from the established ulcers and compelled to evaporate from the skin and discharged through the natural elimination organs with the help of medications and physical methods.[62]

Since the fifth century, mercury had already been well known in Islamic medicine for the treatment of other skin diseases, including scabies and even leprosy. Since European barber-surgeons traditionally dealt with injuries and external diseases, their opinion about the treatment of a new disease carried great weight. As a salve or ointment prepared with "lard of swine" and turpentine as a vehicle, mercury was generously applied and rubbed into the skin of the whole body except for the head and chest by the attending surgeons. With the patient placed supine on a table located in a special room, this messy, painful hands-on approach took place at least once or twice a day for periods of forty days and constituted the accepted therapy. Improvement or disappearance of symptoms was taken for a cure. In addition to the rubbings, patients such as Vázquez were usually kept in closed, small rooms heated by open fireplaces or were frequently brought to the vapor baths. The diuretic effects of these extremely hot chambers were increased by forcing the patients to remain under several layers of blankets to promote further sweating to rid their bodies of the presumed venereal poison causing their skin lesions.[63]

Mercury, meanwhile, not only exhibited diuretic properties but also produced highly iatrogenic reactions of mercurial poisoning, including excessive salivation, malodorous inflammation of tongue, gums, and palate, and the loosening of teeth. Earlier in the century, one contemporary medical author, Paracelsus, had already criticized the irritating mercurial rubbings, arguing that most healers lacked the necessary knowledge regarding proper dosage and could cause great harm. Still, salivation not only was deemed useful in further draining the poison from the affected body but constituted an accurate index for proper dosage. Indeed, the loss of three pints of saliva per day was considered an ideal amount, reflective of an adequate mercury saturation of the sick body. To boot, those locked up in overheated treatment rooms were exposed to a dangerously stuffy environment that could only adversely influence their overall health. Vázquez must also have been regularly visited by the attending barber-surgeon who was in charge of changing dressings while attempting to drain the infected buboes. By 1585 this approach constituted a welcome advance over previous efforts involving the use of hot irons placed over the chronic ulcers.[64]

Given the effects of warfare and the hazards of mining and agriculture, as well as the vicissitudes of contemporary travel, surgical care was in great demand at hospitals. To inform the friars and, at times, barber-surgeons who attended hospital inmates, one barber-surgeon, the Spaniard Alonso López de Hinojosos, published his *Suma y recopilación de cirugía* in 1578. Divided into seven sections, this book examined anatomy, bloodletting, abscesses, wounds, fractures, and syphilitic buboes, all based on the writings of the French surgeon Guy de Chauliac. In the colonies since about 1567, López de Hinojosos had acquired extensive clinical experience at the Hospital Real de los Naturales in Mexico City, cleansing and dressing wounds and ulcers, lancing boils and abscesses, and setting broken bones and dislocated limbs. Fresh wounds benefited from a host of drying agents before being sutured or cauterized. In Europe, a revolution

in the management of gunshot wounds occurred in the 1540s: after the publication of Ambroise Paré's wartime experiences, Europe stopped using scalding oil to treat such wounds.

In New Spain and elsewhere in the colonies, the presence of native healers, who employed an array of local plants with medicinal qualities hitherto unknown to the colonists, added significantly to hospital care.[65] This native practice occurred primarily in institutions dedicated to the native population. Here, early on, both indigenous healers and their patients could continue to employ local preparations in lieu of the costly and unavailable Old World armamentarium of purgatives, analgesics, diuretics, and stimulants according to shared preconquest paradigms of health and disease. Most of the medicinal plants, including some hallucinogens, were inextricably woven together with divinatory shamanistic practices, often cleverly disguised as part of Christian ceremonies.

Stripped of religious meanings, many of these products even found a niche in European medical practices.[66] A second edition of López de Hinojosos's *Suma,* published in 1595, promoted the use of more than fifty native herbs, based on the barber-surgeon's experience at the Hospital Real de los Naturales.[67] The same can be said of another book, the *Tratado breve de medicina* (Mexico City, 1592), by another Spanish physician, now an Augustinian friar, Agustín Farfán.[68] Readily available, the products described by these authors were prepared as powders, syrups, wines, infusions, and ointments and widely administered to the sick.[69] In fact, herbal infusions, plasters, and ointments must have been important components of the treatment dispensed to Juan Manuel before his death.

Hospitals thus provided small but controlled populations for clinical observation and experimentation. When Hernández visited the Hospital de Santa Cruz in about 1574, he was able to learn a great deal about many healing herbs, returning to Mexico City with a rich harvest of information concerning their pharmacological actions. Searching for care of his impaired health, Gregorio López, hermit and author of the *Tesoro de medicinas,* had a similar experience at that institution.[70] Yet a lack of precise measuring techniques and the absence of standardized preparations of such plants may have created variations in dosage that prevented a clear understanding of their clinical effects. Thus, a vigorous program of clinical trials initiated by Franciscan and Augustinian friars and Spanish physicians sought to improve on the existing therapeutic indications.[71] Later, sporadic autopsies of natives were authorized and sought to inform physicians of causes of death.

Epilogue

Despite the care given to him at the hospital in Uruapan, Juan Manuel probably died a few days after admission, another casualty of the fulminating cocoliztli, which is said to have killed eight hundred thousand natives of New Spain during 1545. According to contemporary observers, most of the victims also experienced great fear and anxiety before succumbing to the rapidly lethal disease. Although he was delirious and bleeding, Juan Manuel's last hours could have been somewhat less stressful at the hospital. Possibly treated by a native healer and surrounded by friends and members of his confraternity, Juan Manuel may have died within the newly imposed Christian liturgy of prayers, sacraments, and songs increasingly shared by all inhabitants of the pueblo. On one level, then, the colonial hospital provided inmates with a locus to share their fears and suffering with a valuable support group that included caregivers, priests, and other patients. The extent to which traditional indigenous rituals were added under the guise of Christian symbols probably depended on the level of acculturation already achieved in Uruapan by the native inhabitants in 1545.[72] In general, dying patients such as Juan Manuel became the focus of well-orchestrated and dignified rituals, opportunities for the display of communal bonding and solidarity. What a contrast with the lone and homeless thousands who simply collapsed on city streets and distant mountains!

Xavier Vázquez's stay in the wards of Zumárraga's more medicalized Hospital del Amor de Dios in Mexico City must have lasted several months. In Europe, the average institutional mortality rate for syphilis fluctuated between 16 and 24 percent. During the sixteenth century, the full-fledged therapeutic regimen appeared to be constructed as a Lenten-like forty-day penance in which the sinful patient's body was punished by starvation and heroic methods to eliminate the venereal poison with the aid of copious sweating, purging, and bloodletting. In some patients, the disease's most obvious manifestations retreated, leading physicians to believe that they had achieved a cure.

Vázquez's advanced case, however, characterized by involvement of the cranial bones, healed only slowly, and the facial disfigurement remained. Perhaps he could suspend wearing his velvet face cloth, but now the sustained mercurial poisoning had taken its toll on his teeth and kidneys. For its part, the hospital had fulfilled its medical mission, delivering an aggressive, painful, but possibly efficacious treatment widely interpreted by patients as a retributive corporeal punishment.[73] Penniless and without job prospects, Vázquez faced a grim future following his discharge. However, his long hospitalization may have allowed him to make friends among the other inmates and the caregivers. At this point, the hospital's charitable mission came into play, and the authorities decided to keep the old sinner as a part-time employee in the role of an auxiliary accountant because of his previous background as a seasoned distributor of alms. Earning his keep, Vázquez would live out his few last days at the Hospital del Amor de Dios in the company of other patients and staff actively practicing his religion and possibly convinced of the redemptive quality of his bodily sufferings.[74]

Perhaps the juxtaposition of these two patients with hypothetical case histories admitted to colonial hospitals in New Spain during the sixteenth century facilitates the portrayal of these establishments' full spectrum of conflicting ideologies, patronage, and functions. Given the lack of contemporary clinical records, the full role played by such institutions can only be guessed. As the sixteenth century came to a close, the pressing agendas that had originally fueled hospital foundations were no longer operative. The initial evangelizing effort of Franciscans and Augustinians had succeeded, but the monastic orders were now engaged in a power struggle with the Crown, the colonial administration, and the secular clergy following the rules imposed by the Council of Trent. Most remaining Indians were ostensibly Christianized, harnessed socially and politically into a new network of colonial cities and larger villages.

Their dwindling numbers and the policies of *congregación* prompted many pueblos to be abandoned, their chapels, hospitals, and dwellings razed.[75] Churches and schools fulfilled the remaining acculturation needs.

Although the traditional Christian ideology of charitable works survived, the viability of existing hospitals had to be reassessed. Lacking funds, many could no longer offer services, as personnel were reduced and buildings crumbled for lack of maintenance. More prosperous establishments became overloaded with friars, administrators, and lay brothers, many personally profiting from their employment at the expense of patient services. Tales of corruption surrounded some pueblo-hospitals of Franciscan origin, where dishonest native chieftains, aligned with bishops and clerics, had resumed exploitation of the commoners.

In demanding centralization and accountability of poor relief, the Spanish Crown followed developments in contemporary Europe. A royal decree from Philip II issued in 1596 included instructions to his New Spain and Peru viceroys, enjoining them to visit all hospitals in their capital cities personally or to have judges inspect the remaining hospital services. Reports about the state of their buildings and endowments were requested. In the name of efficiency, consolidation efforts were launched to harness a decaying colonial hospital system that had been allowed to mushroom without proper controls. By 1600, the spectacular wave of hospital foundations in Spanish America had crested. Surviving institutions entered a long period of stagnation and retrenchment until humanistic and mercantilist ideologies linked to the Enlightenment induced new reforms.

NOTES

1. This generic Náhuatl term was employed for a contagious disease variously identified as typhus or typhoid fever, mumps, hepatitis, even bubonic plague. See Elsa Malvido and Carlos Viesca Treviño, "La epidemia de cocoliztli de 1576," *Historias* 11 (1986): 27–33, and Hanns J. Prem, "Disease Outbreaks in Central Mexico during the Sixteenth Century," in *The Secret Judgments of God: Native Peoples and Old World Disease in Colonial Spanish America*, ed. Noble D. Cook and W. G. Lovell (Norman: University of Oklahoma Press, 1992), 22–50. For an overview of sixteenth-century diseases in New Spain, see Carlos Viesca Treviño, "Las enfermedades," in *Medicina novohispana, siglo XVI, historia general de la medicina en México*, ed. Gonzalo Beltrán and Roberto Moreno de los

Arcos (Mexico City: UNAM, 1990), 2:93–109, as well as Enrique Florescano and Elsa Malvido, eds., *Ensayos sobre la historia de las epidemias en México*, 2 vols. (Mexico City: IMSS, 1980), and Noble D. Cook and W. G. Lovell, "Unravelling the Web of Disease," in *Secret Judgments of God*, 215–44. The dramatic impact of these periodic epidemics has been repeatedly recounted in numerous publications, including William H. McNeill's chapter "Transoceanic Exchanges, 1500–1700," in *Plagues and Peoples* (Garden City, N.Y.: Anchor/Doubleday, 1976), 199–234, and Alfred W. Crosby Jr., *The Columbian Exchange: Biological and Cultural Consequences of 1492* (Westport, Conn.: Greenwood Press, 1972). More recent works are Ann F. Ramenofsky, *Vectors of Death: The Archaeology of European Contact* (Albuquerque: University of New Mexico Press, 1987); David E. Stannard, *American Holocaust: Columbus and the Conquest of the New World* (New York: Oxford University Press, 1992); and Noble D. Cook, *Born to Die: Disease and New World Conquest, 1492–1650* (New York: Cambridge University Press, 1998).

2. A good summary account of this particular institution can be found in Josefina Muriel, "Hospital Real de Sanct Joseph de los Naturales," in *Hospitales de la Nueva España*, 2 vols. (Mexico City: Jus, 1956–60), 1:115–36. See also C. Venegas Ramírez, "La asistencia hospitalaria para los indios en la Nueva España," *Anales del Instituto de Antropología y Historia* 19 (1966): 227–40, and Francisco Guerra, "Hospital Real de los Naturales, 1553," in *El Hospital en Hispanoamerica y Filipinas, 1492–1898* (Madrid: Ministerio de Sanidad y Consumo, 1994), 247–50.

3. Carmen Venegas Ramírez, *Régimen hospitalario para Indios en la Nueva España* (Mexico City: Instituto Nacional de Antropología y Historia, 1973).

4. For background information regarding the rationale for Hernández's mission, see David C. Goodman, *Power and Penury: Government, Technology, and Science in Philip II's Spain* (Cambridge: Cambridge University Press, 1988), 209–60. A useful general text concerning the history of this period is John Lynch, *Spain under the Habsburgs*, 2d ed., 2 vols. (New York: New York University Press, 1982).

5. Efrén del Pozo, "Huastepec en la historia de la medicina mexicana," *Boletín de la Sociedad Mexicana de Historia y Filosofía de la Medicina* 3 (September 1974): 51–58.

6. Alonso López de Hinojosos, *Suma y recopilación de chirugía* (Mexico City, 1578), reprinted in Nuestros Clasicos (Mexico City: Academia Nacional de Medicina, 1977). See *Mexican Treasury*, Letter 11: February 10, 1576.

7. G. B. Risse, "Medicine in New Spain," in *Medicine in the New World*, ed. Ronald L. Numbers (Knoxville: University of Tennessee Press, 1987), 12–63.

8. For a comparative analysis, G. B. Risse, "Transcending Cultural Barriers: The European Reception of Medicinal Plants from the Americas," in *Botanical Drugs of the Americas in the Old and the New Worlds*, ed. Wolfgang-Hagen Hein (Stuttgart: Wissenschaftliche Verlagsgesselschaft, 1984), 31–42, and J. Worth Estes, "The European Reception of the First Drugs from the New World," *Pharmacy in History* 37 (1995): 3–23.

9. Among them, James Axtell, *Beyond 1492: Encounters in Colonial North America* (New York: Oxford University Press, 1994), and Anthony Pagden, *European Encounters with the New World: From Renaissance to Romanticism* (New Haven: Yale University Press, 1994).

10. Miguel León-Portilla, "Rewriting History: The Encounter of Two Worlds," *UC Mexus News* 29 (Fall 1992): 1–8.

11. For further details, Brian Catchpole, *The Clash of Cultures* (London: Heinemann Educational, 1981), and Germán Somolinos d'Ardois, "El fenómeno de fusión cultural y su trascendencia

médica," in *Capítulos de historia médica mexicana*, vol. 2 (Mexico City: Sociedad Mexicana de Historia y Filosofía de Medicina, 1978), 99–173.

12. The best source for information about original documents is the catalog of the Archivo General de la Nación, Indice de los ramos hospitales y protomedicato (Mexico City: Departamento de Publicaciones del Archivo General de la Nación, 1977). However, material for the sixteenth century remains scanty.

13. Basic information about this hospital, established in 1540, can be found in Muriel, *Hospitales de la Nueva España*, 1:86–90. See also entry no. 482 in Guerra, *Hospital en Hispanoamerica*, 230–31.

14. This private institution was created in 1539. For more details, see Muriel, *Hospitales de la Nueva España*, 1:147–53, and Guerra, *Hospital en Hispanoamerica*, entry no. 478, p. 229. More historical details are in Jon Arrizabalaga and Roger French, *The Great Pox: The French Disease in Renaissance Europe* (New Haven: Yale University Press, 1997).

15. See John Bossy, *Christianity in the West, 1400–1700* (Oxford: Oxford University Press, 1985), and Charles H. Lippy, Robert Choquette, and Stafford Poole, "Iberian Catholicism Comes to the Americas," in *Christianity Comes to the Americas, 1492–1776* (New York: Paragon House, 1992), 1:1–129.

16. For details, John L. Mecham, *Church and State in Latin America*, rev. ed. (Chapel Hill: University of North Carolina Press, 1966).

17. See Robert Ricard, *The Spiritual Conquest of Mexico*, trans. Lesley Byrd Simpson (Berkeley: University of California Press, 1966), 155–61.

18. John Leddy Phelan, *The Millennial Kingdom of the Franciscans in the New World: A Study of the Writings of Gerónimo de Mendieta (1525–1604)*, University of California Publications in History, 52 (Berkeley: University of California Press, 1956).

19. Quoted in J. Guijarro Oliveras, "Política sanitaria en las Leyes de Indias," *Archivo Iberoamericano de historia de la medicina y antropología médica* 9 (1957): 255–62.

20. See letter of Pedro de Gante, a Franciscan friar, to Charles V in 1532 reproduced in *Cartas de Indias*, no. 8, and quoted in Ricard, *Spiritual Conquest of Mexico*, 350. For details, Pedro Borges, *Métodos misionales en la Cristianización de América, siglo XVI* (Madrid: CSIC, 1960), and Colin M. MacLachlan, *Spain's Empire in the New World: The Role of Ideas in Institutional and Social Change* (Berkeley: University of California Press, 1988).

21. For a general understanding of the geographical contours of the conquest and Spanish settlement, see Peter Gerhard, *A Guide to the Historical Geography of New Spain* (Cambridge: Cambridge University Press, 1972).

22. See James Lockhart, *The Nahuas after the Conquest: A Social and Cultural History of the Indians of Central Mexico, Sixteenth through Eighteenth Centuries* (Stanford: Stanford University Press, 1992), 14–58.

23. Pedro J. Bravo de Lagunas y Castilla, *Discurso histórico-jurídico del origen, fundación . . . del Hospital de San Lázaro* (Lima: Oficina de los Huérfanos, 1761), 4.

24. W. Borah, "Social Welfare and Social Obligation in New Spain: A Tentative Assessment," *Congreso internacional de Americanistas* 36 (1966): 45–57.

25. Serge Gruzinski, "Indian Confraternities, Brotherhoods, and Mayordomías in Central New Spain: A List of Questions for the Historian and the Anthropologist," in *The Indian Community of Colonial Mexico: Fifteen Essays on Land Tenure, Corporate Organizations, Ideology, and Village Politics*, ed. A. Ouweneel and S. Miller (Amsterdam: CEDLA, 1990), 205–23.

26. Lockhart, *Nahuas after the Conquest*, 218–29. For further reading, consult MacLachlan, *Spain's Empire in the New World*, especially the conclusions, 123–35.

27. Although this quotation is from the seventeenth century, it expresses a central function of the confraternities in the earlier period. See Gruzinski, "Indian Confraternities," 221.

28. "We charge and mandate our viceroys, governing bodies, and governors to take special care to ensure that, in all the towns of Spaniards and Indians in their provinces and under their jurisdictions, hospitals are established in which the sick poor are cared for, and Christian charity practiced": law 1, title 4, bk. 1, in *Recopilación de Leyes de los Reynos de Las Indias* (1681), reprinted in 4 vols. (Madrid: Ed. Cultura Hispánica, 1973), 2:159, as quoted in Guijarro Oliveras, "Política sanitaria en las Leyes de Indias," 256.

29. Fortino Hipólito Vera, *Apuntamientos históricos de los concilios provinciales mexicanos y privilegios de América* (Mexico City, 1893), 11, as summarized by Stafford Poole, *Pedro Moya de Contreras: Catholic Reform and Royal Power in New Spain, 1571–1591* (Berkeley: University of California Press, 1987), 128.

30. Thomas More, *Utopia*, ed. Edward Surtz, S.J., and J. H. Hexter, *The Yale Edition of the Complete Works of St. Thomas More*, vol. 4 (New Haven: Yale University Press 1965).

31. M. M. Lacas, "A Social Welfare Organizer in Sixteenth-Century New Spain: Don Vasco de Quiroga, First Bishop of Michoacán," *The Americas* 14 (1957): 57–86.

32. Fintan B. Warren, *Vasco de Quiroga and His Pueblo Hospitals of Santa Fé* (Washington, D.C.: Academy of American Franciscan History, 1963). The original documentation and a valuable biography by Juan José Moreno can be found in Rafael Aguayo Spencer, ed., *Don Vasco de Quiroga: Documentos* (Mexico City, Editorial Polis, 1939).

33. See, for example, an important case study: Daniel T. Reff, *Disease, Depopulation, and Cultural Change in Northwestern New Spain, 1518–1764* (Salt Lake City: University of Utah Press, 1991).

34. The demographic impact of the epidemics in New Spain has produced widely diverging estimates concerning the actual die-off. For a recent update, consult F. J. Brooks, "Revising the Conquest of Mexico: Smallpox, Sources, and Populations," *Journal of Interdisciplinary History* 24 (1993): 1–29.

35. For an overview of colonial medicine, see Francisco Guerra, "Medical Colonization of the New World," *Medical History* 7 (1963): 147–54.

36. Miguel León-Portilla, "Las comunidades mesoamericanas ante la institución de los hospitales para indios," *Boletín de la Sociedad Mexicana de Historia y Filosofía de la Medicina* 44 (1983): 193–217.

37. A good primary source is Alonso de Zorita, *Life and Labor in Ancient Mexico: The Brief and Summary Relation of the Lords of New Spain*, trans. with an introduction by Benjamin Keen (New Brunswick, N.J.: Rutgers University Press, 1963). See Elsa Malvido, "Illness, Epidemics," below.

38. L. Gómez Canedo, "Desarrollo de la metodología misional franciscana en América," *Archivo iberoamericano* 46 (1986): 209–50. The dedication to the Virgin Mary was politically inspired by orders from Bishop Quiroga, designed to provide the institution with access to privileges and indulgences granted to Hernán Cortés's original establishment in Mexico City.

39. C. E. Casteñada, "The Coming of the Augustinians to the New World," *Records of the American Catholic Historical Society of Philadelphia* 60 (1949): 189–96.

40. For more information about the Tarascan Indians, consult Helen P. Pollard, *Tariacuri's Legacy: The Prehispanic Tarascan State* (Norman: University of Oklahoma Press, 1993), and J. Benedict

Warren, *The Conquest of Michoacan: The Spanish Domination of the Tarascan Kingdom in Western Mexico, 1521–1530* (Norman: University of Oklahoma Press, 1985). The Tarascans were famous for their weaving and embroidery skills.

41. The Law of the Indies now permitted private persons to found monasteries, hospitals, hermitages, and churches with their own money and to exercise the patronage over them. See Diego de Encinas, *Provisiones, cédulas y capítulos de ordenanzas . . . tocantes al buen gobierno de las Indias* (1596), reprinted in 4 vols. (Madrid: Cultura Hispánica, 1945), 1:145–47. This publication contains decrees and other documents emanating from the Council of Indies not found in the *Recopilación de Leyes de los Reynos de Indias,* as quoted in Mecham, *Church and State in Latin America,* 24.

42. See Guenter B. Risse, "Hospitals as Segregation and Confinement Tools," in *Mending Bodies—Saving Souls: A History of Hospitals* (New York: Oxford University Press, 1999), 167–229.

43. J. Toscano Moreno, "Los hospitales y la hospitalidad de los Franciscanos en la Nueva Galicia," *Boletín del Instituto de Investigaciones Bibliográficas* 4 (1970): 389–404.

44. For an overview of their role in Spain, consult Maureen Flynn, *Sacred Charity: Confraternities and Social Welfare in Spain, 1400–1700* (Ithaca, N.Y.: Cornell University Press, 1990).

45. A useful case study is presented by Poole, *Pedro Moya de Contreras.*

46. See D. Stanislawski, "Early Spanish Town Planning in the New World," *Geographical Review* 38 (1947): 94–105.

47. For details, Salvador Clavijo y Clavijo, *La obra de la Orden Hospitalaria de San Juan de Dios en América y Filipinas* (Madrid: Arges, 1950). Information about this new brotherhood is provided by Grace Goldin, "Juan de Dios and the Hospital of Christian Charity," *Journal of the History of Medicine* 33 (1978): 6–34.

48. Career patterns of such priests are examined in John F. Schwaller, *The Church and Clergy in Sixteenth-Century Mexico* (Albuquerque: University of New Mexico Press, 1987).

49. Craig Varjabedian and Michael Wallis, *En Divina Luz: The Penitente Moradas of New Mexico* (Albuquerque: University of New Mexico Press, 1994), 55.

50. Muriel, *Hospitales de la Nueva España,* 1:36–48. For Zumárraga's Hospital del Amor de Dios, see also entry no. 478 in Guerra, *Hospital en Hispanoamerica,* 229.

51. Juan de Barrios (1563–c. 1644) was an alumnus of the University of Alcalá de Henares in Spain who had traveled extensively and practiced medicine in Madrid before leaving for the colonies in 1589. Although he apparently had no medical degree, Barrios quickly became a member of the small group of physicians attending the Spanish elite in Mexico City. See also the *Index medicamentorum* in *Mexican Treasury.* More details about Barrios are in Juan Comas, "Influencia de la farmacopía y terapéutica indígenas de Nueva España en la obra de Juan de Barrios," *Anales de antropología* 8 (1971): 125–50. The standard review of early colonial publications in New Spain is Joaquín García Icazbalceta, *Bibliografía mexicana del siglo XVI* (Mexico City: Fondo de Cultura Económica, 1954). [The opening chapter of Francisco Bravo's *Opera medicinalia* discusses tabardete; and see Jaime Vilchis, "Globalizing the Natural History," below—Ed.]

52. C. Viqueira, "Los hospitales para locos e 'inocentes' en Hispanoamérica y sus antecedentes españoles," *Revista española de antropología americana* 5 (1970): 341–84.

53. J. S. Leiby, "San Hipólito's Treatment of the Mentally Ill in Mexico City, 1589–1650," *Historian* 54 (1992): 491–98.

54. Muriel, *Hospitales de la Nueva España,* 86–88.

55. The debate concerning the origin of venereal syphilis continues. For a summary of the arguments, see Francisco Guerra, "The Dispute over Syphilis, Europe versus America," *Clio medica* 13 (1978): 47–55, and J. Baker and G. J. Armelagos, "The Origin and Antiquity of Syphilis: Paleopathological Diagnosis and Interpretation," *Current Anthropology* 29 (1988): 703–37. In that same year, 1585, Ambroise Paré, a French barber-surgeon, published his influential treatise "Of the Lues Venerea," which can be found in the *Collected Works of Ambroise Paré,* translated from Latin by Thomas Johnson (London, 1634). See J. Worth Estes, "American Drugs," below.

56. A primary source about life in Mexico City is Francisco Cervantes de Salazar, *Life in the Imperial and Loyal City of Mexico in New Spain and the Royal and Pontifical University of Mexico,* trans. M. L. Barrett Shepard and ed. C. E. Castañeda (Austin: University of Texas Press, 1953).

57. For details concerning the nature of colonial labor draft and its abuses, see Charles Gibson, *The Aztecs under Spanish Rule: A History of the Indians of the Valley of Mexico, 1519–1810* (Stanford: Stanford University Press, 1964), 387–90.

58. María Luz López Terrada, "El tratamiento de la sífilis en un hospital renacentista: La sala del mal de siment del Hospital General de Valencia," *Asclepio* 41 (1989): 19–50.

59. For a view of the internal organization of a similar hospital, see the "Ordenanzas del hospital de San Cosme y San Damian (vulgo de las Bubas)," *Archivo hispalense* 44 (1967): 67–71.

60. Juan de Cárdenas, *Problemas y secretos maravillosos de las Indias* (1591), facs. repr. ed. by X. Lozoya (Mexico City: Academia Nacional de Medicina, 1980), chap. 5, pp. 264–71.

61. Fray Gerónimo de Mendieta, *Historia eclesiástica indiana,* ed. J. García Icazbalceta (Mexico City, 1870), chap. 36, p. 516.

62. J. G. O'Shea, "Two Minutes with Venus, Two Years with Mercury: Mercury as an Antisyphilitic Chemotherapeutic Agent," *Journal of the Royal Society of Medicine* 83 (1990): 392–95.

63. This preference for mercury reflected the experiences of contemporary European barber-surgeons such as Paré but also the therapeutic failure of guaiacum, the holy wood from the New World employed as a substitute for mercury during the first half of the sixteenth century. See Robert S. Munger, "Guaiacum, the Holy Wood from the New World," *Journal of the History of Medicine and Allied Sciences* 4 (1949): 196–229, and J. Worth Estes, "American Drugs," below.

64. Claude Quétel, "The Great Pox (Sixteenth Century)," in *The History of Syphilis,* trans. Judith Braddock and Brian Pike (Baltimore: Johns Hopkins University Press, 1990), 50–72.

65. N. Quezada, "La herbolaria en el México colonial," in *Estado actual del conocimiento en plantas medicinales mexicanas,* ed. X. Lozoya (Mexico City: IMEPLAM, 1979), 51–70.

66. José L. Valverde and José A. Perez Romero, *Drogas americanas en fuentes de escritores franciscanos y domínicos* (Granada: Universidad de Granada, 1988).

67. López de Hinojosos, *Suma y recopilación de cirugía,* 1595 ed. See Carlos Viesca Treviño, "Alonso López y su *Suma y recopilación de cirugía* (1535–1597)," in *Estudios sobre etnobotánica y antropología médica,* ed. Carlos Viesca Treviño (Mexico City: IMEPLAM, 1976), 29–58. See also Simon Varey and Rafael Chabrán, "Medical Natural History in the Renaissance: The Strange Case of Francisco Hernández," *Huntington Library Quarterly* 57 (1994): 132–33.

68. Juan Comas, "Influencia de la medicina azteca en la obra de Fr. Agustín Farfán," *Proceedings of the International Congress of Americanists* 31 (1955): 27–30, and G. Folch Jou, "Las drogas en la obra de Fray Agustin Farfán," *Actas, Congreso Internacional de Historia de la Medicina* (1956), 2 vols. (Madrid: Instituto

"Arnaldo de Vilanova" de Historia de la Medicina, CSIC, [1958]), 2:165–81.

69. See Debra Hassig, "Transplanted Medicine: Colonial Mexican Herbals of the Sixteenth Century," *Res* 17–18 (Spring–Autumn 1989): 30–53, and Jaime Vilchis, "Medicina novohispana del siglo XVI y la materia médica indígena," *Quipu* 5 (January–April 1988): 19–48.

70. Juan Comas, "Un caso de aculturación farmacológica en la Nueva España del siglo XVI: El 'Tesoro de Medicinas' de Gregorio López," *Anales de antropología* 1 (1964): 145–73. See *Index medicamentorum* and Rafael Chabrán and Simon Varey, "Hernández Texts," in *Mexican Treasury* for connections between López and Hernández.

71. Bernard R. Ortiz de Montellano has published an interesting study concerning the empirical effectiveness of certain Aztec drugs: "Empirical Aztec Medicine," *Science* 188 (April 18, 1975): 215–20, and more recently in his book *Aztec Medicine, Health, and Nutrition* (New Brunswick, N.J.: Rutgers University Press, 1990).

72. For background on this issue, see Gonzalo Aguirre Beltrán, *Medicina y magia: El proceso de aculturación en la estructura colonial* (Mexico City: Instituto Nacional Indigenista, 1963). Further discussions are contained in Serge Gruzinski, *The Conquest of Mexico: The Incorporation of Indian Societies into the Western World,* trans. Eileen Corrigan (Cambridge, England: Polity Press, 1993), 201–28.

73. Paul A. Russell, "Syphilis, God's Scourge or Nature's Vengeance?: The German Printed Response to a Public Problem in the Early Sixteenth Century," *Archiv für Reformationsgeschichte* 80 (1989): 286–307. For more details about the contemporary treatment of syphilis, consult Owsei Temkin, "Therapeutic Trends and the Treatment of Syphilis before 1900," *Bulletin of the History of Medicine* 29 (1955): 309–16.

74. The moral aspects surrounding this disease in the sixteenth century are discussed by Owsei Temkin, "On the History of 'Morality and Syphilis,'" in *The Double Face of Janus* (Baltimore: Johns Hopkins University Press, 1977), 472–84.

75. C. A. Mayo, "La distribución de los hospitales en Hispanoamérica a principios del siglo XVII," *Semana médica* (Buenos Aires) 157 (1980): 178–87.

ILLNESS, EPIDEMICS, AND DISPLACED CLASSES IN SIXTEENTH-CENTURY NEW SPAIN

ELSA MALVIDO

The "celebration" of the quincentennial in 1992 brought into sharper focus one of the most controversial periods of human history. I am thinking especially of the destruction of millions of human beings whose only fault was that they were biologically, culturally, and geographically "other," or alien beings.[1] To facilitate the European attempt to appropriate gold, silver, and souls, the "otherness" of the native inhabitants was enough to justify their being exploited in every sense. And so I think that as we cannot—indeed, should not—celebrate tragedy, there is nothing to go on celebrating, except perhaps a funeral.

Sixteenth-century America had to be invented day by day, as the distinguished Mexican historian Edmundo O'Gorman has brilliantly argued.[2] The process of creating history was difficult for those who stood, without, of course, realizing that they were doing so, at one of the world's historical turning points, one that could be compared only to the achievement of interplanetary travel in our own time. Five centuries later, the idea that to discover something is to possess it continues unchallenged; it is no coincidence that the Spanish words *conquistar* (to conquer) and *inventar* (to invent) can be used synonymously.[3] The

Europeans who invaded the lands they called America and appropriated by force had to continue interpreting faraway lands by inventing them in terms of their own world. The existence of the New World and Europe's discovery of it obliged Europeans to give up the fictions that had survived for centuries about the mythic places beyond the pillars of Hercules, the Antipodes, the lost city of Atlantis, the great void.[4]

The Catholic Church was one of the institutions most seriously affected by this reshaping of myth. The church was actually placed in a serious predicament, since it had to accept the discoveries with a certain degree of benevolence. In so doing, it had to modify its own ideas and teachings about the universe, to confront a world that was really round (even though the Inquisition had already burned many who believed this truth). The church had to understand that the Americas represented another continent, and not the land of the Great Khan. Nonetheless, the Spaniards persisted in referring to their new American territories as the Indies, a land of heretics. But in the end the most difficult task facing the church was to recognize the "other," that is, the native inhabitants, as equals. In certain respects it was convenient for the church to accept them as "children of God" at the cost of inhibiting its own accumulation of wealth; by recognizing any such equality, the church could not reduce the American population to the category of chattel slavery. The contemporary debate over the nature of the indigenous Americans was complicated, long, and tortuous and eventually concluded with a compromise. It was decided that the inhabitants of the New World were people without reason, who did have souls. Since the church found itself in difficult times, its power openly challenged and undermined by the Protestant Reformation, it resolved to use this newfound mass of humanity to its advantage.

My purpose in this essay is to try to sketch the dominant trends in health and illness immediately before and after these new lands came to be known as America, that is, up to the time that Francisco Hernández arrived to carry out his survey of the medicinal plants and the people of New Spain. The only way to reach any understanding of those trends is to examine the documents left by the "men of reason" of the time. I also propose to measure, as far as anyone can, the changes that the "souls without reason" had to undergo in the colonization process.[5] And it is my purpose to recognize the capacity of the human animal to adapt to unfavorable conditions over time and to survive. We should remember that human beings, whether polytheistic or monotheistic, have been able to adapt and survive even without the help of their gods and patron saints.

The new, imported diseases with which I am concerned in this essay can be classified into three different groups: biological, social, and biosocial. *Biological diseases* are those transmitted from human to human but that have evolved from diseases transmitted by animals. Among these are smallpox, measles, chicken pox, mumps, and whooping cough. In fifteenth-century Europe, these diseases had become domesticated or endemic, and thus they affected only those populations that had not been exposed to them previously. Diseases transmitted by humans went through two stages in New Spain. The introductory stage, from 1520 to 1563, produced an extraordinary rate of mortality because it did not meet any biological resistance. The other components of the biological diseases made their entrance as pan-

demics, once the colony had settled into the more recognizable social patterns of its early modern form. By 1563, when contact with Spain had become more frequent and when immigration was more organized and was supposedly selective, biological disease came to the end of its invasive phase. In that year whooping cough spread all over the conquered territories, causing an 80 to 90 percent mortality rate among those infected. The second stage, of domestication, covered the period from 1564 until well into the nineteenth century, affecting only those age groups and more isolated geographical groups that had remained unaffected during previous epidemics.[6]

A second group of maladies and conditions can be classified as *social,* whereby we can relate epidemics to issues of internal cultural development and to specific conditions of the social and economic order. Research into these relationships necessarily involves study of nutrition, the effects of warfare, poverty, famine, and alcoholism among the native population, as well as specific diseases such as typhoid and exanthematic typhus. Diseases could now be communicated in new ways, for instance, by gunpowder, the wheel, metal weapons, ships, horses, and the Catholic religion, all of which were able to separate "the other" by wars of conquest or of extinction.[7] These maladies often entailed hunger and thirst, fear, torture, and losing the will to live.[8] Prior to the process of adapting to the unknown and to imposed conditions, the victims tended to generate resistance, though there were few survivors.

The third classification may be called *biosocial* pathology, which consists of just one disease: the plague, transmitted directly by fleas infesting the black rat. The transmission of biosocial disease needs both biological carriers and harsh conditions. The plague in its three forms appeared after the conquest, transported every time on ships with their black rats, and was spread among all the inhabitants of the continent. The range of contagion increased because of new, imported hosts, such as dogs and people. With every native individual susceptible, there were no natural immunities, irrespective of species, class, ethnicity, color, age or sex, New or Old World descent. Ninety percent of those infected died, so that every time the disease arrived, it created a new incursion.

All three types of disease found the most favorable conditions among dense populations and rapidly expanding cities.[9]

New Spain in the Sixteenth Century

The conquest exposed the indigenous population to pandemics, epidemics, and endemics, all made easier by the imposition of a new socioeconomic system. The unchecked advance of epidemics was made possible by gunpowder, steel, the ship, the horse, and the dog, the last three of which were especially important for the rapid transmission and widening range of illnesses. The most rampant forms of cultural domination thus turned out to be the unexpected forces of sickness and death. Smallpox became, though hardly by design, the first factor to unify the native populations—grotesquely—in the colonization process. Smallpox had a much harsher effect on Americans than on Europeans until the native population developed immunities, but we should not underestimate the deadly pandemic capacity of smallpox, measles, chicken pox, mumps, whooping cough, influenza, and plague in its various forms.[10] All these diseases would teach humankind, some more forcefully and terribly than others, that we all belong to one species—one that is dreadfully weak in the face of disease.

In the pre-Hispanic period, diseases were closely linked to ecology and vagaries of the climate, in what might be called a natural relationship. Social diseases were certainly spread by various types of warfare, but the spread of disease was limited by the social development of native groups. Interactions of all kinds tended to be much more localized than they were after the arrival of the Spanish, and more localized than they were in the Old World, where, over several centuries of traffic between Europe, Asia, and Africa, livestock, human beings, and merchandise continually exchanged strains of disease and generated immunities to them.[11] The diseases exhibited such inexplicable and diverse patterns of occurrence as the following: (1) they became generalized in all ecological niches regardless of the state of the group's previous development; (2) they affected only the native population; (3) they acquired their most virulent, aggressive, or primitive forms as a result of the native

lack of immunity; and (4) they remained endemic throughout the century. This "colonial" morbidity was divided, just as it was in Spain, into biological, social, and biosocial types, even though it would exhibit specific characteristics of its own once it came into contact with a virgin population such as that of the New World.

As has been said often enough before, no one today can suggest plausibly that the native people of the Americas lived in Paradise, even if Columbus wondered about it and Hernández went even further.[12] Rather, the native inhabitants suffered typical illnesses according to their stages of development, especially when climatic conditions played a determinant role and affected their ecological niches and—obviously—their health. The evidence can be found in three kinds of source: documents that refer to the pre-Hispanic period; American skeletal remains, from various periods; documents that were generated at the moment of conquest, and especially those documents that refer to the effects of these diseases. From these materials we can deduce that pre-Hispanic cultures suffered from "natural" diseases, whereby ecological and climatological changes either favored or retarded their growth or survival. Thus the health or sickness of various groups in particular geographic locations could be dependent on such factors as storms, heavy rains, flooding, cyclones, hail storms, periods of frost and snow, and winds or periods of drought, be they short or long term. They were also affected by external infestations such as those of locusts and the *chahuistle* (a parasite that affects grains), which contributed to famine, lack of water, malnutrition, and death.[13] Here we should also include the other zoonoses that affected humans because of ecological changes: for example, yellow fever in the jungles and malaria in marshy areas, or typhus during periods of war and famine. All these have been documented and reported in a range of sources. As P. C. C. Garnham has said, "All infective human diseases must have been zoonoses at one time; that is during the period when the anthropoid ape was being transformed into *Homo sapiens*," to which I would add that this is the clearest expression of humans' animal nature to this day.[14]

One other type of disease active in the pre-Hispanic era was social, caused by humans and including various forms of war, slavery, human sacrifice, the exploitation of one group by another, and the systematic appropriation of the means of production and reproduction.[15] According to the annual calendar—from at least the time of Teotihuacan until the era of the Mexica—no less than one-fourth of the time was devoted to war.[16] This should not surprise us, since in the twentieth century we continued to spend about the same proportion of our time fighting one another.

Our second source consists of information obtained from osteopathology. Research into the skeletal remains of people of the period reveals that they suffered from syphilis, yaws, tuberculosis or other related diseases such as rheumatoid arthritis, various tumors, and skin or bone diseases leading to fractures. Dating from the time of the sixteenth-century conquest of the Valley of Mexico (today Huexotl, state of Mexico) is a newly discovered cemetery—already Christianized—where I have carried out research following the work of Ronald Hare. The evidence of other cultural artifacts at the same site indicates that the people eventually buried there had obtained an equilibrium with nature and had been able to maintain a relatively good state of health.

Both forms of disease, whether natural or social, were conditioned by the sociopolitical and technological situations of each population group. Pre-Hispanic communication was limited to walking or the canoe, so that each of these groups was framed by specific and restricted geo-economic spaces. This was just as applicable to hunter-gatherers and fishermen who migrated at specific seasons of the year, so that the effects of their problems were constrained by the time and space of the regions in which they lived and moved. Famine, infectious diseases, and political crises, then, would not affect people outside specific niches. The only crisis that reached farther afield was war. The constant practice of the ritual bath as a prophylactic by almost all these population groups and their nearly unlimited variety of healthy foods— whatever was fresh and easily available—made transmission and the spread of contagion virtually impossible in normal circumstances, because these conditions did not favor the incubation or spread of disease. Thus these population groups avoided the spread of diseases before they caused death or could be cured.

Nonetheless, some sedentary groups adopted extraordinary strategies in order to confront the problems of famine that resulted from natural disasters. Among the more extreme measures they took in order to survive were migration to other ecological niches; eating foods that were not strictly edible; bartering goods for food at exaggerated prices; and even selling children, either temporarily or permanently, just to keep them alive.

All this leads us to conclude that because of specific stages of development and the forms of expropriation and appropriation of goods in use in specific ecological niches, the diseases acquired the characteristics of epidemics, which were almost always related to natural ecological changes or caused by the spread of humans or temporary zoonoses.

Smallpox, 1518–1521

Smallpox played a special part as one of the fundamental vectors of disease in New Spain. It was because of the spread of smallpox that the population was reduced and New Spain incorporated into Spanish, and more generally European, hegemony. Smallpox is in reality the only disease that can be traced, more or less, from the islands of the Caribbean to Tenochtitlán, the capital of the Aztecs, today's Mexico City. The example of smallpox permits us to observe the route that, with some variations, other imported diseases would follow during the three centuries of Spanish colonizations. It was during the first voyages of discovery led by Columbus between 1492 and 1495 that smallpox was introduced to the inhabitants of the Caribbean islands, but it was not until a second outbreak that had traveled from Spain to Hispaniola in 1518 that smallpox spread to Cuba. From Havana it was transported at the beginning of March 1520 on the punitive expedition led by Pánfilo de Narváez, who was sent by Governor Velázquez to arrest Hernán Cortés. On board the nineteen ships was an army of nine hundred Spanish men, accompanied by some native and black slaves: among this group there was at least one man infected with smallpox, probably in the presymptomatic stage. Although no one died on the journey, at least seven men showed symptoms during the voyage and were ill when they landed on the Mexican coast.[17]

They reportedly dropped anchor at San Juan Ulúa on April 19. From there they sailed to Cempoala, where, while they waited for Cortés, they infected the population of the whole town. This is how López de Gómara described it:

> It happened that among the men of Narváez was a Negro sick with the smallpox, and he infected the household in Cempoala where he was quartered; and it spread from one Indian to another, and they, being so numerous and eating and sleeping together, quickly infected the whole country. In most houses all the occupants died, for, since it was their custom to bathe as a cure for all diseases, they bathed for the smallpox and were struck down. They had the custom, or vice, of taking cold baths after hot ones, so a man sick with the smallpox only escaped by a miracle. Those who did survive, having scratched themselves, were left in such a condition that they frightened the others with the many deep pits on their faces, hands, and bodies. And then came famine, not because of a want of bread, but of meal, for the women do nothing but grind maize between two stones and bake it. The women, then, fell sick of the smallpox, bread failed, and many died of hunger. The corpses stank so horribly that no one would bury them; the streets were filled with them; and it is even said that the officials, in order to remedy this situation, pulled the houses down to cover the corpses.[18]

It is interesting to note that the blame was placed on a black slave accused of being the carrier.

If Pánfilo de Narváez expected the inhabitants of Cempoala to join him in his fight against Cortés, we can only suppose that the pandemic thwarted his expectation. This was surely the reason that the battle between the two white leaders took place on May 29 in Cempoala and not near Tenochtitlán, that is, a month and ten days after Narváez's arrival on the coast of Mexico. This event would be pivotal for the propagation of smallpox, since Narváez's defeated soldiers joined Cortés and returned to Mexico with him, spreading the disease among native allies who were now either survivors or carriers. When Cortés returned to the Aztec capital, he found that the previously friendly Mexica had turned against the Spaniards.

Cortés was eventually defeated in Tenochtitlán between June 8 and June 30, 1520, the latter date known by Cortés as the Night of Sorrows. After that night the Mexica would tell their story of lining up the Spaniards and robbing them.[19] With this act, the pandemic would claim its first quota of victims among the Mexica, remaining in Tenochtitlán and continuing to collect victims until September. If the dates are correct, the pandemic took approximately two years to travel from Hispaniola to Tenochtitlán. The disease traveled more rapidly over land; it took from April 19 to May 29 to travel from San Juan de Ulúa to Cempoala. Then it took two more months to reach the center of Tenochtitlán. Smallpox took six months to travel about 280 miles.

The Indian enemies of the Mexica were obviously the ones who carried the disease, and it is probable that, during the battle on the Night of Sorrows, the Spaniards did not realize that their Tlaxcalan and other native allies were already ill or that many of them were already dying from disease. The reason that the Spaniards did not recognize the presence of the disease among their native allies was that the symptoms were different in this virgin population. In other words, as yet there were no typical external symptoms. And there were several other factors distracting the invaders: among these were Cortés's attempts to grapple with his own failure to keep control of the Aztec empire; the destructive greediness and the ransacking of Tenochtitlán; and, lastly, the Spaniards' struggle for their own survival.

My hypothesis, then, is that during this struggle and unknown to anyone, smallpox became a tremendous ally of the Mexica by infecting the Tlaxcalans and other allies of Cortés. Without even knowing it, the native people from Cempoala were direct carriers of the disease. In the absence of any native record by the vanquished about this battle, no one has been able to confirm (or deny) this hypothesis definitively. Thus we can offer the following explanation. Despite their numbers and the vast array of arms, the Spaniards and their allies lost the battle against the Mexica, but the price of the Mexican victory was infection. Infection was generated by various means: bodies, clothing, arms, animals, and other possessions of the enemies, as well as prisoners taken during the long skirmish. It was said at the time that Spanish corpses were tossed aside, but we do not know whether they were burned or simply left abandoned for scavenging animals and birds. According to López de Gómara, "450 Spaniards died, 4,000 Indian friends, 46 horses, and, I believe, all the prisoners. Some say more, some less, but this is the truest number."[20] We now know that the smallpox virus can thrive in the clothing, hair, and beards of the dead as well as in animals that are in contact with those infected. Thus the likelihood of contagion must, if anything, have increased after the battle.

Warfare, smallpox, hunger, and thirst came and went through the towns that surrounded the city on the route to Chalco. By December 1520, many towns had been stricken, and their leaders had died. According to the native chronicles, among the distinguished who died in this first epidemic of 1520 were not only the brave Cuitlahuac, the Mexica king, but also many other rulers of the surrounding towns. As a result, Cortés was asked to name their successors, and as he did so, he specified that the cause of death had been smallpox. Among the dead was his friend Maxixca, Lord of Tlaxcala.[21]

I have attempted to follow the routes of smallpox contagion as they corresponded with the arrival of Pánfilo de Narváez's ships in San Juan de Ulúa and his journey through the new lands. Unfortunately the chroniclers neglected to explain what was happening to the "others" in terms of disease, largely because they were consumed by other priorities and their own self-interest. The Spaniards now recognized that the disease had not been present in the New World before their arrival. What they did not fully understand was the actual impact that it would have on other cultures and on a population more dense and concentrated than that of the Caribbean islands. But even less could the Spanish imagine that smallpox would become their greatest ally in the conquest of Tenochtitlán, a city that they would find depopulated and terrorized by the effects of smallpox when they returned in 1521.[22]

Many years after the Spanish reconquered Tenochtitlán in 1521, smallpox continued to bring destruction as the conquerors, now playing the role of discoverers, advanced throughout the kingdom that the Spaniards now called New Spain. This slow and long process of invasion of smallpox has caused confusion of the dates and consequently mistaken chronologies of smallpox epidemics. Although historians customarily identify many different epidemics, in reality it was the original epidemic manifesting itself in different places at different times.[23]

The first epidemic of smallpox brought by the Spaniards constitutes the watershed in the new disease history of America. It was a monumentally important event that changed the lives of the entire native population. The destruction of the native peoples was so catastrophic that those who survived became literally the first generation of a new era. It is important to note that because the victims of the epidemic constituted a virgin population, the smallpox strain was atypical. That is to say, it acquired a more aggressive, hemorrhagic form, prompting a higher mortality and several characteristics that differed from those experienced in Europe. The characteristics may have been similar to those that were exhibited in the stricken Caribbean populations between 1492 and 1495.

Even though we cannot follow the paths of smallpox with absolute certainty, we can say that between the end of 1519 and 1520, it traveled slowly, at the same speed that the enemies of the Mexica were advancing with their horses, wheels, and ships. It is from this moment that smallpox can be considered the first unifying element of the species, without regard to stages of development, and no respecter of social class or any other factor besides the immunological virginity it encountered. The one exception to this generalization is that virgin populations will be more susceptible to this disease. For more than a century, smallpox remained endemic, traveling through villages at the same rate that they were being conquered. So it was that even from the very beginning of the conquest of Mexico, those diseases transmitted only from human to human flourished.

Possibly because smallpox had been the first disease imported into New Spain, and so the most virulent of all, the rhythm of its cycle was slower. It took the susceptible population a century to recover, from 1518 to 1615. In his discussion of acute infections in which "the organisms disappear upon recovery or death," Ronald Hare comments: "Whether the patient dies or recovers from these diseases, the organisms are usually available for transfer to other persons for no longer than the acute phase of the disease, that is, about seven to fourteen days, and except for the virus of smallpox which can remain alive for some months, those that have reached the external environment usually die within a day or so."[24] Viruses that were endemic in Spain could travel on almost every crossing to America, carried by one or more infected persons.

Mumps is an unusual case, since it occurred as a pandemic in 1550 and a second time in 1595–97, these being apparently the only two outbreaks in the sixteenth century. However, it is well documented in the medical texts from the sixteenth century to the nineteenth as a common disease, although it may not always have been correctly identified.

Cycles of social and biosocial diseases occurred at first in significant epidemic outbreaks, remaining endemic throughout the sixteenth century and into the following one, until the colonial system was established and had changed the structure of society. Only then did these lose some of their strength, although they became more acute with major climatic changes that were responsible for the rising price of corn, control of the crop, and famine among the native people in general and among the poorest of them in particular. Biosocial diseases went through similar cycles in Europe and America, making remorseless and devastating invasions of the population every twenty-five years. They affected not just men and women but all animal species. This cycle persisted throughout the colonial period.

Conclusion

America was invented as a poor copy of the mother country and became a place where alien beings invaded a different ecological niche, converting Noah's ark into Pandora's box.[25] It is clear that the Spaniards "invented" the native people according to their own needs. To the colonizers, the native people lacked reason but, unfortunately, also lacked the defenses necessary to ward off the infectious diseases brought from Europe and so fell victim to all the Old World's illnesses. However, each agent of infection was attached to one form of human disease that today we codify individually according to the symptoms: those that produce immunity among victims who survive; those that do not stimulate the production of any defenses; and, lastly, those that never generate immunity but occur in different strains every time.

A large proportion of the native population of New Spain had died by the middle of the sixteenth century. Some historical demographers call this genocide, referring to what were known in New Spain as the Wars of Extinction—military campaigns against specific native groups such as the Cholulteca and the Mexica.[26] These campaigns functioned effectively as the equivalents of epidemics. Yet Europeans, Americans, Asians, and Africans demonstrate that all human beings have the capacity to survive and to adapt to new circumstances. The species, through the process of reproduction, has created a newly adapted human being who is more resistant to sickness and death. That ability to survive should be celebrated today—and for as long as the species, we mere human beings, remains on earth. It is clear, then, that to discover and to conquer have been synonymous for centuries, words that have coincided as they do for historians, who continually seek to discover the past and to reinvent it.

NOTES

1. The locus classicus for discussion of the "other" is Tzvetan Todorov, *La conquête de l'Amérique: La question de l'autre* (Paris: Seuil, 1982); English edition, *The Conquest of America* (New York: Harper & Row, 1984), reprinted in various formats in 1985, 1987, 1992. I refer to the 1992 English edition.

2. Edmundo O'Gorman, *The Invention of America* (Bloomington: Indiana University Press, 1961), a considerably revised version of *La invención de América: El universalismo de la cultura del Occidente* (Mexico City: Fondo de Cultura Económica, 1958). See also his important study *La idea del descubrimiento de América: Historia de esa interpretacion y crítica de sus fundamentos* (Mexico City: Centro de Estudios Filosóficos, 1951) and *Cuatro historiadores de Indias* (Mexico City: SEP/Setentas, 1972).

3. [Because we tend to associate invention with an act of creation, we might remember that the Latin root of *inventar* is *invenio, -ire*, whose radical meaning is to come upon, hence to discover. An inventor is thus a discoverer.—Ed.]

4. See Bartolomé de las Casas's commentary on Columbus (*Historia de las Indias*, ed. Agustín Millares, 2d ed. [Mexico City: Fondo de Cultura Económica, 1965]) and O'Gorman's critique of it (*Invention of America*, 20–21). Columbus himself thought he had found "the earthly Paradise," which "the sacred theologians and learned philosophers" had placed "at the end of the Orient," exactly the location of "those lands which I have now discovered" (*A Synoptic Edition of the Log of Columbus's First Voyage*, ed. Francesca Lardici, textual ed. Valeria Bertolucci Pizzorusso, trans. Cynthia L. Chamberlin and Blair Sullivan, Repertorium Columbianum, vol. 6 [Turnhout, Belgium: Brepols, 1999], 131.

5. See Fernando Benítez, *El libro de los desastres* (Mexico City: Era, 1988), 14–15.

6. See Elsa Malvido, "Cronología de las epidemias y crisis agrícolas en la época colonial," in *Ensayos sobre la historia de las epidemias en México*, ed. Enrique Florescano and Elsa Malvido, 2 vols. (Mexico City: Instituto Mexicano del Seguro Social, 1982), 1:171–76.

7. [For an unusual and stimulating perspective, see Jared Diamond, "Why Did Human History Unfold Differently on Different Continents for the Last 13,000 Years?" UCLA Faculty Research Lecture, April 11, 1996, <http://www.bruin.ucla.edu/FRL/Diamond/001.html>, and Diamond's full-length study *Guns, Germs, and Steel: The Fates of Human Societies* (New York: Norton, 1997).—Ed.]

8. Desgano vital (translated here as losing the will to live) is general demoralization that sometimes results in impotence and suicide. In the face of a seemingly invincible invading power, many Mexicans simply gave up.

9. See José María López Piñero, *Historia de la medicina* (Madrid: Historia 16, [1991]), 84–86.

10. On smallpox's harsher effect on Americans, see the model proposed by Russell Thornton, Tim Miller, and Jonathan Warren, "American Indian Population Recovery following Smallpox Epidemics," *American Anthropologist* 93, no. 1 (1991): 28–41. On the pandemic capacity of these diseases, see the wide range of essays in Florescano and Malvido, *Ensayos sobre la historia de las epidemias,* esp. vol. 1.

11. See William H. McNeill, *Plagues and Peoples* (Garden City, N.Y.: Anchor/Doubleday, 1976), 199.

12. See V. I. Polunin, "Health and Disease in Contemporary Primitive Societies," in *Diseases in Antiquity: A Survey of the Diseases, Injuries, and Surgery of Early Populations,* ed. Don Brothwell and A. T. Sandison (Springfield, Ill.: Charles C. Thomas, 1967), 69. Also, Columbus's *Log,* February 21, 1493 (n. 4 above), and "Account of the Third Voyage," in *Textos y documentos completos,* ed. Consuelo Varela and Juan Gil, 2d ed. (Madrid: Alianza, 1992), 380–81. The connection is maintained by the very title of Kirkpatrick Sale's *The Conquest of Paradise: Christopher Columbus and the Columbian Legacy* (New York: Knopf, 1990). Hernández invoked Paradise in his essay on cacao (see *Mexican Treasury,* "Five Special Texts").

13. See Rosaura Hernández Rodríguez, "Epidemias y calamidades en el México prehispánico," in Florescano and Malvida, *Ensayos sobre historia de las epidemias,* 1:139–56. See also André Gunder Frank, *La agricultura mexicana: Transformación del modo de producción, 1521–1630* (Mexico City: Era, 1982).

14. Zoonosis is an animal that is a reservoir of a human disease (P. C. C. Garnham, "Zoonoses or Infections Common to Man and Animals," *Journal of Tropical Medicine and Hygiene* 61 [1958]: 92).

15. E. Noguera et al., *Los señoríos y estados militares* (Mexico City: SEP-INAH, 1976), is useful on this last topic.

16. The sacking, burning, and partial destruction of Teotihuacan occurred at the end of the eighth century. The Mexica were one of three dominant population groups that conquered the "Aztec" empire and are usually considered Aztecs.

17. Francisco López de Gómara, *Cortés: The Life of the Conqueror by His Secretary,* trans. Lesley Byrd Simpson (Berkeley: University of California Press, 1964), 192–94, 204–5, which is based on Cortés's testimony, not on its author's experience (López de Gómara was in Spain at the time). My summary of the movements of Cortés is drawn mainly from two sources: this work by López de Gómara (originally *Istoria de la conquista de México* [Zaragoza, 1552]) and Cortés, *Cartas de relación,* trans. Anthony Pagden as *Letters from Mexico,* rev. ed. [New Haven: Yale University Press, 1986]). Further contemporary sources that I have consulted include the *Codice Ramírez,* printed in Hernando Alvarado Tezozomoc, *Crónica mexicana* (Mexico City: UNAM, 1943), also separately published (Mexico City: Innovación, 1979); Bernal Díaz del Castillo, *The Discovery and Conquest of Mexico,* trans. Irving A. Leonard (New York: Farrar, Straus and Cudahy, 1956); and Juan Ginés de Sepúlveda, *Democrates segundo o De las justas causas de la guerra contra los Indios,* with parallel texts in Latin and Spanish, trans. and ed. Angel Losada (Madrid: Instituto Francisco de Vitoria, CSIC, 1951).

18. López de Gómara, *Cortés,* 204–5; and see Juan de Torquemada, *Monarquía indiana* (Mexico City: UNAM, 1975), vol. 2, chap. 66.

19. G. R. G. Conway, *La noche triste* (Mexico City: Robredo/Porrua, 1943). See Diego Muñoz Camargo, *Historia de Tlaxcala,* 2d ed. (Mexico: Ateneo Nacional de Ciencias y Artes, 1947), esp. 236–37.

20. López de Gómara, *Cortés,* 221.

21. Ibid., 238, and Cortés, *Letters from Mexico,* 165.

22. Cortés, *Letters from Mexico,* 263–64, and Pagden's useful bibliographical and critical note on the smallpox at 491 n. 77.

23. One serious problem with the early sources is that the dates presented in the documents differ according to which conqueror, priest, or Amerindian group provides them. The Spanish sources contradict one another, and native calendars, which do not coincide with Western ones, are difficult to reconcile. Neither are recollections often consistent with one another. All of this leads me to conclude that the dates of the events are, ultimately, mythical and are more likely to relate, in the cases of Spaniards and Indians, to their deities, saints, and celebrations than to actual dates.

24. Ronald Hare, "The Antiquity of Diseases Caused by Bacteria and Viruses: A Review of the Problem from a Bacteriologist's Point of View," in Brothwell and Sandison, *Diseases in Antiquity,* 119.

25. See Elsa Malvido, "El arca de Noe o la caja de Pandora?" in *Pandemias, epidemias, y endemias en la Nueva España, 1519–1810* (Mexico: Pedro Domecq, IMSS, 1992).

26. See, for example, Todorov, *Conquest of America:* "The sixteenth century perpetrated the greatest genocide in human history" (5) and again, 133. See also such sources as Sepúlveda, *Democrates segundo.*

ANTHROPOLOGY, REASON, AND THE DICTATES OF FAITH IN THE ANTIQUITIES OF FRANCISCO HERNÁNDEZ

DAVID A. BORUCHOFF

When the newlywed woman reached the seventh month of her pregnancy, her close relatives, after eating and drinking, would discuss the choice of a midwife, with whose art and advice the delivery would be safe and easy. Then they would go to one whom they knew to be the most skilled in the city and the most diligent in the practice of her art, so that she would care for the health of the woman in labor, and assist her at the moment of childbirth, and they begged her assistance with fervent supplication. She replied with reasons that she would do so, with all the diligence and care of which she was capable, all for their satisfaction, the health of the child, and the health of the mother. And after frequent visits to the pregnant woman, she would not only take her to the baths known as temazcal in their native country, which they used a great deal for pregnant women, mothers of young children, and convalescents, but she would also lay down a set of rules for living which were to be observed carefully and religiously at the time of delivery.[1]

With these words, Francisco Hernández begins the second chapter of his account of the "antiquities of New Spain," the old ways and practices of the Mexican people. In a manner more discursive than analytic, Hernández leads the reader through the rites of birth, consecration, marriage, and death to show that from first to last, through law and education, the lives of the Nahua are guided by the wisdom of the elders and by a sense of their community. Though the ceremonies and values described in these pages are expressly pagan, still they should not be regarded as superstition, the mark of a backward and barbaric people, for in Hernández's view there is a logical, if not transcendent, purpose that governs the transmission of native custom and belief. Both men and women learn to act and speak, to think and live and be what prudence and the social good have determined. A Mexican is made and molded by traditions handed down through the generations. He or she is the product of social and cultural forces refined by convention but born under the sign of reason.

Given the emphasis that other historians of the sixteenth century place on the Mexicans' belief in astrological determinism or the fateful influence of one's day sign, it is curious that Hernández should choose to omit this aspect from his initial description of the rituals that accompany childbirth. Whereas Bernardino de Sahagún devotes an entire chapter of his *Historia general de las cosas de la Nueva*

España to the complicated process by which the new parents would enlist the aid of a soothsayer to divine the fortune of their child, Hernández merely comments: "But if the birth went well, the midwife would talk to the baby, as if he were already capable of reason and could understand what was said to him. She would invoke the gods to ensure that his birth gave him a prime place among the gods, and access to a good augury at his birth. She would ask what fate or destiny had been assigned to him from the beginning of the world."[2] From Hernández's words, it would seem that the midwife's science, and the "customary little prayers" that she recites as she goes about her duties, may serve to ensure a happy life. And the infant himself, to whom the midwife speaks, according to Hernández, "as if he were already capable of reason," appears to possess knowledge of his own destiny, the "luck or inborn fate" to which he is bound by birth. Hernández does not tell us to whom the midwife directs her questions, save to say that their intent is to ensure the gods' favor. He makes no mention of the learned seers and their books or of the day signs and their meaning. Rather, it is dialogue itself that receives the author's attention, as the mother and her newborn child are greeted by a succession of relations, who offer solace and guidance to both.

Like other Spanish texts of the mid- to late sixteenth century, Hernández's account of the "antiquities of New Spain" is based in large part on the *huehuetlahtolli* of the Mexican people, the rhetorical set pieces that served to transmit knowledge and social values among the Nahua.[3] Literally "the sayings of the ancients," this patterned form of speech was commonly assigned a regulatory function by European writers, who saw the huehuetlahtolli as an affective or ceremonial mode of discourse, helpful in maintaining the public order and indicative of cultural values but fundamentally independent of day-to-day relations within the Mexican community.[4] In the words of Sahagún's informants, the declamatory language of the huehuetlahtolli is "characteristic of [the Mexican people's] forefathers and of the works that *they* had done," a feature that would appear to diminish the usefulness of these sayings as a true indication of the Nahua's convictions and understanding as an individual.[5] It is thus logical that Sahagún, among others, would choose to describe the huehuetlahtolli as "the

Rhetoric and Moral Philosophy and Theology of the Mexican People" and to observe that "all nations, no matter how barbarous and low their character, have always fixed their gaze upon the wise and powerful to speak on their behalf, and upon illustrious men for their moral virtues."[6]

In contrast to this perspective, Francisco Hernández assimilates the huehuetlahtolli within the fabric of everyday life, refashioning the oratory of the Nahua into dialogue and their erudition into conversation. The "sayings of the ancients" structure human relations in Hernández's narration and produce an oddly dramatic and formal, yet lucid, form of interaction between key members of Mexican society: parents and children, husband and wife, teachers and students, and so on. To return to the initial example that Hernández offers of the "antiquities of New Spain," we see that the decision to engage a midwife is taken following the meal, and presumably while the family is still gathered for dinner. By personalizing the ways of tradition, Hernández conflates the attributes of ceremonial discourse and rational discussion; the birthing ritual becomes a tribute to the benefits of dialogue and to the intellectual predisposition of the Mexican people. The family seeks out the counsel of an expert midwife who can guide the expectant mother through each step of pregnancy and birth, alternating medical and social prescriptions with comfort and assurance, in short, with the application of scientific and human understanding. When the mother-to-be responds favorably to this regime, meeting instruction with diligence, the midwife then turns her attention to the newborn child and asks that he too receive "a passage of good omen to this light," that is, the right of entry to life in the Mexican community and perhaps, metaphorically, to reason. And so, from the first, Hernández reports that midwife and family treat the infant boy as though he were endowed with understanding, telling him of the adversity and hardship that await him as he enters society[7] and of the manner in which he must serve his gods and people: "'It is important for you, newborn baby, to go to war, to die in battle, so that in the end you will go to heaven, to serve the sun, and to live a life of peace and happiness, among the bravest of men who lived, lost once they fell in combat.' With these words they demonstrated that every boy was destined to go to war in obeisance to the sun."[8]

Indoctrination begins at birth. Tradition is a logical, rational, and meaningful process by virtue of which the individual can assume his correct place in the Nahua world.[9]

It is fitting, then, that Hernández would begin his account of the "antiquities of New Spain" with a series of decisive moments, or rites of passage, in the development of Nahua men and women, since his aim is to show that human behavior results from tutelage, rather than from the accident of one's birth. From his narration we learn that in Mexico, newborn boys would be presented with "a small shield, a bow, and four small arrows appropriate to the child's age, and a small mantle like the Mexicans' cape."[10] In contrast, an infant girl would receive the *huepilli* and *cueitl*, the attire characteristic of Mexican women, as well as the various instruments that she will use later in life as part of her domestic routine.[11] This attention to symbolic action and to the reinforcement of sexual and cultural identity continues in subsequent chapters of Hernández's *Antiquities*, which describe the ceremonial bathing of newborn children and the different forms of education that they receive in accordance with their sex and social standing, a process that culminates in the depiction of courtship, marriage, and death among the Nahua. If Hernández describes phenomena that are not significantly different from those found in the works of Sahagún, Diego Durán, José Acosta, and others, still he does so with a curious attention to the individual's capacity for rational belief and expression and to the role of native traditions in achieving this end. So too does Hernández reorder the Nahua's rites of passage in accordance with medical and scientific criteria, so as to make ceremony parallel the Europeans' understanding of the chronology of human development, in contradistinction to the more authentic or symbolic ranking assigned to them by native informants.[12] By inserting the Nahua's cultural practices into an analytic framework, the huehuetlahtolli that Hernández cites appeal both to the speaker's good sense and discretion, as a member of the indigenous community, and to the intellect of those who listen. It is rhetoric as persuasion, rather than ritual, that comes to the fore in these pages.

More telling yet, however, is the process of selection that dictates which of the "sayings of the ancients" Hernández will transcribe in the form of direct quotation. In contrast to the fundamentally religious criteria of Sahagún, who offers examples of the words that accompany both good and bad day signs so as to underscore the importance of the notion of fate among the Nahua—and, thus, the necessary opposition of free will to human nature—Hernández restricts his attention to more generic formulas that express collective fears and aspirations. The practice of what he terms "lavation" (*lauatio*) appears in this way to equalize the potential of all newborn children across certain broad categories related to sex and nobility and, in short, to deny those features that would limit the development of reason or value within Nahua society. The midwife's huehuetlahtolli initiate the child's education but do not address the question of aptitude or promise, for these will be determined by his schooling. It follows that Hernández would choose systematically to transcribe each of the various orations that may help to cleanse the child of inborn defects or adversity, as we see in the following passage:

> Then, she sprinkled some more of the same water on the infant's breast, saying, "Receive this celestial water which washes impurity from your heart," then, sprinkling water on his head again, she said, "Son, receive this divine water, which must be drunk that all may live, that it may wash you and wash away all your misfortunes, part of your life since the beginning of the world: this water in truth has a unique power to oppose misfortune." At the same time she washed the baby's little body all over, exclaiming, "In which part of you is unhappiness hidden, or in which part are you hiding? Leave this child; today he is born again in the healthful waters in which he has been bathed, according to the will of Chalchiutlicue, the goddess of the sea."[13]

Although other writers relate similar examples, it is not with the same intensity or with the singular purpose of providing a new beginning for the child, who may then grow through the exercise of reason.[14] This is Hernández's aim in opening his account of the "antiquities of New Spain" with an enactment of birth and baptism in Nahua culture. And this, too, is the metaphorical sense of his historiographical exercise.

———

If I have chosen to describe in detail a Latin text with which so few are conversant, it is, quite simply, because the work of Francisco Hernández illustrates the interdependence of natural and moral history, as well as the contradictions that arise when the methodology of scientific analysis is applied to socioreligious phenomena. The period in which Hernández was emerging from the University of Alcalá de Henares was noteworthy for Spain's growing intolerance of ideological and social difference. While in Spain this tendency is perhaps most clearly encapsulated in the passage of legislation curbing vagrancy on the one hand and the nobiliary aspirations of the bourgeoisie on the other, it is accompanied, with reference to the New World, by the debate on the just causes of war against the Amerindians. Given the close professional ties that Hernández maintained with the court of Philip II and, moreover, his awareness that previous works of natural history had been used to define both the moral and spiritual constitution of the New World's inhabitants, it is beyond doubt that Hernández was conscious of the pressures to which his own Latin treatise would be subject. In the prologue to the *Antiquities,* Hernández takes great pains to justify the inclusion of native traditions and rituals in a work that was commissioned to deal only with natural phenomena, a contradiction that he resolves by arguing that the former may serve to reveal what he terms "the usefulness of the Indian people."[15]

During the seven years that Hernández spent in the New World, from 1571 to 1577, he compiled a wealth of data relating to the geography, agriculture, and climate of New Spain, as well as the medicinal value of the plants and minerals that he found there. The titles of physician to King Philip II and *protomédico general* of the Indies certainly should have facilitated his entry into all levels of colonial society. In addition, and more important, his royal commission to write a natural history of the New World brought Hernández into contact with the work of the Franciscan missionaries fray Toribio de Benavente (or Motolinía) and Bernardino de Sahagún, whose studies of the Mexican people would provide him with access to the testimony of native informants. It is understandable, therefore, that the information presented in the *Antiquities* should coincide, at times verbatim, with other contemporaneous accounts. Nor is it surprising to find that Hernández tends toward a more general or synthetic treatment of his subject, since a lack of

familiarity with the Náhuatl language forced him to work primarily through interpreters and intermediate sources. All the same, it is significant that Hernández should frame his narrative in the language of Christian humanism rather than that of missionary censure. That is to say, where Sahagún and Durán will insist that a knowledge of indigenous practices is necessary to their eradication—since, as the latter asserts, "we shall never succeed in teaching them to know the true God, if first the superstitions, ceremonies and false worship of the false gods, whom they are accustomed to worship, are not worn down and erased completely from their memory"—Hernández is far more concerned with the principles that govern the constitution and, more significant, the transmission of indigenous scholarship.[16] Although he, too, will argue for the necessity of implanting the Christian faith, it is with the understanding that traditional practices embody cultural and scientific knowledge as well as religious convictions. In this regard, one may establish a direct correlation between Hernández's concern for the intellectual capacity of the Mexican people and his advocacy of what, in the terminology of the sixteenth century, were called "sweet and gentle medicines." Indeed, as Acosta argues in a treatise written in the same years as Hernández's *Antiquities* and titled *De Procuranda Indorum Salute,* the goal of conversion is facilitated, rather than impeded, by an understanding of "the customs and personal habits" of the native peoples, and especially their achievements in the fields of public administration and science. As Acosta explains: "⟨All these nations⟩ are powerful and do not want for human wisdom, and for this reason they should be defeated and made subject to the Gospel by means of their own reason, with the grace of God at work internally; and if one should attempt to subject them to Christ by force and with arms, one will accomplish nothing more than to transform them into great enemies of the Christian faith."[17]

It is logical that, with this philosophy as a guide, Hernández's discussion of the "antiquities of New Spain" would attempt to distinguish between the rational organization of Nahua society on the one hand and the irrational or superstitious beliefs that ritual and ceremony may serve to perpetuate on the other. In large part this goal is achieved through the division of his work into three parts or books dealing with the customs and social institutions of the Mexican people, the course of their history, and, finally, their religion and calendar. At best this grouping is imprecise, if not misleading, since it is clear today that one cannot speak of a people's customs apart from the religious convictions that provide a sense of collective purpose. Nevertheless, this is what Hernández attempts in his *Antiquities*, and only partly out of an obligation, shared by other authors of the period, to conform to the principles of scientific writing first set forth by the Romans.[18] More important, his concern is for the inherent worth of native thought and institutions. Given the linguistic barriers to direct examination and his evident mistrust of the testimony of individual Nahua, Hernández directs his attention to the deep structures of Mexican culture in an effort to reach what he characterizes in Latin as the *arcana,* or hidden mysteries, of native wisdom. The terminology that Hernández employs in this regard is significant in its perhaps unconscious repetition of a key phrase from the Second Epistle to the Corinthians, in which Saint Paul recalls the problematic experience of a man who has had knowledge of Paradise: "He heard secret words, which it is not permitted for a man to utter."[19] By observing that the Nahua "hide away in arcana what they have come to know and have found out," Hernández suggests the ineffable nature of their traditional wisdom, a form of knowledge beyond the scope of everyday language.

In this fashion, the huehuetlahtolli of the Nahua may be seen to comprise a body of learning purposefully obscured within the fabric of daily life and to which Hernández, as a student of physical and moral anatomy, seeks access. As he observes of this endeavor: "What has been most difficult and kept me from this work is that the rites of these people are so varied and inconstant that it is barely possible to make a firm and complete account of their habits. . . . Either to protect themselves or due to their hatred of us, they hide away in arcana what they have come to know and have found out, or because they have forgotten the ways of their elders (for such is their simplicity and laziness) they can say nothing worthy of record."[20] Leaving aside Hernández's final, parenthetical comment for reasons that I shall explain in due order, it is clear that in his view consideration of traditional practices and discourse may serve to unlock the secrets of what the Nahua have learned over the course of their existence. In this way, the huehuetlahtolli define the architecture of collective experience and cognition, the human dimension of a more comprehensive study of the natural history of New Spain. In contrast, although the perspective of both Sahagún and Durán may also be characterized by their distrust of the testimony of indigenous informants, this is invariably directed toward the capacity of rote knowledge and patterned discourse to disguise the individual's own psychology. Their presentation of native traditions conforms to the needs of the confessional, that is to say, the missionary priest's objective of differentiating between collective values and personal convictions. The study that Sahagún and Durán undertake of the huehuetlahtolli may be seen, therefore, as a direct complement to the contemporaneous translation into Náhuatl of handbooks for use in the spiritual examination of the Indians, a human "science," as Sahagún makes clear in his contention that since "preachers and confessors are physicians of the soul, . . . it is appropriate that they have practical knowledge of medicine and of spiritual illnesses."[21]

On the basis of the preceding discussion, one may rightly conclude that antithetical intellectual concerns and methodologies dictate the relative value given to the individual and society by each author in his discussion of Mexican culture. Whereas Sahagún and Durán seek to examine the spiritual health of individual Nahua and, thus, to determine the degree to which missionaries have had success in their efforts to instill the Christian faith, Hernández looks beyond individuals and their beliefs, so as to understand the constitution of Nahua society as a whole. One must recognize, however, that in pursuing truth of a structural or systemic nature, Hernández, like many scientific writers of the sixteenth century, has run the risk of censure, since the application of profane or "objective" criteria to human subjects, without regard for the orthodoxy of their beliefs, was strictly proscribed by both religious and civil authorities. Although Hernández attempts to calm this fear by asserting his own subscription to the Christian doctrine of free will, his words do not, in fact, address the propriety of associating the rational behavior of the Nahua with their ancient traditions and practices. Nor does he account for the goodness that he sees in their social relations. On the contrary, his justification for writing on the "antiquities of New Spain" appears to equate the perpetuation of native customs with the incidental, and often "dishonest," effect that the heavens exert on the body. Thus, in defense of his own interest in the Nahua, he will contend, implausibly and with little conviction, that cultural practices are a product of nature, as are unconscious traits and movements. As he explains to King Philip II in his prologue:

> Although you have commissioned me only to pursue the history of natural and earthly matters, . . . nevertheless, it is my judgment that the customs and rites of the people are not so distant from this type of history. Because even if in large measure these customs and rites should not be attributed to the heavens and the stars, since the human will is free and not obliged to anyone . . . still the most learned of the philosophers are of the opinion that the body and the soul act in agreement, and that there exists a mutual correspondence between the body and the stars; so that by setting aside what is honest and just, we are often left to follow the inclinations of the heavens and the body, and only rarely is anyone to be found who can firmly and calmly resist these pressures and this force of nature.[22]

Were Hernández to restrict his attention to superficial phenomena and instinctual actions, this initial statement of purpose might strike the reader as credible, albeit somewhat confused in its presentation of a paradigm found in other natural histories of the period. However, given that the chapters that follow deal instead with the interaction of ritual and reason in Mexican society, one must conclude that the justification that Hernández supplies in the prologue does not apply to his analysis of the New World as a whole. If this is true of book 1, his "natural" history, it is more characteristic yet of Hernández's attitude when discussing religious matters, for even when he speaks explicitly of the importance of astrology and omens among the Nahua, it is merely to decry the general ignorance and stupidity of these native people, who consider these to be signs that foretell God's will.[23]

It is clear that the scientific methodology employed by Hernández has yielded conclusions at odds with the moral justification that he offers when dedicating his work to Philip II. Whereas Sahagún and Durán may assert without pause their belief in free will, since this is a central tenet of the missionary's doctrine, Hernández feels the need to create an artificial link between this theological precept and the postulation of causality central to the discipline of natural history. The result is a vague and rambling exposition of generic pronouncements whose ideology is meant to comfort, rather than to explain. This, I would argue, is precisely Hernández's intention, since he, too, is aware of the dangers implicit in his finding that the Mexicans' ancient ways and practices have advanced the cause of rational behavior. Although Christian orthodoxy may accept the association of environmental stimuli and human temperament, this tolerance does not extend to the beneficial influence that one may find in pagan institutions and socioreligious discourse, such as the huehuetlahtolli. It is not sufficient to denounce the Mexicans' habitual observances as mistaken or superstitious or even as the convictions of "that people misled and miserably deceived by the arts of Satan."[24] One must also show that these "antiquities" have been perpetuated in an inherently detrimental or subversive fashion, something that Hernández himself is not prepared to do. On the contrary, when writing of the "sayings with which the Nahua would speak to their gods and to one another," Hernández takes care to leave the task of passing judgment to his reader, even as he provides evidence that virtues have arisen in the New World independently of Christian and European standards of conduct.[25] Rather than account for this discrepancy, which easily might be taken as praise for the native people's religion, Hernández argues that any reader of even moderate intelligence may see the truth of his own observations. He writes:

> I have concluded that I should not completely omit discussion of such matters, with which I show how virtuous these people were even when they were idolaters and cannibals, and how much care they took to educate their children, and how great was the power of their sayings; but, by the same token, I have not seen fit to relate everything from top to bottom, partly because these matters do not in my eyes belong to the writing of history, and also because what might be said and shown in support of how the prudent and upright men of those times would practice virtue and condemn vice may easily be

surmised by anyone with even medium intelligence or comprehension.[26]

As an illustration of Hernández's refusal to conflate the civic and moral dimensions of the institutions that, for him, sustain Nahua society, it may be opportune to consider his perspective in a passage from the *Antiquities* in which he does, in fact, find fault with the knowledge passed down from generation to generation by native experts, here in the field of medicine. In this example, one may clearly discern Hernández's adherence to scientific criteria, a feature that distinguishes his work from that of the majority of his contemporaries. At the outset of book 2, which deals with the wisdom, ceremonies, and history of the inhabitants of the Valley of Mexico, Hernández discusses the limitations of empiricism, examining first "knowledge of the heavens and heavenly bodies, as well as meteorological phenomena and celestial omens" (chap. 1) and then the practices of "the doctors called Titici" (chap. 2), described as follows:

Among the Indians, men and women alike practice medicine and are called Titici. These do not study the nature of illnesses and the differences between them. Instead, without knowing the cause or accident of an illness, they are accustomed to prescribe medicines, but without recourse to method in the treatment of the illnesses that they must cure. They are merely empirical healers and use, for any illness whatsoever, only those herbs, minerals, or animal parts that they have received, passed from hand to hand, as a birthright from their elders, and this they also teach to those who follow.

Practically all that they do is to prescribe a diet for their patients. They never cut anyone's veins, not even when, through an incision in the skin, they take out blood and burn the body. Wounds are treated with simple medicines or by covering them with their flours; with these things they are usually helped, but only rarely are compound or mixed medicines used. There are no surgeons or pharmacists among the Titici but rather only physicians, who by themselves dispense all manners of treatment. And it is amazing how ineptly and artlessly they do so and how dangerous this is for the people. For not only do they oblige recently delivered women to take steam baths, they also instruct them to bathe themselves and their newborn children in icy water after these baths, which they call temaxcálli. But what am I saying? They

sprinkle icy water even upon those who have fevers with eruptions and other types of outbreaks. Such actions are no less imprudent than when they rub their patients' bodies with very hot things, replying haughtily to anyone who would question them that heat is defeated by heat.[27]

Although dismissive of the Nahua's grasp of medical knowledge, Hernández approaches their actions from a clinician's perspective, grounding his judgment in rational, rather than moral or racial, arguments. His scorn is reserved for the practices of the Titici, and not for their intentions and cultural identity: if the Nahua's ways are imprudent, this is because they are unfamiliar with the principles of medicine (as regards the body's humors) set down by European authorities, such as Galen.

Quite a different viewpoint is found in the work of other writers who deal with the "antiquities" of New Spain, especially those writers whose works were published in the first decades of the seventeenth century, at a time when it could no longer be argued that the mistaken practices of the Indians were due to the recentness of their conversion to Christianity. In contrast to the culturally neutral language with which Hernández presents the false erudition of the Titici, Hernando Ruiz de Alarcón begins his sixth treatise, "On the superstitious doctors and their tricks," by saying that "the word tiçitl is commonly construed as what one would call a doctor in Spanish, but when examined more closely, it is held by the natives to signify a wise man, a doctor, a soothsayer, a witch, or perhaps one who has made a pact with the devil."[28] This is a judgment both shared and advanced, as regards the "diabolic" pretensions of the Titici, by Dr. Jacinto de la Serna in his contemporaneous *Manual de ministros de indios para el conocimiento de sus idolatrias, y extirpación de ellas*:

There is no likeness so exact, nor a portrait so lifelike of a doctor that they call titzitl, or dogmatic charlatan of the Indians, than that of a wolf, since a wolf is the color of the earth, with frightening hair and varied movements. He is dirty, disgusting, lowly and cruel in his self-defense. And when out of the reach of harm, he is insolent, much as he is fearful and standoffish when he sees danger. He is a traitor, false, bloodthirsty and fond of flesh, because he is always enraged with hunger and no one can be sure of his wiles nor escape his betrayal. . . . There is no quality of these ⟨creatures⟩ that does not suit well and truly these false dogmatics (the Titici), for in appearance they are abominable. They are lowly and insolent when they act without being seen; and in public, they are fearful and deceptive. They thirst for blood and flesh, and never do they perform their duties unless those who consult with them pay dearly for this service, which consists in tearing asunder the souls of those so unfortunate as to seek their advice, and whom they deceive, dividing them from the teachings of our Holy Mother Church.[29]

Clearly, as the use of the words *superstitious, witchcraft,* and *idolatry* displaced the term *antiquities* in the treatises written in New Spain in the final part of the sixteenth century, so too did tolerance for indigenous culture, as an independent phenomenon, diminish. To judge by Juan de Cárdenas's *Problemas y secretos maravillosos de las Indias* (1591), the writing of natural history seems also to have been motivated by the desire to adduce a rational explanation for the singularities of life in the New World, much as has been seen in the *Antiquities*. After dedicating the first two books of his *Problemas y secretos* to the climate, geography, plants, and minerals of the Americas, Cárdenas turns his attention in book 3 to what he terms "the properties and qualities of the men and animals born in the Indies," and more specifically to the question of "why the Spaniards who are born in this land are without exception of lively and delicate intellect, and if it is true that they live less than those born in Europe, and why they become greyhaired so quickly, why there are so many with ills of the stomach, why the women experience such great pain when they menstruate, why the Indians do not grow facial hair, why there are none who suffer from tuberculosis in the Indies, why the animals here do not suffer from rabies, etc."[30] Although today's reader may have difficulty in accepting that there is a scientific basis for Cárdenas's findings, it is clear, nevertheless, that his analysis conforms to orthodox notions of taxonomy, placing natural phenomena and physical attributes on the one hand and social organization and morality on the other. Furthermore, except as regards external traits, Cárdenas does not discriminate between the effect that nature has on the Spaniards and on the native Mexicans. If there are differences in character and outlook, these are inborn, since both Spaniard and Mexican respond equally to environmental stimuli. In this

fashion, Cárdenas adheres to Saint Isidore's distinction between the inner and outer facets of the human condition and to his assertion that the "complete man" is formed "by the union of the spirit and the body."[31] Insofar as it is possible, Cárdenas restricts his attention to the latter. The apparent singularity of the New World is explained by traditional scholarship, and his natural history participates in what one may term the folkloric mode, as the title *Problemas y secretos maravillosos* so well illustrates.

In an analogous fashion, the *Apologética historia sumaria* of fray Bartolomé de las Casas sets forth the Christian position on the issues of free will and the effects of the celestial bodies. Following Aristotle and the Old Testament, Las Casas argues that natural phenomena can have only an indirect influence on human behavior because the application of free will can arrest this natural inclination, or as he terms it, "causality." The examples that Las Casas cites merit careful examination because they reveal at least in part the author's motive in making this theological question a facet of his New World history. He writes: "The gentile poets called the planet Mars the god of war because that planet is by its very nature disproportionately hot and dry. The hotness or heat incites and arouses anger, and the dryness incites impatience. Hence it is that the great thirst that proceeds from great dryness is the cause of impatience. Anger, then, and impatience are the causes of quarrels and war, and since quarrels and wars are not caused by the celestial bodies except indirectly, by giving off incentives, these bodies cannot have influence upon free will."[32] Las Casas disposes of astrology and other disingenuous means of divination in an equally summary fashion, by stating that natural portents can reveal only the material dimension of existence, on which the celestial bodies do indeed appear to have a direct bearing. Thus, he argues that such traditional omens as the croaking of frogs or the unaccustomed movements of other animals will always have a rational explanation: they respond to changes in the level of humidity.[33] If people can read the future in these actions, it is because they have learned to understand the relationship that exists between instinctual movements and circumstance. Las Casas opposes the certainty of scientific knowledge to the false beliefs of superstition, so as to uphold the supremacy of religious doctrine and the distinction that it makes between the natural and moral facets of human behavior.[34] Hence, his contention that both the idolatry of the Indians and the ferocity of the Spaniards represent a similar lack of self-restraint, that is, the misapplication of free will.

But as Las Casas rejects in this fashion the singularity of the people of the New World, he unconsciously gives voice to the ideological prejudices that animate the writing of natural history in these same lands. By choosing to illustrate the limited reach of the celestial bodies through reference to but four elements—heat, humidity, dryness, and cold—Las Casas frames the question of causality in the same terms as had earlier authorities in speaking of the *ecumene* and the habitability of the Tropics.[35] As Las Casas himself observes when explaining Columbus's motives for believing that there must exist uncharted yet inhabited lands to the southwest: "It is a general and natural law that since the life of men and their health consists of humid and temperate warmth, according to physicians, and finally in equality, however much more temperate the location or part of the world, and however much the sites are near or distant as regards their temperateness, so much better and more favorable, or worse, will be the ⟨prospect for⟩ habitation."[36] Although this reasoning permits Las Casas to extol time and again the natural goodness of the island of Hispaniola, it also of necessity underscores the negative sense of the examples that he cites when speaking of the secondary influence that the celestial bodies appear to exert on people's behavior.[37] If the equilibrium of basic elements through "equality, or temperateness, or mediocrity" is seen by Las Casas to constitute what he refers to as "the root of happiness and fertility and habitation," then the excess of any single agent would diminish the quality of life in this region.[38] Indeed, the extreme heat and dryness that Las Casas associates with the planet Mars, and thus with warlike tendencies, are the principal characteristics of the lands that the ancients had deemed unfit for human settlement. In like fashion, the immoderate humidity that serves to induce the ominous movements of lesser animals also contributes to pestilence and corruption among humans.[39] In this way, and perhaps unconsciously, Las Casas defines the constraint of free will by nature as the mark of subhuman

existence; Christianity and ecumene are synonymous in his discourse.

It follows that, to the extent that the climate of the New World should contravene traditional notions of habitability, a dark shadow would be cast on the moral constitution of the people and cultures that are to be found there. If the island of Hispaniola provides a propitious setting for civilized existence, in Las Casas's judgment, this most clearly is not the case in all parts of the Indies, nor is it the only perspective offered by contemporaneous writers. Indeed, it would seem that in his own descriptions, Las Casas is far less concerned with physical reality than with revealing the benevolence of the native people, whose freedoms he would seek to protect. By stressing that the land of Hispaniola is "fertile, well-drained, cleared and bathed in favorable airs or winds, as well as free of marshes and pestilence or rot and other unfit elements," Las Casas not only certifies its fitness for habitation—"this aforementioned region is very much temperate and quite apt and ready for human habitation, and most worthy of being frequented and settled by men"—but also, and most conspicuously, suggests the spiritual worth of the Spaniards' discoveries. He adds: "And thus it is likely that this must be the land of earthly Paradise."[40] Las Casas conjoins the concerns of natural history and the language of moral judgment, but as he does so, his narrative systematically excludes those two natural attributes—extreme heat and humidity—that other European writers of the same period underscore in their own descriptions of Hispaniola and the New World.

In contrast, when Juan de Cárdenas begins his explication of the "problems and marvelous secrets" that provide the title for his work, he does so by stating that "the singular and strange effects that we shall later recount of this western land may be reduced to the heat and the humidity that reign over this Indian soil."[41] Although most other writers of the sixteenth century, from Oviedo to Acosta, concur with Cárdenas in this assessment, Las Casas is quite adamant in denying it, and this for reasons that expose the intrinsic interrelationship of natural and moral history. By defining earthly Paradise as that land that is "fertile, well-drained, cleared and bathed in favorable airs or winds, as well as free of marshes and pestilence or rot and other unfit elements,"

Las Casas suggests the degenerative influence of excessive heat and humidity. To judge by the series of terms just mentioned, the "happiness and fertility and habitation" sought by Las Casas are possible only in those regions where humans have tamed nature. Free will must defeat the menace of excess humidity by draining and clearing the land to rid it of "marshes and pestilence or rot and other unfit elements," in Las Casas's terminology. For all its beauty, the New World must be made civilized, and this quite clearly has a Christian dimension, as the pairing of "happiness and fertility" with "habitation" makes plain.

Lest one conclude that Las Casas is alone in this conception, one should consider as well the comments of Gonzalo Fernández de Oviedo, who states: "As is known to all those of us who have spent some time here, the lands of the Indies where Christians have set foot and settled . . . appear to have been transformed, as I see in those provinces through which I have traveled; and with each new day, they change more, as regards the onset of tempests both hot and cold, and each day, as more Spaniards arrive and time passes, we find the heat to be more temperate and the cold to be less severe. This opinion is held in common by all Spaniards who have lived here for some time; on this they agree and have said so."[42]

While Oviedo will argue that it is the presence of the Spaniards that has served to transform nature and permit civilized life on Hispaniola, since before and in general "this land is extremely humid, and was not tramped down or open as now, but rather covered by trees and hidden, and for so many years possessed by savage people," Las Casas attributes the domestication of this same region to the efforts of the native people.[43] It is evident, nevertheless, that both authors understand the ways in which the natural history of the Americas may serve to project the spiritual measure of their inhabitants. In fact, Oviedo explicitly associates the destructive force of the hurricanes found in the New World with the pernicious actions of the Devil. If these natural phenomena imperil civilized existence, uprooting trees and houses alike, once again it is European culture, in the unambiguous form of the Christian sacraments, that will restore order and vouchsafe future settlement. As Oviedo explains:

When the Devil wishes to put fear ⟨into the inhabitants of these lands⟩, he sends forth a hurricane, which is a kind of tempest, but so powerfully made that it can tear down houses and uproot many and very sizable trees. In the mountains, which as a rule are densely packed with tall timber, I have seen everything upset for the space of a league, with all the trees, both great and small, laid flat, many with their roots extended upwards. Such sights are terrifying, and without doubt they seem to be the Devil's doing, for no one can look upon them without great fear. And so it is that all Christians should pay heed and understand that wherever the Holy Sacrament has been brought to bear in these lands, never again has there been such an abundance of these hurricanes and great tempests, nor have they been dangerous as was their wont.[44]

To judge by Oviedo's words, it would seem that only the power of God might serve to set the New World and its inhabitants on the secure foundation of civilized existence. Indeed, for all his efforts to praise the valor of the Spanish conquistadores, even Hernán Cortés's secretary, Francisco López de Gómara, is obliged to reach much the same conclusion in the final pages of his history, *La conquista de México* (Zaragoza, 1552). If, for Gómara, the Spaniards' efforts to convert the native people of New Spain to Christianity found success only when "our people placed the Holy Sacrament in many places, chasing away the devil as the latter himself confessed to the [native] priests who inquired as to his absence and aloofness," so too did the processions organized by Christian missionaries restore order to the natural world and, thus, facilitate the campaign to dismantle the vestiges of pre-Columbian worship.[45] As Gómara explains: "Many times there has been too little water to grow cereal crops, but through collective prayers and processions, it was made to rain. ⟨In contrast,⟩ it rained so much in 1528 that these crops, the livestock and even the houses of the people were lost. They held a procession and prayers in Mexico, and in Texcoco and other towns, and the rains ended, which was a great confirmation of the Faith. It rained, and then it cleared, and there was health, this despite the threats of the Devil, for at this time idols were being destroyed and temples were being torn down."[46]

On the basis of such evidence, found not only in the works of professional historians but also in the accounts of

Spanish missionaries, such as fray Toribio de Benavente, one may conclude that, in the sixteenth century, the practice of New World historiography was animated by the imperfect adaptation of European culture to an environment whose excesses it had yet fully to master.[47] If, for Las Casas, the intervention of Spanish settlers was unnatural, to the extent that it was moved by ambition and other worldly values, this is clearly not the opinion expressed in more official works.[48] Rather, in these, the question of healthful settlement is most usually construed as the reduction of natural obstacles, so as to permit a European way of life. It is little wonder, then, that Juan de Cárdenas should ascribe the shortened life span of the Spaniards born in the Americas to the same, apparently scientific, causes that more generally imperil the establishment of civilization. As Cárdenas reasons, in accordance with Galen: "Because of the immoderate climate of the Indian region, which itself is hot and humid, the heat of the air consumes and disperses our own heat; and it is truly thus, that the greater the heat of the land, the less heat that man has in his stomach and internal organs. Humidity also bloats the body with wastes, which little by little, without illness, drown man's natural heat and shorten his life."[49] Although a resident of the Mexican capital, Cárdenas assiduously upholds the validity of European scholarship, and, in this way, differences in the natural constitution of the New World render it inferior to the ideal model proffered by classical authorities. The "problems and marvelous secrets" of which he writes consist largely of phenomena adverse to human health and well-being. His science can offer no escape from the ravages of nature, save the fond memory of a childhood spent in another climate, far removed from the problems of America. So it is that Cárdenas begins the prologue to the third and final book of his New World history with these words: "If it is permitted that man give praise to his country, with such an obligation and just cause must I then praise my sweet and dear homeland Constantina, the refreshment of Seville, the garden of Spain, pleasant and delightful woodland of Europe."[50]

Although some seventy years have passed since Cortés first set foot in the Valley of Mexico, it would appear that European writers, like Juan de Cárdenas, had yet to accord this region of the New World an identity independent from the intellectual prejudices of Europe or to consider the natural history of America apart from the threat of physical and moral corruption that this continent may pose to European settlers. Lest one conclude that Cárdenas is alone in citing the dangers of the Mexican capital—and, more particularly, the unhealthfulness of its location amid the waters of Lake Texcoco, to say nothing of the diet and habits of its residents—one should heed the words of Enrico Martínez, who, in a treatise published shortly thereafter, in the first years of the seventeenth century, presents the following analysis of why disease is so prevalent among the inhabitants of the Valley of Mexico:

> If one carefully examines the location of the city of Mexico and the temperament of the sky in this region, one finds present all of the factors cited [by Albertus Magnus, Avicenna and Hippocrates in their respective treatises]. Indeed, the great quantity of unclean matter and dead animals that is thrown into its canals is more harmful than the stagnant waters [of which these authorities have written], much as the mud left on the shores of the lagoon when its waters recede to their normal level after the rainy season is the breeding ground of worms and vermin. From the latter, and from the mud in which they live, there arises a foul stench which, finding the air receptive, corrupts it. In addition, whereas this city is situated in the western part of the lagoon (to the contrary to what is mandated by the Royal Ordinances that govern the foundation of new settlements), it is susceptible to poor health. This is because the vapors that arise from the lake and its shore during the day, when not consumed or transformed into rain, are wont to fall back upon the city at night, due to the westerly movement of the sky and because these vapors are raised by the heat of the sun which, when absent at night, is replaced by the heat of the city, which brings down and draws in these vapors. For this reason, when observed in the morning hours from the neighboring heights, Mexico has a kind of fog of vapors above it, although everything else about it is clear and calm. This is the situation as regards the land and sky, to which is added the vice of eating many and different foods, the pampered and idle life of some, the little physical exercise that they do, and other things of this sort, with which their bodies are disposed to illness.
>
> Given that the conditions of this city are disposed as has been said, it is logical that whenever the air is upset or put out of balance by an unusual conjunction of the

planets, so too are the bodies of those who live here put out of balance and made susceptible to illness. For as Galen observes in his book *De febribus*, the human body does not suffer from corruption, unless the material of which it is formed has been prepared and in some fashion subjected to a corruptive force.[51]

How different the perspective of Francisco Hernández: not only does he vent his hope that those who are born today amid the humidity of the Mexican capital will not succumb to the apparently pernicious effect of their surroundings, but he also suggests that the ancient ways and practices of the Nahua had served, in their own fashion, better to balance the forces of nature in the Valley of Mexico. Just as he sees "all the greatness one could meet in the most prosperous cities of Spain" within the various institutions that the Spaniards brought to the Mexican capital of the 1570s, so too does he cite the ingenuity with which the Nahua had built their own city of Tenochtitlán, conquered by Cortés and his men some fifty years before.[52] If one may judge by the praise that Hernández expresses for the canals and aqueducts of Tenochtitlán, it would appear that the Nahua were once as well at ease with the world of water as the Spaniards are with that of dry land. Like the rituals that animate Mexican culture within Hernández's account, the design of Tenochtitlán suggests the rational approach that the Nahua commonly adopt to natural phenomena that are incompatible with the Spanish-Christian worldview. It would appear, then, that the native Mexicans were indeed masters of their surroundings, but through means ill appreciated by the European tradition. In fact, because of this adaptation to a world of antagonistic values, the Nahua would be perceived as an inferior or barbaric people.

In this way, the rituals and discourse described by Hernández can be presented only as "antiquities" or vestiges of past greatness, for when judged in terms of postconquest, Christian precepts, they connote an unhealthful way of life and knowledge of little use to the Spanish public. It is in this light that one must understand the need that Hernández feels to bemoan the "simplicity and laziness" of the Mexican people, even as he lauds the rational structure of their society. As one finds in the final chapter of the first book of the *Antiquities*, without recourse to the standard

explanation that knowledge "of the true God and of the doctrine and practices of the true religion" is needed if one is to "experience, happily and without sin, the life of the body and spirit," Hernández is at a loss to explain how a people endowed with all the basic components of civilization could, nevertheless, "so many centuries after the creation of the world, have remained in such simplicity."[53] Such are the perils of scientific writing in the sixteenth century, and, indeed, it is tragic that the learning contained in the ancient ways and practices of the Nahua will be forever lost to all those who, like Francisco Hernández, are obliged to place moral judgment before the truths of nature.

NOTES

1. See *Mexican Treasury, Antiquities of New Spain,* 1.2. I acknowledge the benefit that I have derived from Joaquín García Pimentel's Spanish translation of *De antiquitatibus Novae Hispaniae* (published posthumously by Pedro Robredo [Mexico, 1945] and incorporated into the UNAM edition of Hernández's *Obras completas,* vol. 6).

2. Fray Bernardino de Sahagún, *Historia general de las cosas de la Nueva España,* bk. 6, chap. 36, ed. Angel María Garibay Kintana, 7th ed. (Mexico City: Porrúa, 1989), 397–98. The complete title of this chapter is: "On how the parents of the child would call for the soothsayers to tell them the fortune or fate that the child brought with him, according to the sign in which he was born; once they had arrived these [soothsayers] would diligently ask at what hour he had been born, and if he had been born before midnight, they would attribute to him the sign of the previous day; and if he had been born after midnight, they would attribute to him the sign of the next day; and if he had been born at midnight, they would attribute to him both signs; and then they would consult their books, and they would foretell his fate, be this good or bad, in accordance with the quality of the sign in which he was born." For Hernández quotation, see *Mexican Treasury, Antiquities,* 1.2.

3. The marginal annotations left by Joaquín García Pimentel when making his Spanish translation of *De antiquitatibus Novae Hispaniae* reveal the close correspondence between the material contained in bk. 1, chaps. 2–7 of Hernández's *De antiquitatibus* and what was likely his primary source, Sahagún's *Historia general de las cosas de la Nueva España.* It is worthy of note that Hernández himself prepared a Latin translation of several sections of Sahagún's manuscript, including the majority of the appendixes that appear at the conclusion of bk. 2 of Sahagún's *Historia general.*

4. It is perhaps due to the affinities between classical poetics and this aspect of the huehuetlahtolli that the latter captured the attention of Spanish intellectuals trained in the humanist tradition. In a passage whose relevance would be evident to the first European students of the huehuetlahtolli, Aristotle observes: "The orator has . . . to guess the subjects on which his hearers really hold views already, and what those views are, and then must express, as general truths, these same views on these same subjects. This is one advantage of using maxims. There is another which is more important—it invests a speech with moral character. There is moral character in every speech in which the moral purpose is conspicuous: and maxims always produce this effect, because the utterance of them amounts to a general declaration of moral principles: so that,

if the maxims are sound, they display the speaker as a man of sound moral character" (Aristotle, *Rhetoric*, bk. 2, chap. 21, trans. W. Rhys Roberts, in *The Rhetoric and the Poetics of Aristotle*, ed. Friedrich Solmsen, Modern Library Edition [New York: Random House, 1954], 139). Although the social benefits of patterned discourse are addressed at length by Aristotle (for example, in bk. 1, chap. 8 of his *Rhetoric*), it was common for the missionaries to view the huehuetlahtolli as a threat to the sacrament of confession, insofar as the Nahua were wont to employ the "sayings of the ancients" in an equivocal fashion, both to conceal their own beliefs and to suggest the sanctity of ancient ways and practices.

5. Quotation from Sahagún, *Historia general*, 297.

6. Ibid.

7. "As she cut the umbilical cord, almost shedding tears [the midwife] predicted menacing disasters, and she foretold what unfortunate circumstances and toil had been reserved for his lot" (*Mexican Treasury, Antiquities*, 1.2).

8. Ibid.

9. It is interesting to note the similarities between the notion of sacrifice called for in this passage and the virtues described in the section of Hernández's *Christian Doctrine* (c. 1574) that deals with the sacrament of baptism. As the following verses indicate, in both texts signs and ritual are accompanied by exhortation, rational discussion, and leading questions:

> The priest then asks, do you abhor the tempter,
> The old serpent? the show and shining surface
> Of this poor world? and in one God do you
> Have faith, as holy mother Church instructs?
> And last, do you desire to be made pure
> In clear baptismal crystal lucence?
>
> —
>
> The answer yes, the priest pours holy water,
> Anoints at once the head with mystic oil,
> Then invests him with a robe of white
> And last confers this gift, a sainted name.
>
> —
>
> As fittest athletes still must follow leaders,
> And those who gain the laurels in their victory
> Do not oppose the fiercest foe unarmed,
> Expect not the converted, by this rite
> Become now faithful warriors of Christ,
> To triumph o'er this world, the flesh, the devil,
> If first their heads have not anointed been
> With sacred confirmation's holy oil.
>
> (*Mexican Treasury, The Christian Doctrine*, lines 881–98)

10. *Mexican Treasury, Antiquities*, 1.2.

11. Ibid. "If it was a girl, a *huepilli* and *cueitl*, girls' clothes, as well as a case, a distaff, and a spindle—and all things concerned with sewing—would be given to her."

12. James Lockhart, *The Nahuas after the Conquest* (Stanford: Stanford University Press, 1992), 255, observes: "At the level of the individual . . . the documents the Nahuas wrote emphasize rites of passage, above all the basic ceremonies associated with death, birth, and marriage. It is my impression that the order just given corresponds to the relative importance that the Nahuas gave to these rites." Although it is Lockhart's purpose to explore the interaction of native and Christian beliefs in postconquest Nahua society, his observations, with reference to the religious culture of the Nahua before the arrival of the Spaniards, are borne out in the testimony transcribed by Sahagún and Durán.

13. *Mexican Treasury, Antiquities*, 1.2.

14. On other writers, see, for example, bk. 6, chaps. 37–38 of Sahagún's *Historia general*, 398–401.

15. *Mexican Treasury, Antiquities*, 1.2.

16. Diego Durán, *Historia de las Indias de Nueva España e islas de la Tierra Firme*, ed. Angel María Garibay Kintana (Mexico: Porrúa, 1967), 1:3.

17. José Acosta, *De Procuranda Indorum Salute*, ed. and trans. Francisco Mateos (Madrid: Ediciones España Misionera, 1952), 46.

18. It is significant in this regard that Hernández continued to translate Pliny's *Natural History* into Spanish while in New Spain.

19. 2 Cor. 12:4.

20. *Antiquities*, prologue (*OC* 6.47).

21. Sahagún, *Historia general*, 17.

22. *De Antiquitatibus*, facs. ed. (Mexico City: Talleres Gráficos del Museo Nacional de Arqueología, Historia y Etnografía, 1926).

23. *Mexican Treasury, Antiquities*, 2.1 and 2.18.

24. Ibid., 3.1.

25. Quotation from *Antiquities*, 1.17, chapter heading (*OC* 6.79).

26. Ibid. (*OC* 6.81).

27. *Mexican Treasury, Antiquities*, 2.2.

28. Hernando Ruiz de Alarcón, *Tratado de las supersticiones y costumbres gentilicas que oy viuen entre los indios desta Nueua España* (Mexico, 1629), in *Anales del Museo Nacional de México* 6 (1892): 195. [See Michael D. Coe and Gordon Whittaker, *Aztec Sorcerers in Seventeenth Century Mexico: The Treatise on Superstitions by Hernando Ruiz de Alarcón* (Albany: Institute for Mesoamerican Studies, State University of New York, 1982).—Ed.]

29. Jacinto de la Serna, *Manual de ministros de indios para el conocimiento de sus idolatrias, y extirpacion de ellas*, in *Anales del Museo Nacional de México* 6 (1892): 454.

30. Juan de Cárdenas, *Problemas y secretos maravillosos de las Indias*, ed. Angeles Durán (Madrid: Alianza, 1988), 22.

31. Saint Isidore of Seville, *Etymologiarum sive originum*, bk. XI, pt. 1, sec. 4, ed. W. M. Lindsay (Oxford: Clarendon Press, 1911), vol. 2, n.p. (The pages of this edition are not numbered.)

32. Bartolomé de las Casas, *Apologética historia sumaria*, ed. Juan Pérez de Tudela Bueso, *Biblioteca de Autores Españoles*, nos. 105–6 (Madrid: Atlas, 1958), 1:283.

33. Ibid., 1:285–86.

34. For example, in ibid., 1:73, Las Casas observes: "The celestial bodies can, however, indirectly cause changes in the spirit, insofar as in influencing the body, they make it more or less, better or worse, more able or less able to receive the spirit; and in the moment of its infusion, the spirit is determined in its level of goodness, or of not such good as far as natural being (not moral being, but natural, I say) is concerned."

35. In this regard, Las Casas, like Cárdenas, appears to draw on the *Etymologiarum* of Saint Isidore. It is interesting to note that in several editions from the late Middle Ages, Isidore's text is accompanied by a series of explanatory diagrams patterned on those of Isidore himself and that represent the constituent features of the world, the seasons, and humans (*mundus, annus, homo*). In an illustration from the 1473 Strasbourg edition of the *Etymologiarum* (reproduced by Anthony Grafton, with April Shelford and Nancy Siraisi, in *New Worlds, Ancient Texts: The Power of Tradition and the Shock of Discovery* [Cambridge: Harvard University Press, 1992], 3), the four seasons and the four humors are inscribed within a circle defined by the four prime elements (fire, air, water, and earth) and the four basic qualities (hotness, dryness, humidity, and coldness) with which these may interact.

36. Bartolomé de las Casas, *Historia de las Indias,* ed. Agustín Millares Carlo, 2d ed. (Mexico: Fondo de Cultura Económica, 1965), 1:48

37. On extolling the natural goodness of the island: for example, Las Casas declares in the *Apologética historia,* 1.55: "The position of the heavens and the favorable distance of the sun, and thus the superior and universal agent, comes together in the salubriousness, fertility, healthfulness, happiness and population of this island of Hispaniola, and in its being by its nature most habitable."

38. Quotation at ibid., 1.55.

39. Ibid., 1.99–101.

40. Ibid., 1.54–55.

41. Cárdenas, *Problemas y secretos,* 37.

42. Gonzalo Fernández de Oviedo y Valdés, *Historia general y natural de las Indias,* ed. Juan Pérez de Tudela Bueso, Biblioteca de Autores Españoles, nos. 117–21 (Madrid: Atlas, 1959), 1:206.

43. Quotation from ibid., 1:206.

44. Gonzalo Fernández de Oviedo y Valdés, *Sumario de la natural historia de las Indias,* ed. Manuel Ballesteros (Madrid: Historia 16, 1986), 85.

45. Quotation from Francisco López de Gómara, *La conquista de México,* ed. José Luis de Rojas (Madrid: Historia 16, 1986), 481.

46. Ibid.

47. Regarding the accounts of Spanish missionaries: it would appear that Gómara's version of the events of 1528 was drawn from the opening passage of bk. 2, chap. 2 of fray Toribio de Benavente's *Historia de los indios de la Nueva España* (c. 1541), ed. Claudio Esteva (Madrid: Historia 16, 1985), 155: "The fourth year after the arrival of the ⟨twelve⟩ friars to this land was one of great rains, so much so that the cornfields were lost and many houses fell down. There had never been, until then, processions among the Indians, and in Texcoco they set out with a poor cross; and whereas it had not ceased to rain for many days, it pleased Our Lord due to his clemency, and due to the pleas of his Most Holy Mother, and of Saint Anthony, whose worship is foremost in that town, that from that same day forward the rains did stop, in confirmation of the weak and tender faith of those who had newly been converted."

48. See Las Casas's comments as he concludes bk. 2, chap. 1 of the *Historia de las Indias,* 2:207–8, particularly with regard to the effect of Spanish rule on agricultural production.

49. Cárdenas, *Problemas y secretos,* 206–7.

50. The irony of his words is increased by the heading that appears immediately before: "The Third Book of the Problems and Admirable Secrets of *This Land*" [*Libro tercero de los problemas y admirables secretos* desta tierra], 201 (my emphasis).

51. For Cárdenas citing the unhealthfulness of the location of the Mexican capital, see *Problemas y secretos,* 207–8. Enrico Martínez, *Repertorio de los tiempos, y historia natural desta Nueua España* (Mexico City, 1606), ed. Francisco de la Maza (Mexico: Secretaria de Educación Pública, 1948), 179–80. A similar perspective on the threat of contagion, posed by the canals and waters about the city of Mexico, is found in the selections from Juan Barrios, *Verdadera medicina, cirugía y astrología* (Mexico City, 1607) reproduced by Joaquín García Icazbalceta in his *Biblioteca mexicana del siglo XVI,* ed. and rev. Agustín Millares Carlo, 2d ed. (Mexico: Fondo de Cultura Económica, 1981), 239–40.

52. Quotation from *Antiquities,* 1.22.

53. Ibid., 1.28.

ENTR'ACTE

RAFAEL CHABRÁN

SIMON VAREY

The essays in the first part of this volume have established who Hernández was and have described the intellectual environments in which his characteristic thinking was nurtured and developed. The authors have also explained the appropriate conditions—legal, practical, and cultural—in which Hernández found himself once he arrived in New Spain. The essays in the second part of the volume explain what happened to the work of Hernández, how it became known, how it was disseminated, and how it was put to use. In this brief sketch at the midpoint of the volume, we aim to spell out just what it was that Hernández did during his seven years in New Spain and how he did it. We know what Hernández was supposed to do, because we have the royal instructions, but instructions, like speed limits, are often disregarded.

Within four months of Hernández's arrival at Veracruz, he was confronted by the Inquisition in the famous but scantily documented case of Dr. Pedro López. In a parallel but apparently unrelated series of confrontations, the local bureaucracies prevented Hernández from exercising his duties as *protomédico*. The part of the royal instructions that required Hernández to examine local doctors was therefore ignored, almost from the start.

After seven or eight months of preparation, the expedition began with Hernández's departure from Seville in August 1570. He wasted no opportunities, studying plants in the Canaries when his ship made a routine stop there for two weeks. On the other side of the Atlantic, Hernández apparently carried out similar surveys of the plants of Haiti and Cuba and wrote descriptions of them.[1] Hernández spent the first two years of his time in New Spain examining plants, the next four writing and revising, and the last year or so tending to the victims of the *cocoliztli* and dissecting the bodies of those who died from it. In those early years when he was examining plants, we do not know whether he examined animals and minerals at the same time, though it seems likely that he did. Yet when he wrote to Philip II eight months after his work in New Spain had begun, he mentioned only plants—more than eight hundred new species, he said. By the time the expedition was over, he had written descriptions of thousands of plants and hundreds of mammals, birds, reptiles, fish, insects, and minerals.

The corrected manuscripts and the resulting formulaic descriptions indicate his methods of gathering information. As specified in the instructions, Hernández did consult local healers, physicians, apothecaries, and anyone else involved with the business of caring for the sick. Hernández's method of gathering information thus depended on native informants, who sometimes cooperated, sometimes—to his chagrin—not.[2] Most of the Spanish chroniclers were known locally as "the interrogator" or "questioner," and Hernández was probably no exception. It is most likely that he used something like a questionnaire or at least asked his informants the same kinds of questions, in the same order, everywhere he went. No copy of any questionnaire has survived, but there were precedents for it, one of which he certainly knew.[3] Fray Bernadino de Sahagún, some two decades earlier, had used this method to gather information about plants. Sahagún's sequence was: (1) what kind of plant is this? (2) what does it look like? (3) which parts are useful (medicinally)? (4) which illnesses does it cure? (5) how is a medication prepared from it? (6) how is it administered? (7) where is it found? Descriptions based on answers to these queries produce formulaic essays. Hernández clearly used a method very much like Sahagún's with the addition, at the beginning of the sequence of questions, of a much greater interest in nomenclature, which would eventually lead Hernández to rethink his taxonomy.

Hernández clearly did not find very many plants growing within the confines of Mexico City itself, though some of his descriptions speak of varieties grown, then as now, in gardens (especially hospital gardens), in window boxes, and on patios. He was more interested in seeing and examining the plants in the wild, so that he could make an informed judgment about the terrain in which they flourished and thus could decide whether or not they would be likely to thrive in the Spanish climate. Consequently, the majority of the plants that Hernández described came from all over the Valley of Mexico. He was supposed to go on to Peru and carry out a similar survey there, but he claimed sickness, fatigue, and advancing old age as reasons not to carry out this part of his mission.

Once in New Spain in February 1571, Hernández seems to have hurried from Veracruz straight to Mexico City. He kept no diary of his subsequent travels, and the organization of his written materials gives no indication of when he traveled anywhere. But his botanical descriptions frequently tell us where a plant grows—although sometimes the location he cites is topographical rather than cartographically precise ("warm and mild regions," or even "Mexico," which covers wide and diverse territory), and just as frequently he tells us that a plant grows (say) in Michoacán even though he admits he has not actually seen it himself—yet we know that he did spend some time in Michoacán. Equally, Hernández clearly bases some descriptions on firsthand evidence, and in many of those cases the plants are known to grow in one region of Mexico but not another, and so on. Somolinos did a fine job of extrapolating from the Hernández texts, so that he was able to project the range of his travels in Mexico with a fair degree of accuracy and to list the 240 or so places mentioned by Hernández.[4]

Over the course of the next seven years, Hernández traveled to the handful of principal botanical gardens, most obviously those at Cuernavaca and Huaxtepec, and all the major hospitals, attached to convents, within a radius of about sixty miles from Mexico City. Accompanied at least some of the time by his son Juan, who assisted with the field research, he did visit other places that were farther afield, such as Jiquilpan, Jilotlan, Colima, and Motines to the west of Mexico City. There is evidence that he went as far northwest as Guanajuato and Queretaro; similarly, he seems to have reached Huejutla to the north, which would take him through another seven or eight convents. As he traveled through the difficult and demanding terrain to the southeast of Mexico City, he seems to have gone on one looping circuit, down to Tecuanapa on the Pacific coast, then along the coastline and slightly inland to Tututepec, across to Coatlan and Nexapa, and then back to Mexico City via Oaxaca and Yanguitlan, with a side trip to Iztlan and Papalotipac. Somolinos painstakingly describes each of five journeys that Hernández made, each one in a loop.[5]

One important place in which Hernández resided and worked was the hospital at Huaxtepec, where Gregorio López would follow him in the decade of the 1580s, the two men having met there (probably) in 1576. The surviving textual evidence of a manuscript copy of López strongly suggests that Hernández left a copy of his *Index medicamentorum*, in Latin, at Huaxtepec and that López translated it into Spanish, though until now no one has ever recognized López's text for what it is.[6] We cannot be absolutely certain how long Hernández spent in any of these places, or even if he definitely visited all of them, because his many allusions to these regions and their inhabitants occur in descriptions of plants: his purpose is not to tell us where he has been but to note the climate in which the plants thrive. We do know that he had himself carried in a litter, with a retinue of bearers and painters, that he hated the food, the climate, and the terrain, and that he was bitten half to death by insects.[7] He was accompanied on these journeys by his son Juan and presumably by Francisco Domínguez and his successors, at least sometimes. Each arduous journey would take the travelers to a hospital, which meant staying at a monastery and making daily journeys into the surrounding country. On these journeys he was accompanied by native artists, three of whom—Pedro Vasquez and Anton and Baltasar Elias— he named in his will and to whom he bequeathed sixty ducats each. We do not know for certain if native informants joined the party and traveled together or if Hernández sought them out in the vicinity of each monastery. We also cannot be certain that Hernández wrote notes in the field and corrected them later, at the monastery, but in view of the overwhelming mass of detailed information that he was collecting, it seems probable that he must have done something like that.

The sheer scale of Hernández's research was breathtaking. In the course of the expedition, Hernández wrote down thousands of descriptions without traveling as far as Guatemala, never mind Peru. It is clear that he could not observe every species and every specimen, as his descriptions occasionally demonstrate. Yet it was important to Hernández that his descriptions should, if at all possible, be based on firsthand observation, because he wanted to see and describe plants during different stages of their annual cycles. In this way he succeeded in informing himself about the medicinal uses of different parts of a plant at different times of year. If for no other reason, his firsthand observations set him apart from Monardes, who had to rely on derivative information brought back to Spain.

An important part of the process of recording information about the plants was to have the artists make paintings of them. The *Codex Pomar* gives us an idea of what the original paintings must have been like. That manuscript shows two distinct styles of perception and representation, mostly demonstrated in differences of perspective.[8] The later illustrations that we know from the Rome edition of Hernández are thoroughly European. Hernández supervised the artists, and although his will shows that he appreciated their work, his poem to Arias Montano gives a different view:

> I cannot begin to count the mistakes of the artists, who
> were to illustrate my work, and yet were the greatest
>   part of my care,
> so that nothing, from the point of view of a fat thumb,
>   would be different
> from what was being copied, but rather all would be as
>   it was in reality.

These lines also show that his goal was to have the artists render everything in proportion, by using the thumb as a simple measuring device. His intention was to represent "reality."

The main botanical work undertaken by Hernández was to combine his own observation with information about plants from local people who had some involvement with care for the sick. Hernández thus became the vehicle for native information, written in the form he adopted by following Sahagún: the framework of each description was thus Spanish, the main body of content Mexican. The organization of the manuscript would eventually be Mexican, too, though subsequent publication of Recchi's selection would obscure Hernández's intention in that respect.

As we know, Hernández was also at work in New Spain on his translation of Pliny's *Natural History* and his own *Antiquities*, in addition to a number of other works that are now lost. These included *A Method of Identifying the Plants of Both Worlds; Table of Illnesses and Remedies of This Land; New World Plants That Grow in Europe and Their Benefits to the Native Population; Experiments and Antidotes from the New World;* a work on the topography of New Spain; his commentary on Pliny; *A Book of Stoic Questions* and *A Book of Stoic Problems;* and *The Christian Doctrine.* Of the lost works, one that catches the eye is his *Table of Illnesses and Remedies,* which we think was probably the *Index medicamentorum* that he left at Huaxtepec and which turns up in translated and edited forms in the work of Barrios and López. But of the others, the comparative treatise on European and Mexican methods of describing plants is revealing even in its absence. We know that Hernández rewrote the *Antiquities* and that he felt that his own *Natural History* was the New World complement to Pliny. If there is one thread that holds all these apparently diverse works together, it might be their author's ability to recognize the differences between the practices of Spain and New Spain, to see that both had numerous strong points, to look for ways in which they could be blended, and to blend them himself.

Hernández's years in New Spain were the most productive of his life, and his writings from this period show how he viewed medicine and plants. Medicinal botany was not, in the end, his major concern. The *Antiquities* belong together with Hernández's remarkable poem *The Christian Doctrine,* as these two works bring together two contrasting but complementary "worlds." The thinking behind the religious beliefs and practices of those worlds provides concepts of the body and the life cycle, which, of course, lead to differing methods of preserving and extending lives. Hernández examined plants and animals—and patients—with care and precision, but when he wrote down his findings, he interpreted "natural" and "history" as broadly as possible and created a natural history of the world.

NOTES

1. He alludes to these works throughout his surviving manuscripts, but they are long lost.

2. Epistle to Arias Montano, in *Mexican Treasury,* "Spain, 1790." Somolinos, "Vida y obra," 196, points out the reluctance of native peoples throughout Spanish America to yield their secrets to the pale men with beards. The comment by Pedro de Osma in his letter to Monardes is probably typical: "And we did aske of certaine Indians that went to serve us, where these beastes had their stones [i.e., bezoars], and as they are our enemies and would not that we should knowe their secretes, they answered unto us that they knewe nothing of these stones" (*Joyfull Newes Out of the Newe Founde Worlde,* trans. John Frampton [1577, 1580, 1596; reprint, London: Constable, 1925], 1:136).

3. The one that Hernández evidently did not know was the Cruz/Badianus manuscript.

4. For the full list, see *OC* 1:377–91.

5. Somolinos, "Vida y obra," 197–229, based on his earlier article "El viaje del doctor Francisco Hernández por la Nueva España," *Anales del Instituto de Biología* 22 (1951): 435–84.

6. See our introduction, "Hernández Texts," in *Mexican Treasury.* Most writing about López hovers above hagiography. One important article that does not is by Juan Comas, "El caso de aculturación farmacológica en la Nueva España del siglo XVI: El 'Tesoro de Medicinas' de Gregorio López," *Anales de Antropología* 1 (1964): 145–73.

7. Somolinos, "Vida y obra," 175, 195, and our text of the *Epistle to Arias Montano* in *Mexican Treasury,* "Spain, 1790."

8. *Medicinas, drogas* contains a small representative selection of images from this codex.

PART III ⁓ THE DISSEMINATION OF HERNÁNDEZ'S KNOWLEDGE

THE RECEPTION OF AMERICAN DRUGS IN EUROPE, 1500-1650

J . W O R T H E S T E S

Although Christopher Columbus looked for spices and drug plants, as well as gold, in the West Indies, he failed to identify any of them correctly, even when a physician accompanied him.[1] In 1519, Hernán Cortés saw a huge marketplace in Tenochtitlán where, he estimated, more than sixty thousand people were buying and selling all kinds of goods. He had already seen an immense market in the provincial capital Tlaxcala, where "they sell a great deal of . . . medicinal and cooking herbs," but he was astonished to find in the Aztec capital "streets of herbalists where all the medicinal herbs and roots found in the land are sold. There are shops like apothecaries', where they sell ready-made medicines as well as liquid ointments and plasters." Cortés wrote to Charles V about the agricultural promise of Mexico for growing Spanish plants, but the conquistador foresaw no market for Mexican plant products in the Old World.[2]

Cortés's comrades, too, were astounded by the botanical wonders they saw in Tenochtitlán. One was impressed by Moctezuma's gardens of medicinal herbs and by the city's many herb sellers. Another wrote that "in this street they lay out the peppers, in that medicinal roots and herbs, of which the natives know an infinite variety." Both men com-

mented on the value and reverence attached to chocolate and on its healthful properties.[3]

Several sixteenth-century works describe Mexican drugs. The earliest is probably the Cruz/Badianus manuscript, written in 1552 by Martin de la Cruz, an Aztec healer who taught medicine at a Franciscan college near the Mexico City, and translated into Latin by Johannes Badianus, who taught Latin at the same school. Although intended as a gift to Charles V, the manuscript disappeared from view soon after it arrived in Europe and did not resurface until 1929, when it was found in the Vatican Library. Thus, it exerted little or no influence on European medicine in the sixteenth century.[4] Bernardino de Sahagún went to Mexico as a Franciscan missionary in 1529 and compiled, from carefully constructed questionnaires, information about the Aztecs' life in general, including their health and medical practices. His final report, completed by 1580, was not widely read in Europe, either.[5]

The person most responsible for introducing American drugs to Europe was a Spanish physician, Nicolás Monardes. Born a year after Columbus first visited the New World, Monardes completed his medical degree at Alcalá de Henares

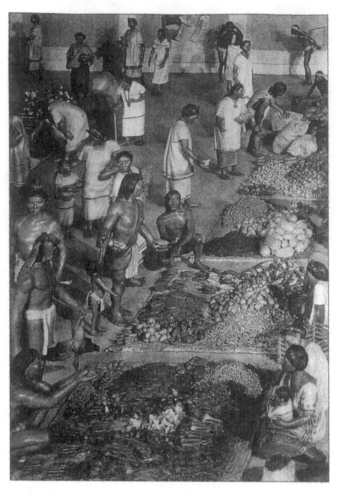

Reconstruction of a pre-Columbian
herb and spice market in Tenochtitlán.

"rare profite" from selling the drugs. By 1600, Frampton's translation, and others in Italian and Latin, had made Monardes the best-known Spanish physician in Europe. Inasmuch as he never visited the New World, it is ironic that it was his work, not that of firsthand observers such as Cruz, Sahagún, and Hernández, that was most frequently cited in European descriptions of American drugs before 1650.[7]

Monardes and his contemporaries thought that health depended on maintaining balances between four putative fluids—the "four humors"—of the body: blood, phlegm, black bile, and yellow bile. In the tradition established by Galen in the second century A.D., Monardes associated blood with heat and moisture; phlegm with moisture and cold; black bile with cold and dryness; and yellow bile with dryness and heat. Each humor was further associated with a season of the year and with a corresponding behavioral type: blood with spring and the sanguine temperament, water with winter and the phlegmatic temperament, black bile with autumn and melancholy, and yellow bile with summer and the choleric or bilious temperament. This ancient theory satisfactorily explained the physiological imbalances that had to be rectified in order to restore health and stability to the sick body. At the bedside, physicians assessed illness in terms of the four correlate qualities—heat, cold, moisture, and dryness—when making a diagnosis. Then they chose remedies with appropriately opposite properties that could be expected to counteract the underlying cause of the illness by restoring the humors to their normal balanced state, thereby correcting the associated symptoms.

The works of the French military surgeon Ambroise Paré, a near contemporary of Monardes, exemplify humoral medical practices. He wrote that hot drugs help remove the causes of illness because they open obstructed internal passageways for the humors, feces, urine, sweat, and other fluids. The same drugs also thin the humors, and in large amounts they redden, scar, and mortify tissues. Dry drugs, too, thin and rarefy the humors, but in large doses they are astringent because they contract and shrink tissues. By contrast, cooling drugs constrict dilated passages and condense the humors, while excessive doses congeal, stupefy, and mortify. Moist drugs lubricate the body's passages, but in excess they, too, obstruct the flow of humors.[8]

in 1533 and returned home to practice in Seville until he died, in 1588. His interest in Mexican and Peruvian drugs was guided not only by his profession but also by his investments and businesses, including drug merchandising, which fostered his contacts among merchants and clergy returning from the New World. According to his own account, he tried on his own patients many of the drugs his contacts brought to the wharves of Seville.[6]

Monardes published his first book on American medicines in 1569 and his second two years later; he combined them into one volume in 1574. It appeared in some fifty editions in several languages, including an English version by John Frampton, a Dorset merchant who had traveled in Spain. He called his 1577 edition of Monardes's work *Joyfull Newes Out of the Newe Founde Worlde,* not only because both men predicted that the newfound drugs would cure heretofore incurable diseases but also because they anticipated

Several American drugs were considered only as New World examples of ancient medicines long familiar to European physicians, such as peppers from the East, which were used to stimulate the appetite and improve digestion. Monardes, who described chili peppers as hot and dry in the fourth degree—that is, maximally hot and dry—said they settle the stomach and are good for ailments of the breast and for weak arms and legs.[9]

Resinous balsams were used as wound ointments because, as Paré and other physicians said, they soften scar tissue.[10] Monardes especially praised balsam of Peru. Conquistadores probably first applied it to their wounds simply because its aroma resembled that of familiar European balms. The high price of American balms was partly justified in the natural history of South America by José Acosta, who was in Peru in 1571: "And although all plants are medicinall when they are well known and applied, yet there are some things especially, which wee see directly ordained by the Creator for phisicke; and for the health of man. . . . Above all, Baulme is with reason esteemed for the excellent smell, but much more for the exquisite effect it hath to cure woundes." However, Acosta thought that New World balms were less effective than those from the Old World. Indeed, American Indians had told him that they did not place much therapeutic faith in their own balms.[11]

Hernández ascribed even more Galenic virtues to the balsam of Peru (which he called "molle"): "In nature it is hot and dry in the third degree. . . . It strengthens and gives heat to the upper intestine, binds the lower one. . . . It moves the urine, heals old or recent wounds, stops bloody fluxes, cures hemorrhoids, alleviates arthritis, makes films disappear from the eyes, clears flatulence and strengthens the limbs; it dries moist humors; mixed with lotions it resolves phlegmatic swellings. . . . This tree exudes a hot and astringent resin, which, besides being useful in all the above ways, purges phlegmatic and mixed humors if it is dissolved in water."[12] However, Hernández probably learned this information before he left for Mexico; it is not of obvious American origin.

Monardes said that balsam of Tolu (in modern Colombia) was equally effective in promoting wound healing because it prevents inflammation, and he agreed with Hernández that it was also useful for respiratory ailments when taken by mouth.[13] An important English apothecary sent some to Clusius in 1581, and it appeared in Germany about 1614, but the syrup made with the balsam achieved little prominence in medical practice;[14] its reputation was probably due to its fragrance alone.

Europeans applied the term *dragon's blood* to the bright red sap of an East Indian palm.[15] The Cruz/Badianus manuscript shows a plant labeled "dragon's blood" (from the Spanish *sangre de drago*). Although Cruz did not specify its medical uses, later observers said the Aztecs used it for pain in the chest.[16] On the other hand, Monardes—and Frampton—depicted little lizardlike dragons in the leaves of what he called "dragon's blood." Monardes reported that the red sap was effective against diarrhea and hemorrhage in his own patients and as a wound ointment.[17]

It might be thought surprising that Spanish physicians adopted no Mexican species of *Datura*—the genus that includes the Jimsonweed, *Datura stramonium,* which contains compounds that have several distinctive effects on the body, including, in high doses, hallucinations. According to Cruz/Badianus, Aztec healers administered *Datura* species for many conditions, and among Sahagún's eleven "herbs that madden" are several species of the genus.[18] However, virtually no American medicines made with any species of *Datura* entered European medical practice, most likely because they are hallucinogenic. Not only might such drugs have disastrously disruptive consequences, but the clergy associated them with witchcraft because the Aztecs used them in divination rituals.[19] Besides, European physicians already had a number of related drug plants that produce similar effects.

Although the balsams and a number of other American drugs gained only minor shares of the transatlantic drug market, several won major roles in European therapeutics during the 150 years after 1492. The most celebrated was guaiacum, which had entered European medicine by 1517, perhaps as early as 1508. In 1519, Ulrich von Hutten, a German writer—but not a physician—published the single most influential book about the wondrous remedy. Others had written about it by then, but von Hutten's was the bestseller; it was available in French and English by 1540.[20]

Guaiacum's popularity rested on its reputation as a cure for syphilis, which many agreed had been brought to Europe in the 1490s by sailors who had accompanied Columbus to the New World. It is not certain today that syphilis did originate in the New World, but in the sixteenth century it seemed a good possibility.[21] The chief reason for von Hutten's enthusiasm for guaiacum was that it had cured him of the new disease a year before he wrote his book, whereas repeated courses of mercurial drugs had been ineffective. Ironically, four years later he died of syphilis.[22]

Mercurial ointments for syphilis—the treatments that had failed von Hutten—had been introduced in 1497, because they had long been used for other skin diseases.[23] Guaiacum seems to have been prescribed primarily by physicians who treated those who could pay most for it, whereas the cheaper mercurials were more likely to be prescribed by barbers for the less affluent. For the elite who could afford the new drug, its effects were less unpleasant than those of mercury, whose side effects were often regarded as the patient's punishment for having contracted a venereal disease in the first place.[24]

Monardes said that guaiacum was the best remedy for syphilis—unless "the sicke man doe returne to tumble in the same bosome, where he tooke the firste [attack]"—because, he explained, "Our Lord God [willed that] from whence the evil of the Poxe came, from thence should come the remedy for them."[25] That is, remedies can be found near places where the diseases they cure arise.

Guaiacum therapy involved a complex schedule of sweating and purging, a salt-free diet that included half a chicken and five ounces of bread at lunch but no dinner until late in the course of treatment, and repeated doses of the wondrous new medicine.[26] Von Hutten explained how it removes syphilitic humors via sweat, urine, and feces:

> The doctors gather that it has a heating and drying effect and they say that it cures the defects of the blood and the liver.... Therefore it delays fluxes, either by its drying effect removing noxious humors or eradicating their original causes.... It loosens phlegm, it opens the obstructed passages of the urine ... and it stimulates and impels the urine.... It most violently draws off so-called black bile; and so it makes the patient more cheerful and checks iras-

cibility.... It removes catarrh; and it frees the blood from fluxes and, ... by warming the brain it relieves the heaviness of the head.... [It] entirely renews [the stomach], and it makes the bowels as good as ever before. Its effect on emaciated and dwarfed limbs is excellent, for it increases them and fills them out, it expands contracted muscles and hardens and strengthens relaxed ones.[27]

Monardes agreed that, because guaiacum is hot and dry in the second degree, it unclogs the excretory and secretory channels of the body, thereby purifying corrupted blood. Hernández, too, said it is hot to the second degree, "with a noted dryness," but added little else about the drug's properties; presumably they would be perceived as logical consequences of the first.[28]

Guaiacum's reputation spread quickly. Vesalius thought it was the most valuable of all the drugs introduced from the Americas.[29] Benvenuto Cellini was a typical advocate of guaiacum. When he took it against his doctor's advice in the 1530s, he wrote, it cured him of a bad case of secondary syphilis.[30]

Von Hutten sneered that, after guaiacum entered European commerce, "the doctors would not recommend it, seeing only a loss to their income" if all their syphilitic patients recovered.[31] After his book appeared, demand for guaiacum soared. So did its price, because its importation and distribution were a monopoly awarded by Charles V to the banking house of Fugger, headquartered in Augsburg, in return for a large loan. At the height of its popularity, guaiacum sold there for three gold florins a pound.[32] Moreover, whenever its price rose, the wonder drug was counterfeited. When demand fell, so did its price, as happened when the Fuggers lost their monopoly in 1525.[33]

In the 1540s physicians began to report patients who had failed to respond to guaiacum. Paré thought it "hath not strength to extinguish the venome of the venereous virulency," as an alliterating translator put it, although he did agree that it promotes sweating and diuresis because, as a heating drug, it sublimates ill humors.[34] Even Girolamo Fracastoro, who named syphilis in 1530, had lost faith in guaiacum by 1546.[35] Although its reputation had waned by the time Hernández went to New Spain, it remained in European and American pharmacopoeias until it gradually faded into total obscurity in the early nineteenth century.

The next most popular remedy from the New World was probably sarsaparilla. Monardes said it entered Spain about 1545 and, because, like guaiacum, it was hot and dry in the second degree, it was useful in treating "any maner of Reumes or runnynges" and whatever he meant by the "evill of women" (*mal de mugeres*). Francisco Bravo, a Spanish physician who had been to New Spain, agreed that it was hot and dry. In 1570 he compared it favorably with guaiacum as a blood purifier suitable for syphilis, rheumatism, and other inflammatory diseases. Hernández attributed the same properties to sarsaparilla, although he seems to have been less sure about its mechanism of action when he explained that it is "cold and dry, although it has mixed hot and subtle parts." Physicians had proclaimed it better for syphilis than guaiacum as early as 1553, but sarsaparilla, too, lost favor. In 1649, Culpeper said only that it is "somewhat hot and dry, helpful against pains in the head, and joynts[. The roots] provoke sweat, and are used familiarly in drying Diet-drinks."[36]

Another long-term survivor in European medicine was *mechoacan,* or jalap, the moderately strong cathartic that Monardes called "Rhubarb of Michoacán" and "Rhubarb of the Indies," although it is not related to the true cathartic rhubarb.[37] In 1597 the English herbalist John Gerard said its medical quality was between hot and cold, but also dry.[38] It was known in Europe as jalap by 1610, and at midcentury Culpeper expanded on its cathartic and diuretic properties: "[It] is temperate, yet drying, purgeth flegm chiefly from the head and joynts, it is good for old [i.e., chronic] diseases in the head, and may safely be given even to Feaverish bodies, because of its [cool] temperature; it is also profitable against Coughs and pains in the [kidneys], as also against [syphilis]."[39]

Sassafras bark from Florida could "comfort" the liver and stomach and dissolve obstructions in the body "to ingender good humors," wrote Monardes, because it moves both the stool and urine. Culpeper explained that these effects were due to the drug's hot and dry qualities. Therefore, it was recommended for stomachache, lameness, gout, dropsy, scurvy, jaundice, and syphilis, among other illnesses,

and to promote pregnancy because it promoted menstrual flow.[40]

From Seville, Monardes relayed travelers' tales of Peruvian Indians chewing a mixture of coca leaves and burned cockle shells to allay hunger and thirst or for pleasure. He said that the Indians mix it with tobacco "when thei [wish to] make themselves dronke, and bee out of judgemente . . . to have their wittes taken from them." Although Hernández's account of coca is secondhand, it resembles that of Monardes.[41] However, European physicians took almost no notice of coca, presumably because they could find no therapeutic use for it.

Monardes reported that tobacco came to Spain as an ornamental flower. Hot and dry in the second degree, it had entered medical practice by the 1570s as a medicine that opens obstructed passages to remove cold humors that cause shortness of breath, kidney stones, and stomachaches. It could also expel intestinal worms and, when applied topically, relieve joint pains and toothaches. Monardes said that the excellent royal physician Dr. Bernardo had experimented successfully with tobacco on a dog intentionally given a "venomous wound." Washing the wound with wine and the crude debridement that Monardes says was usually performed were just as likely to have helped the wound heal.[42]

Culpeper based his description of tobacco on those of Monardes and Clusius: "Neither is there any better salve in the world for wounds than may be made of it, for it cleanseth, fetcheth out the filth though it lie in the bones, brings up the flesh from the bottom [of the wound], and all this it doth speedily, it cures wounds made with poysoned weapons." Because, like sarsaparilla, sassafras, and guaiacum, tobacco is hot and dry in the second degree, Culpeper regarded it as equally good for cleansing patients with illnesses as diverse as headaches, asthma, and stomachaches. Moreover, he reported: "Taken in a pipe it hath almost as many vertues, it easeth weariness, takes away the sence of hunger and thirst, provokes to stool [and] easeth the body of superfluous humors, opens stoppings." Although tobacco achieved a modest medical reputation, its popularity rested chiefly on its pleasurable effects when smoked. England prohibited its cultivation in 1660, but the settlers of Virginia and their principals in London grew rich on it.[43]

The Aztecs dried fermented cocoa beans (correctly, cacao nibs) and ground them as part of the process of making powdered chocolate. A soldier who accompanied Cortés considered chocolate "the most healthful and most nutritious aliment of all known to the world, for one who takes a cup of it, though he may make a long journey, can pass all day without taking another thing, and being cold of its nature, it is better in hot weather than in cold."[44] On the other hand, Acosta disliked the chocolate drink that the Aztecs—and the Spanish—made from cocoa, "for it is loathsome to such as are not acquainted with it, having a skumme or froth that is very unpleasant to taste." He was probably even more critical of his compatriots who made a paste of chocolate mixed with chili peppers that they said was "good for the stomacke, and against the catarre."[45]

Not all medical wonders from the New World were of botanical origin. In 1568, a Spanish soldier named Pedro de Osma sent Monardes a dozen bezoars taken from Peruvian llamas.[46] Bezoars are concretions that form in saccules in the first of the three compartments of llama stomachs. Because the saccules are everted during normal gastric contractions, expelling their contents into the stomach cavity, the pathogenesis of the stones is unknown, and they do not impair gastric function.[47] Bezoars from male goats had long been imported into Europe from Persia as antidotes to poison and as remedies for other illnesses, especially of the skin.[48]

Because of the great demand for bezoars to sell to Spanish soldiers and colonists in Peru, Acosta said that some Indians made them artificially by inserting a nidus for their growth into the stomachs of llamas and vicuñas, even if, in his opinion, those from Peru were less effective as medicines than those from the East Indies. Besides, he said, "there is no medicine that doth alwaies cure infallibly."[49]

Monardes reported that Peruvian bezoars were effective in his own patients, as did other physicians. Although Paré said they were valuable therapeutic agents, he had reservations about them.[50] In 1599 Vargas Manchuca, the author of a vade mecum for Spanish conquistadores, recommended the inclusion of bezoars in military medicine chests destined for use in the Americas.[51] In his 1605 description of medicines from the New World, Clusius included pictures of Peruvian bezoars in a lengthy note to his Latin translation of Monardes.[52] As Friedrich Hoffmann wrote in 1695, bezoars "restore the disturbed or impaired mixture of the blood, and maintain the union of serum and blood."[53] Nevertheless, American bezoars did not win a large market even in Spain, perhaps because the Fuggers judged even the traditionally high-quality Eastern bezoars to be bad investments because they were costly and not reliably effective as medicines, and by the 1690s all bezoars had lost the confidence of European healers.[54]

Although Monardes enthusiastically promoted drugs from the New World, fewer than half of those he described in 1574 were widely accepted in the Old World during the 150 years after 1492. On the whole, American plants contributed little to scientific botany for many years. Some students of natural history continually tried to identify medicinal plants from the New World among those that Dioscorides had described around A.D. 70. Seldom could American species be made to fit the mold he had constructed, although—somehow—sarsaparilla was repeatedly identified (even by Hernández) among the plants that he had described.[55]

Some xenophobic writers thought American remedies were unnecessary. For instance, in 1580 Timothy Bright of London published *A Treatise wherein Is Declared the Sufficiencie of English Medicines for the Cure of All Diseases.* However, others continued to assume that the New World could provide drugs for the tropical and other exotic diseases that were indigenous to the West Indies.

One possible reason for not using the new American remedies was doubt about their efficacy. Not only did physicians and apothecaries lack sure methods for testing any drug, but they knew they had to differentiate among drugs that were inherently ineffective, those that had lost potency during the long transatlantic voyage, and those that had just rotted away while awaiting shipment on the convoys that sailed for Spain only once a year.[56]

It has been hypothesized that another barrier to European acceptance of many drugs from the New World was the difficulty of adding new remedies to the tried and true Galenic medicinal roster. That is, many American drugs might have been seen merely as alternatives to classical remedies, as options that offered little that was really new to the doctor's therapeutic choices.[57] Monardes ascribed traditional Galenic properties, chiefly heat, to the drugs he described in the same proportion (about 74 percent) as contemporary European herbalists did to conventional medicines. This suggests that European physicians could have concluded that little was to be gained by adding more hot drugs to a pharmacopoeia that was already top-heavy with them. In addition, warming drugs would not be expected to help patients with the most common illnesses of Europeans, the fevers, characterized by excessive heat. Moreover, the Aztecs thought that about half their drugs could cure fevers and that another fifth could cure abscesses, sores, and other inflammations. Europeans categorized most fevers together with inflammations as consequences of pathologically increased heat that required cooling remedies in the Galenic tradition. Thus, the Aztecs' opinions about how their drugs affected the body might have made them seem superfluous to observers from the Old World.[58] However, if such arguments against the adoption of remedies from the New World were used, they do not appear in sixteenth-century therapeutic compendiums. (On the other hand, it is possible that European physicians simply favored heating drugs, but it is not yet possible to support this hypothesis.)[59]

Although the Aztecs had extensive repertoires of magical remedies, they had their own hot-cold theory of disease and its treatment (but not a Galenic dry-wet differentiation).[60] Many of the remedies described by Cruz/Badianus and Sahagún were clearly associated with magic, especially stones, animal parts, and Sahagún's "herbs that madden." Only 12 of the 133 medicinal herbs (i.e., 9 percent) mentioned by Sahagún were said to produce catharsis. Because about one-fourth of contemporary European drugs shared this effect, its relative scarcity among American drugs might have discouraged their rapid adoption in the Old World.[61]

Spaniards living in Mexico used traditional local remedies when conventional European drugs were in short supply or when the actions of Mexican drugs could be satisfactorily explained in familiar humoral terms.[62] Agustín Farfán, a Spanish physician who joined the Augustinian order in Mexico, wrote about Aztec remedies that laymen could use when no physician or apothecary was available.[63]

Medicine chests loaded aboard ships in Seville in 1590 and 1600 contained fifty drugs that had been commonplace in European medicine for centuries; none came from the Americas. Although in 1581 a Spanish captain carried mechoacan among twenty-seven drugs he delivered to a garrison in Florida, he may have acquired it en route.[64] One can only speculate why Spanish maritime medical authorities were not infected by Monardes's enthusiasm.

Two lines of evidence suggest that American drugs were more widely adopted in Europe during the 150 years after 1492 than might be inferred from the indirect negative evidence outlined above. More positive deductions can be drawn from European herbals and from Spanish customs records for the port of Seville.

Herbals were compendiums of botanical information that included remedies that had become acceptable as healing agents over a period of time; rarely, if ever, did they include reports of newly introduced drugs still being evaluated for their therapeutic worth. That only a few American drugs are described in Europe's important herbals published before 1590 probably reflects something about both the slow rate of collecting information about the new remedies and their acceptance by European medical practitioners. For instance, no drugs from the New World are described in *The Grete Herball* of Treveris (1526) or the *Kruydeboeck* of Dodoens (1554), and tobacco was the only drug from the New World shown in the herbals of Matthiolus (1586) and L'Obel (1576); L'Obel's "guaiac" was actually ebony. The *Neuw und Volkommenlich Kreuterbuch* of Tabernaemontanus (1591) included mechoacan, tobacco, and other drugs from the New World, but his 1588 edition had not. Gesner included only guaiacum in his books on the distillation of medicines (1565) and general medicine (1599).[65]

The first major English herbal to describe more than one or two medicinal plants from the New World was published in 1597 by John Gerard, a barber-surgeon of London; Thomas Johnson published a posthumous expansion in 1633 (reissued in 1636). Both editions relied heavily on Monardes for American drugs. The first included substantial articles on mechoacan, tobacco, and sassafras, as well as a Caribbean version of mastic.[66] The 1636 edition added articles on guaiacum, sarsaparilla, and minor drugs such as balsam of Peru and dragon's blood, but Johnson was most effusive in praising tobacco.[67]

José Acosta's book was not an herbal but a collection of his observations on the natural history of the New World. Although an English edition appeared in 1604, there is no good internal evidence that Johnson used it in preparing his edition of Gerard's herbal. Not only did the Spanish missionary give lengthy descriptions of bezoars, Peruvian balsam, cacao, and coca (but only as a nonmedical curiosity); he also included brief notes on others, such as tobacco, mechoacan, guaiacum, and sarsaparilla.[68]

Clusius is often cited by later herbalists. *His Exoticorum libri decem* of 1605 includes a long chapter on American medicines that is nearly a new edition of Monardes.[69] John Parkinson relied just as heavily on Monardes in his herbal of 1640, in which he described tobacco, sarsaparilla, sassafras, and medical curiosities such as coca. More enthusiastic about jalap than others, Parkinson lamented that it was no longer prescribed as often as when it was first introduced to England (probably via Frampton's edition of Monardes).[70]

The appearance of several American drugs in European herbals published between 1590 and 1650 is evidence that they had by then been accepted into the medical practices of the Old World after a period of empirical assessment that probably began before 1520. For whatever reasons, many others were rejected sooner or later: no more than half the fifty-one American drugs that Monardes described can be found in herbals and medical texts published between 1600 and 1800, and none appears to have been as prominent among the medical practices of those years as much older Galenic remedies.

Data pertaining to sales of American drugs provide more immediate evidence of their acceptability, inasmuch as their supply must have been in some measure a more rapid response to demand for them than can be discerned in contemporary medical texts. For instance, Monardes said that balsam of Peru was so effective that in Rome it initially commanded a price of one hundred ducats an ounce, but the price fell to ten ducats as imports grew over the fifty years after its European debut in 1524.[71]

Spanish merchants hoped the discovery of the New World would free their country from dependence on Venice and Portugal, Spain's maritime rivals, for drugs from the Near and Far East, and from fear that the Ottoman Empire could imperil traditional drug supply routes from the East. Several Spaniards emigrated to the New World to engage in the potentially lucrative transatlantic drug trade.[72] Indeed, it may have engendered a few fortunes, including the probable rewards of the Fuggers' temporary monopoly on guaiacum. Other bankers tried to monopolize imports of healing balsams, and one obtained a monopoly on exporting them from Santo Domingo. For a time, American balsams were among the most expensive drugs in Europe, at least until Dutch and English sea power had broken the Spanish drug monopolies, by about 1600.[73]

The risks to American raw materials intended for European pharmacies were considerable. The trip from Caribbean ports required 77 to 110 days (the average was 86 days) but could be as long as seven months.[74] In the 1520s, about a hundred Spanish ships, totaling 4,500 tons, were engaged in transatlantic trade each year. Both the number of ships and their average size doubled over the next eighty years, quadrupling the total carrying capacity.[75] Data for measuring profits made by shipping any commodity are rare for the early modern period, and little is known about how drug plants were harvested and prepared for shipment to Seville.[76]

Nevertheless, surviving records show that nearly 670 tons of sarsaparilla were unloaded at Seville in twenty-five years between 1568 and 1619. Similarly, 930 tons of guaiacum were imported in thirteen of the forty years following 1568, long after its popularity had begun to wane. (It is not possible to determine if these data are complete, but they probably do represent a nearly complete inventory of sarsaparilla imports in light of the vicissitudes of transatlantic shipping in the sixteenth century and the uncertainty that suitable harvests even occurred in any given year.) It is puzzling that the cash value of guaiacum was less than that of sarsaparilla in the years for which data are available. One might assume that it was because physicians had already lost faith in the efficacy of guaiacum by the 1550s, but it could also be because the Fuggers' earlier monopoly had simply stabilized its price at Seville, even if others had been transshipping it on to northern Europe since 1525.[77]

However one looks at the few available import data (comparable data for other indigenous American drugs are not available), it is hard to agree that drugs were only incidental imports from the New World, arriving merely as practical ballast, as has been postulated. Indeed, medicinal plants ranked just after cochineal, indigo, hides, and sugar in terms of both taxable values and amounts unloaded at Seville.[78]

English traders, too, tried to capitalize on American drugs. Sassafras, for instance, was among the commodities sent from Virginia after Jamestown was settled in 1607. Demand for it was so great that expeditions were sent to New England in 1602 and 1603 to collect it for English entrepreneurs, who hoped to sell it for £50 a ton.[79] Although the price of sassafras had fallen by 1620, as late as 1770 England imported more than 76 tons, valued at £2,142. Other drug plants harvested in Bermuda, Virginia, and the Carolinas included sarsaparilla, mechoacan, ipecac, Jimsonweed, and sassafras. Not only did colonial planters and entrepreneurs send new drug plants for evaluation or as articles of trade, but British physicians and naturalists actively sought new species to introduce into medical practice.[80]

——

In summary, it was chiefly the secondhand reports of Nicolás Monardes that supported the entry of several American drugs into European medical practice during the 150 years after Columbus found the New World. The earliest firsthand accounts, including those of Francisco Hernández, remained unpublished—but not unknown—in Europe until long after they were written, as did less systematic accounts by Franciscan and Dominican friars who had worked in the Americas.[81] Acosta's book may have had some slight influence, but he was more interested in natural history than in therapeutics.

It seems likely that a few merchants and apothecaries made substantial short-term profits from American drugs in the sixteenth century and perhaps afterward. The most profitable drugs, at least for a few years, were probably guaiacum, sarsaparilla, sassafras, and tobacco, but the only ones that are still important in medical practice were introduced much later: cinchona and ipecac in the seventeenth century, cocaine in 1884, and curare in 1942.

Of 218 plant drugs available in England in 1874, twenty-five (12.4 percent), came from the New World.[82] Three hundred years earlier, in 1574, Monardes had described forty-seven drugs from the New World, and perhaps twenty others were added to European pharmacopoeias over the next fifty years.

Some did not survive even Monardes's century. Others, such as the balsams of Peru and Tolu, dragon's blood, and pepper, remained in use until physicians finally recognized their lack of efficacy in the nineteenth century. Guaiacum and jalap had all but disappeared from medical practice by 1830, although guaiacum extracts are still used as expectorants and for identifying blood in the stool. In the late nineteenth century, sarsaparilla probably commanded a larger market than any other drug native to Spanish America, as a major ingredient of many home remedies. Sassafras degenerated into a folk remedy and flavoring until it was banned as unsafe; cocoa butter is still used in ointments and cosmetics; and tobacco is now a major health problem.

In the end, little of truly lasting therapeutic value came from the New World, save for the four drugs that achieved prominence only 150 years or more *after* Columbus's last voyage to the Americas. Others survived for decades, even centuries, in the pharmacies of Europe and North America, but only a few were sources of significant financial profit in the sixteenth century. It should not, of course, be surprising that many American drugs were prescribed for as long as they were during all the centuries before it was widely recognized that the body can often heal itself.[83]

NOTES

1. Samuel Eliot Morison, trans. and ed., *Journals and Other Documents on the Life and Voyages of Christopher Columbus* (New York: Heritage Press, 1963); Cecil Jane, trans., *The Four Voyages of Columbus*, 2 vols. in 1 (1930, 1933; reprint, New York: Dover, 1988), 1:68–69, 76; William D. Phillips Jr., "Columbus and European Views of the World," *American Neptune* 53 (1993): 260–67. Also see George B. Griffenhagen, "The Materia Medica of Christopher Columbus," *Pharmacy in History* 34 (1992): 131–45.

2. Hernán Cortés, *Letter from Mexico*, trans. Anthony Pagden (New Haven: Yale University Press, 1986), 67–68, 103, 336.

3. Bernal Díaz del Castillo, *The Discovery and Conquest of Mexico*, trans. Irving A. Leonard (New York: Farrar, Straus, Cudahy, 1956), 211, 214; The Anonymous Conqueror, *Narrative of Some Things of New Spain and of the Great City of Temestitan [i.e., Tenochtitlán], Mexico*, trans. Marshall H. Saville (New York: Cortés Society, 1917), 39–41, 66.

4. Emily Walcott Emmart, trans., *The Badianus Manuscript (Codex Barberini, Latin 241), Vatican Library: An Aztec Herbal of 1552* (Baltimore: Johns Hopkins University Press, 1940), 4–5, 8–9, 17–18, 184.

5. Bernard R. Ortiz de Montellano, *Aztec Medicine, Health, and Nutrition* (New Brunswick, N.J.: Rutgers University Press, 1990), 17–20; Bernardino de Sahagún, *Florentine Codex: General History of the Things of New Spain,* trans. by C. E. Dibble and A. J. O. Anderson, 13 vols. (Santa Fe, N.M.: School of American Research and University of Utah, 1950–63).

6. Francisco Guerra's entry on Monardes in *Dictionary of Scientific Biography,* 9:466.

7. Nicolás Monardes, *Joyfull Newes Out of the Newe Founde Worlde,* trans. John Frampton, 2 vols. (1577; reprint, London: Constable, 1925), introduction by Stephen Gaselee, 1:v–xii, and 1:3, 10–11. The edition of Monardes that Frampton translated is *Primera y segunda y tercera partes de la historia medicinal de las cosas que se traen nuestras Indias occidentales que siruen en medicina* (Sevilla: Alonso Escrivano, 1574).

8. [Ambroise Paré], *Works of That Famous Chirurgion Ambrose Parey,* trans. Thomas Johnson (London, 1634; reprint, Pound Ridge, N.Y.: Milford House, 1968), 1029–30, 1034–35.

9. Monardes, *Joyfull Newes,* 1:47–48.

10. Friedrich Hoffmann, *Fundamenta Medicinae* [1695], trans. Lester S. King (New York: American Elsevier, 1971), 135.

11. José Acosta, *The Naturall and Morall Historie of the East and West Indies,* trans. E[dward] G[rimestone] (London, 1604), 285–87.

12. *Mexican Treasury,* QL 1.2.15.

13. Monardes, *Joyfull Newes,* 2:42–46, and *Mexican Treasury,* QL 1.2.14.

14. Friedrich A. Flückiger, *Pharmacographia: A History of the Principal Drugs of Vegetable Origin,* rev. Daniel Hanbury (London: Macmillan, 1874), 177–79.

15. J. Worth Estes, *Dictionary of Protopharmacology: Therapeutic Practices, 1700–1850* (Canton, Mass.: Science History Publications, 1990), 171.

16. Emmart, *Badianus Manuscript,* 238, 274.

17. Monardes, *Joyfull Newes,* 1:149; Monardes, *La historia medicinal,* facs. ed. with intro. by José M. López Piñero (Madrid: Ministerio de Sanidad y Consumo, 1992), fol. 64r.

18. Emmart, *Badianus Manuscript,* 245, 253; Sahagún, *Florentine Codex,* 11:129–220, esp. 129–31.

19. On disruptive consequences, Robert Beverley, "The Jamestown Weed" [1705], in *America Begins: Early American Writings,* ed. Richard M. Dorson (Greenwich, Conn.: Fawcett, 1966), 110. On their use in divination rituals, Ortiz de Montellano, *Aztec Medicine,* 23.

20. Thomas G. Benedek, "The Influence of Ulrich von Hutten's Medical Descriptions and Metaphorical Use of Medicine," *Bulletin of the History of Medicine* 66 (1992): 355–75; Ulrich von Hutten, "The Remarkable Medicine Guaiacum and the Cure of the Gallic Disease," trans. Clarence W. Mendell, *Archives of Dermatology and Syphilology* 23 (1931): 409–28, 681–704, 1045–63.

21. Robert S. Munger, "Guaiacum, the Holy Wood from the New World," *Journal of the History of Medicine and Allied Sciences* 4 (1949): 196–229; Jon Arrizabalaga, "Syphilis," in *The Cambridge World History of Human Disease,* ed. Kenneth F. Kiple (New York: Cambridge University Press, 1993), 1025–33; Claude Quétel, *The History of Syphilis,* trans. Judith Braddock and Brian Pike (Baltimore: Johns Hopkins University Press, 1990), 10–51; von Hutten, "Remarkable Medicine," 413.

22. Von Hutten, "Remarkable Medicine," 416.

23. Paul A. Russell, "Syphilis, God's Scourge or Nature's Vengeance?: The German Printed Response to a Public Problem in the Early Sixteenth Century," *Archiv für Reformationsgeschichte* 80 (1989): 286–307; Owsei Temkin, "Therapeutic Trends and the Treatment of Syphilis before 1900," *Bulletin of the History of Medicine* 29 (1955): 309–16.

24. Owsei Temkin, "On the History of 'Morality and Syphilis'" (1927), in Owsei Temkin, *The Double Face of Janus* (Baltimore: Johns Hopkins University Press, 1977), 472–84.

25. Monardes, *Joyfull Newes,* 1:28.

26. Benedek, "Influence of Ulrich von Hutten"; von Hutten, "Remarkable Medicine," 422–27.

27. Von Hutten, "Remarkable Medicine," 1050–51.

28. Monardes, *Joyfull Newes,* 1:28–33; *Mexican Treasury,* QL 1.2.29.

29. Harvey Cushing, *A Bio-Bibliography of Andreas Vesalius* (New York: Schuman's, 1943), 160–62; C. D. O'Malley, *Andreas Vesalius of Brussels, 1514–1564* (Berkeley: University of California Press, 1964), 189, 383–89.

30. Benvenuto Cellini, *The Autobiography,* translated by George Bull (Harmondsworth, England: Penguin, 1956), 111–12.

31. Von Hutten, "Remarkable Medicine," 418.

32. Russell, "Syphilis, God's Scourge."

33. Munger, "Guaiacum"; Alfred W. Crosby Jr., *The Columbian Exchange: Biological and Cultural Consequences of 1492* (Westport, Conn.: Greenwood, 1972), 154–55.

34. [Paré], *Works,* 725, 728; Crosby, *Columbian Exchange,* 155.

35. George Sarton, "The Strange Fame of Demetrio Canevari, Philosopher and Physician, Genoese Patrician (1559–1625)," *Journal of the History of Medicine* 1 (1946): 398–418; Monardes, *Joyfull Newes,* 1:38–44. See Geoffrey Eatough, *Fracastoro's "Syphilis"* (Liverpool: Francis Cairns, 1984).

36. Monardes, *Joyfull Newes,* 1:38–44; Flückiger and Hanbury, *Pharmacographia,* 639–47; Nich[olas] Culpeper, *A Physicall Directory or a Translation of the London Dispensatory* (London, 1649), 24; Saul Jarcho, "Medicine in Sixteenth Century New Spain as Illustrated by the Writings of Bravo, Farfán, and Vargas Machuca," *Bulletin of the History of Medicine* 31 (1957): 425–41; Germán Somolinos d'Ardois, "Francisco Bravo y su 'Opera Medicinalia,'" *Anales de la Sociedad Mexicana de Historia de la Ciencia y de la Tecnología,* 2 (1970): 117–45.

37. Monardes, *Joyfull Newes,* 1:54–67.

38. John Gerard, *The Herball or Generall Histories of Plantes* (London, 1597), 723–24; Hoffmann, *Fundamenta,* 124.

39. Culpeper, *Physicall Directory,* 13.

40. Monardes, *Joyfull Newes,* 1:99–120; Gerard, *Herball* (1597), 340–41; Culpeper, *Physicall Directory,* 24.

41. Monardes, *Joyfull Newes,* 2:31–32, and see 1.90; *Mexican Treasury,* T 8.59.

42. Monardes, *Joyfull Newes,* 1:75–98.

43. Culpeper, *Physicall Directory,* 46–47; Berthold Laufer, *Introduction of Tobacco into Europe,* Anthropology Leaflet 19 (Chicago: Field Museum of Natural History, 1924), 6–8, 23–24; David Harley, "The Beginnings of the Tobacco Controversy: Puritanism, James I, and the Royal Physicians," *Bulletin of the History of Medicine* 67 (1993): 28–50.

44. Anonymous Conqueror, *Narrative,* 39–41.

45. Acosta, *Naturall and Morall Historie,* 270–72.

46. Monardes, *Joyfull Newes,* 1:135–45; 2:25–30.

47. Murray E. Fowler, *Medicine and Surgery of South American Camelids: Llama, Alpaca, Vicuña, Guanaco* (Ames: Iowa State University Press, 1989), 10–17, 253.

48. Lynn Thorndike, *A History of Magic and Experimental Science,* 8 vols. (New York: Columbia University Press, 1923–58), vol. 5 (1941): 249, 316, 474, 476; vol. 6 (1941): 315, 420.

49. Acosta, *Naturall and Morall Historie,* 322–26.

50. Monardes, *Joyfull Newes,* 2:25–30; Thorndike, *History of Magic,* 6:315; [Paré], *Works,* 808–9.

51. Jarcho, "Medicine in Sixteenth Century New Spain," 440.

52. Clusius, *Exoticorum libri decem* (Antwerp, 1605), 327–29.

53. Hoffmann, *Fundamenta medicinae,* 122.

54. Thorndike, *History of Magic,* vol. 6 (1941): 315; vol. 7 (1958): 245–49; Francisco Guerra, "Drugs from the Indies and the Political Economy of the Sixteenth Century," *Analecta MedicoHistorica* 1 (1966): 29–54.

55. Joseph Ewan, "The Columbian Discoveries and the Growth of Botanical Ideas with Special Reference to the Sixteenth Century," in *First Images of America,* ed. Fredi Chiappelli, 2 vols. (Berkeley: University of California Press, 1976), 2:807–12; Thorndike, *History of Magic,* 6:266, 271–72, 296, 595–98; A. C. Crombie, *Augustine to Galileo,* 2 vols. in 1 (Cambridge: Harvard University Press, 1961), 2:267–68; Nancy G. Siraisi, *Medieval and Early Renaissance Medicine* (Chicago: University of Chicago Press, 1990), 191. But cf. José M. López Piñero and José Pardo Tomás, "Contribution of Hernández," and Chabrán and Varey, "Hernández in the Netherlands and England," below.

56. Charles H. Talbot, "America and the European Drug Trade," in Chiappelli, *First Images of America,* 2:833–44.

57. Guenter B. Risse, "Transcending Cultural Barriers: The European Reception of Medicinal Plants from the Americas," in *Botanical Drugs of the Americas in the Old and New Worlds,* ed. Wolfgang-Hagen Hein (Stuttgart: Wissenschaftliche Verlagsgesellschaft, 1984), 31–42.

58. P. M. Teigen, "Taste and Quality in Fifteenth- and Sixteenth-Century Galenic Pharmacology," *Pharmacy in History* 29 (1987): 60–68; J. Worth Estes, "The European Reception of the First Drugs from the New World," *Pharmacy in History* 37 (1995): 3–23.

59. Estes, "European Reception," 12.

60. Efrén C. del Pozo, "Aztec Pharmacology," *Annual Review of Pharmacology* 6 (1966): 9–18; Efrén C. del Pozo, "Empiricism and Magic in Aztec Pharmacology," in *Ethnopharmacologic Search for Psychoactive Drugs,* ed. Daniel H. Efron (Washington, D.C.: U.S. Department of Health, Education, and Welfare, 1967), 59–76; Ortiz de Montellano, *Aztec Medicine,* 165–81, 205–9; Estes, "European Reception," 12.

61. Estes, "European Reception," 12.

62. Risse, "Medicine in New Spain," 44–50.

63. Jarcho, "Medicine in Sixteenth Century New Spain," 431–39.

64. Jonathan W. Bream generously provided his translations of two lists he found in the Archives of the Indies in Seville: Account of medicines for the fleet of 1590, Seville, July 16, 1590 (AGI, Contratación 4879), and Account of medicines for the fleet of 1600 (AGI, Indiferente General 1249). Eugene Lyon kindly furnished his translation of the medicines that Rodrigo de Junco took to Florida (AGI Contaduria 944, no. 7).

65. Peter Treveris, *The Grete Herball* (London, 1526); Rembert Dodoens, *A Niewe Herball, or Historie of Plantes,* trans. Henry Lyte (London, 1578); Petrus Andreas Matthiolus, *De Plantis Epitome Utilissima* (Frankfurt am Main, 1586); Matthias L'Obel, *Plantarum seu Stirpium Historia* (Antwerp, 1576); Jacobus Theodorus Tabernaemontanus, *Neuw und Volkommenlich Kreuterbuch* (Frankfurt am Main, 1591); Conrad Gesner, *A New Booke of Destillatyon of Waters, Called the Treasure of Euonymus* (London, 1565), 256; Conrad Gesner, *The Practice of the New and Old Phisicke,* trans. George Baker (London, 1599), 166.

66. Gerard, *Herball* (1597), 285–89, 340–41, 723–24, 1243–44.

67. Gerard, *Herball,* ed. Thomas Johnson (London, 1636), 357–61, 859–61, 872–74, 1523–25, 1529–31, 1611–12.

68. Acosta, *Naturall and Morall Historie,* 174–75, 288–89.

69. Clusius, *Exoticorum libri decem,* 297–354, 329.

70. John Parkinson, *Theatrum Botanicum, The Theater of Plants, or An Universall and Complete Herball* (London, 1640), 173–75, 178–81, 711–12, 1586–87, 1606–8, 1662–63.

71. Monardes, *Joyfull Newes,* 1:23.

72. M. Fernández-Carrión and J. L. Valverde, "Research Note on the Spanish-American Drug Trade," *Pharmacy in History* 30 (1988): 27–32; Monardes, *Joyfull Newes,* 1:xv.

73. Guerra, "Drugs from the Indies"; Talbot, "America and the European Drug Trade."

74. Huguette Chaunu and Pierre Chaunu, *Séville et l'Atlantique (1504–1650),* 8 vols. in 12 (Paris: A. Colin, 1955–59), vol. 5 (1956): 178–79, 256.

75. Richard W. Unger, "The Tonnage of Europe's Merchant Fleets, 1300–1800," *American Neptune* 52 (1992): 247–61.

76. W. Brulez, "Shipping Profits in the Early Modern Period," *Acta historiae neerlandicae* 14 (1981): 65–84; Ross Hassig, *Trade, Tribute, and Transportation: The Sixteenth-Century Political Economy of the Valley of Mexico* (Norman: University of Oklahoma Press, 1985).

77. Estes, "European Reception," 18.

78. Fernández-Carrión and Valverde, "Research Note"; Chaunu and Chaunu, *Séville et l'Atlantique,* vol. 7 (1957):142–43.

79. Douglas McManis, *European Impressions of the New England Coast, 1497–1620,* University of Chicago, Department of Geography, Research Paper 139 (Chicago: Department of Geography, University of Chicago, 1972), 1–147; Flückiger and Hanbury, *Pharmacographia,* 483–85.

80. David L. Cowen, "The British North American Colonies as a Source of Drugs," *Veröffentlichungen der Internationalen Gesellschaft für Geschichte der Pharmazie,* new ser., 28 (1966): 47–58; Wesley Frank Craven, *An Introduction to the History of Bermuda,* 2d ed. (Bermuda: Bermuda Maritime Museum Press, 1990), 86–89. See also Chabrán and Varey, "Hernández in the Netherlands and England," below.

81. José Luis Valverde and José A. Pérez Romero, *Drogas americanas en fuentes de escritores franciscanos y dominicos,* Estudios de la Cátedra de Historia de la Farmacia y Legislación Farmacéutica 8 (Granada: Universidad de Granada, 1988).

82. Estes, "European Reception," 19.

83. I am grateful for many kinds of help to Rafael Chabrán, John H. Elliott, Paul E. Hoffman, LaRue Johnson, Mary Rose Paradis, Richard Wolfe, and Virginia Steele Wood.

THE CONTRIBUTION OF HERNÁNDEZ TO EUROPEAN BOTANY AND MATERIA MEDICA

JOSÉ M. LÓPEZ PIÑERO

JOSÉ PARDO TOMÁS

The true character of the influence of the *Natural History of New Spain* has been distorted by a series of repeated errors and misconceptions about Francisco Hernández and his work. No one denies the exceptional importance of Hernández's expedition to Mexico, and yet it is a widely held—albeit erroneous—belief that the results of the expedition were scarcely circulated and that they were known only partially and long after the fact, even among the best informed. That such a belief can take hold at all suggests unawareness of the circumstances and the content of the printed texts that appeared in the first half of the seventeenth century, not to mention the important role played by those texts in the development of modern botany and materia medica.

The work of Nardo Antonio Recchi has generated all kinds of howls of protest, usually on the grounds that what Recchi did to the manuscript work of Hernández was deform it, when in truth all he did was make a selection, whose limitations we discuss later. Furthermore, the date of Recchi's selection is usually given as the date of publication (1651), well over half a century after the actual date of composition, which, as we shall see, was prior to March 1582.

Misconceptions about the circumstances surrounding the other printed texts of Hernández in the seventeenth century are also, unfortunately, common. In particular, the relationships between the *Quatro libros*, the Rome edition, and the 160 chapters included by Nieremberg in his *Historia naturae* have become confused. After a decade of research on Hernández, his texts, and his influence in Europe from the seventeenth century to the nineteenth, we have recently devoted an entire volume to a discussion of new materials and information about the *Natural History* and its influence on botanical and medical history.[1] In this essay we limit ourselves to an account of the material that is most directly relevant to the purpose of this volume.

The unearthing of a copy of the alphabetical index to Hernández's *Natural History* has enabled us to reconstruct the organization of the "second version" of the whole work, that is, the one that was presented to Philip II and deposited in the library of the Escorial. The extant manuscript copy of this index was made in 1626 by Andrés de los Reyes, then librarian of the Escorial, for Cassiano dal Pozzo, a member of the Accademia dei Lincei. That index, arranged according to Náhuatl etymology, can be compared in detail with the different printed texts (discussed by Rafael Chabrán and Simon Varey in the text volume) as well as the surviving drafts (discussed by Jesús Bustamante in the text volume), and the results are revealing. In the winter of 1575–76, hounded by repeated demands from King Philip, Hernández drew up a copy of his work on the natural history, which he was still in the process of expanding. He did not make a verbatim copy but instead revised the text carefully and thoughtfully, if not definitively, as he went along. This, the "second version," became a sixteen-book work, with a text of 893 pages and another 2,071 pages of paintings of plants. Afterward, Recchi used this copy to make his selection; it was then placed once again in the Escorial, where it was destroyed by the terrible fire in 1671. We have also been able to clear up the doubts that have lingered to this day about the survival or partial survival of the texts, by locating the manuscripts and herbaria that did survive the fire and subsequently gave rise to those doubts. We have found several direct copies of the paintings in the *Codex Pomar*, almost all with titles in Náhuatl and other Amerindian languages. The images include tobacco (*Nicotiana tabacum* L.), the mamey or Haitian zapote (*Lucuma domingensis* Gaertner), the quauhchchioalli or breast tree (*Rhus terebinthifolia* Schlecht and Ham.), the tozcuitlapilxochitl or "cana de cuentas" (*Canna indica* L.), the armadillo (*Dasypus novemcinctus*), the coyote (*Canis latrans*), and the bird of paradise (*Paradisa apoda*). The *Codex Pomar* was given by Philip II to Jaime Honorato Pomar, holder of the chair of "simples," or medical natural history, at the University of Valencia, the most important chair anywhere in the Hispanic world in the sixteenth century. Pomar was one of the king's principal counselors and in April 1598 was named royal botanist.[2]

On February 21, 1580, almost four years after the arrival of the texts that Hernández had sent from Mexico, and two and a half years after he himself had returned from his long stay there, the Neapolitan Nardo Antonio Recchi was commissioned by Philip to "consolidate and put in order" the contents of those volumes, "in order to make them useful and advantageous."[3] This charge was accompanied by Recchi's nomination to the same post of royal botanist that Pomar would fill later. The position included the responsibility of directing the planting and cultivation of medicinal plants in the royal gardens, among which Aranjuez stood out on account of its scientific orientation. Recchi was also required to teach botany to the physicians of the royal household and to supervise distilling, especially at the great laboratory at the Escorial.

The fact that Recchi was given the task of working with the *Natural History* when its author was still alive and residing in Madrid need not mean that Hernández had lost royal favor despite the major changes that had occurred at the court during his absence. In fact, Philip conferred honors on Hernández that show his continued esteem for him. The main reason was, without question, the serious deterioration of Hernández's health, which was also the reason that he had not prolonged his scientific expedition by going on to Peru as originally planned. In mid-1578 he was so close to dying that he made his will, but he overcame this crisis and lived another nine years, until January 28, 1587, even though, according to his children, he never enjoyed a single day's health.

Recchi's efforts are usually dismissed, unjustifiably, as nothing more than a "summary" or "compendium," whereas actually he made a selection, consisting almost exclusively of chapters from Hernández that needed editing; the intellectual criterion for selection was their medical usefulness. He introduced changes of minor importance, most frequently altering the internal order of individual chapters. Occasionally he deleted phrases, very rarely reduced the original chapter to a summary, and equally rarely added the odd phrase of his own usually referring to his observation in Spain of Mexican plants that Hernández had described. Of three new chapters, two deal with balsams that are not Mexican in origin and had already been described by González Fernández de Oviedo. Recchi did not adhere to the original arrangement of the *Natural History,* preferring the traditional Theophrastan categories of trees, shrubs, and herbs. Thus he eliminated at a stroke Hernández's taxonomic innovations, which were, as we shall see, based in part on Amerindian terminology. Just in terms of numbers, Recchi selected about four hundred plants, or about 12 percent of the whole work. He did include most of the descriptions of really outstanding value, although some important ones that he omitted became known in the seventeenth century only from the literal transcriptions of the relevant chapters in Nieremberg's *Historia naturae*.

Recchi is often accused of having taken his time completing the task of editing Hernández's work, but we can show that he finished the work before March 1582. Two letters from Juan de Herrera to Mateo Vázquez, the king's secretary, dated March 24 and May 5 enable us to chart Recchi's project precisely. Herrera warmly defended the project and urged that Recchi's selection of Hernández, which had just been finished, be published as soon as possible. Herrera supported his case by enclosing in one letter a copy of an engraving of the *ahoapatli* (*Galinsoga parviflora* Cavanilles), a plant that Hernández had described. A comparison between this engraving and the corresponding one that appeared in the Lincei's edition shows how much better the quality of engraving would have been if Hernández had been published the way Herrera wished. However, Herrera did not get his way, undoubtedly for economic reasons.

The Contributions of Hernández's *Natural History*

One of the main features of the *Natural History of New Spain* is that the work was conceived from the wide perspective of a natural historian and not just as a contribution to, or application of, materia medica. This explains why Hernández's approach was not primarily pharmacological, as was the case with Monardes, and also why he did not group his descriptions under therapeutic headings similar to those used by Monardes. Hernández's descriptions were based on firsthand observation, with the exception (which he duly noted) of some plants from Peru and the Philippines: his brief notes on these plants were based, he said, on reliable eyewitness accounts. The advanced nature of his version of the Renaissance concept of *experientia* is also manifested very clearly in the way he carried out his botanical research according to a very exact methodology. Hernández's work falls under the rubric of natural history according to the definition of the term during the sixteenth century, that is, the knowledge of nature from a descriptive point of view, in keeping with the meaning of *historia* from antiquity to the nineteenth century. Hernández belonged to a group of

Renaissance naturalists who began to introduce analytical elements into their work. In his case, these elements came mainly from new morphological approaches, which in some instances led Hernández, like other authors sharing the same tendency, to incipient attempts at experimentation.

Hernández's perspective as a natural historian led him to develop the categories of his *Natural History* according to purely botanical criteria. Underlying those categories is the unusual fact that he used Náhuatl names of plants as his taxonomic base, and to a lesser extent Tarascan and Otomí and even other native American languages that are not native to New Spain, such as Arawak and Taino. We should remember that at the beginning of the sixteenth century Otto Brunfels had coined the term *herbae nudae* for plants with no scientific name when he referred to species that were not included in Dioscorides' treatise. During the sixteenth century European botanists made numerous attempts to identify or at least relate these new species—some of them from the Americas—to those studied by Dioscorides and other classical authorities, such as Theophrastus and Pliny. Within this context, Hernández's description of more than three thousand Mexican plants signifies a clean break with the past. Just to get some idea of the vastness of this figure, we should note that Dioscorides' *Materia medica* includes about six hundred species and the medieval Islamic botany about five hundred. Existing European botanical terminology was thus not equipped to integrate a contribution of such enormous proportions, as Hernández was quick to point out throughout his work. Consequently he had to use native names as a principle of nomenclature for this work and his other efforts in taxonomy. In his commentary on Pliny's *Natural History*, Hernández commented with great amazement that of the "great number of herbs [from New Spain] almost none with a particular name remains unnamed or unidentified there."[4] Náhuatl botanical taxonomy, which was studied at the end of the past century by Paso y Troncoso and more systematically later, turns out to have been more advanced in some respects than European taxonomy of the same era.[5] Unlike contemporary writers of botanical treatises and those of the following century, among them Recchi and Ray, as we shall see later, Hernández rejected traditional categories as general organizing principles. Instead of trees, shrubs, and herbs, Hernández's taxonomic criteria consisted of native names or comparison of native plants with those of the Old World, or a combination of the two.

Comparison with European plants was limited to those plants that correspond to the order Euphilicales and the family Ciperaceae. Hernández combined native and European names for members of the Araceae, Urticaceae, Umbelliferae, and Labiadae and the genres Smilax and Croton. The remainder, including the most important ones, were categorized solely by their native names. These include the order Fungi, the families Orchidaceae, Moraceae, Leguminosae, Burseraceae, Cactaceae, Sapotaceae and Cucurbitae, and the genera *Agave, Euphorbia, Asclepia, Ipomoea, Arundo,* and *Pinus.* The category of Fungi included the "teyhointi seu fungus inebrians" (*Psilocibe mexicana* Hen.), whose hallucinogenic effects Hernández distinguished from those of the peyote. Yet vanilla (*Vanilla planifolia* Andr.) does not appear in the family of Orchidaceae, even though Hernández's description of it was the first ever written and was one of his most important contributions. It remained unrecognized even by such a specialist as Patiño, perhaps because Hernández referred to it by its Náhuatl name, "tlilxochitl," which also served as the relevant chapter title in his *Natural History.*

Let us look briefly at two of the most interesting examples of Hernández's categories, the Cactaceae and Solanaceae. To the Cactaceae Hernández devoted a series of fourteen chapters, all of which used the Arawak word *tuna,* while the Náhuatl terms *nopal* or *nochtli* occur in only six. The chapter entitled "nochtli or genus of tunas" is designed to "enumerate its distinct varieties, examine its properties, list the places and climates where it grows, when it should be planted, when it flowers and when it bears fruit." Its types are distinguished by differences among flowers, leaves, and fruits. Consequently, Hernández states that "in Mexico there are, as far as I know, seven species of tunas," which he describes, giving them their Náhuatl names.[6] One of them, "tzapo nochtli yztac," corresponds to the common prickly pear (*Opuntia ficus-indica* [L.] Mill.), and the other six refer to varieties of Opuntia and Cylindropuntia. At the end of the chapter he refers to "tetzihoactli" (*Cereus* sp.) and, in the other chapters, to other varieties of the genera cited and of *Aporocactus, Echinocactus, Epiphyllum, Mammillaria, Myr-*

tillocactus, and *Nopalxochia.* The botanical description and hallucinogenic effects of the *Anhalonium lewini* Hen., with the title "peyotl çacatensis seu radix mollis et lanuginosa" (with a pliant and downy root), are not included by Hernández in this series of chapters on Cactaceae but appear later in the *Natural History.*

Hernández arranged the Solanaceae in four groups. The first was a series of nine chapters, beginning with one entitled "tomatl seu planta acinosa" (berrylike plant). Based on his identification of "species of solano" native to the New World, his descriptions bring together some twenty-one different species of *Lycopersicum, Nicandra, Physalis, Saracha,* and *Solanum.* His treatment contrasts with the vague or erroneous information prevailing in seventeenth- and eighteenth-century Europe. In the first chapter of this series, besides explaining his conception of the group, he refers to "xitomame seu tomame magna" (*Lycopersicum esculentum* Mill.) and to several "tomames" which, among other varieties, correspond to *Physalis peruviana, P. pubescens,* and *P. philadelphica.* In the subsequent chapters Hernández finishes his survey with studies of other types of "tomatl" belonging to these genera. The second group, devoted to the genus *Capsicum,* comprises mainly the chilis, *Capsicum annuum* L. and its varieties—*longum* Sendt, *grossum* Sendt, and *cerasiforme* Mill., *violaceum* D.C., *frutescens* L., and its variety *baccatum* Ir. This important contribution clarifies another confused chapter in the history of sixteenth-century European botany, as the words *piper* and *pimienta* were then applied to the fruits of a wide range of plants, because of which the original Asian "peppers" came to subsume categories of Asian, African, and American species that actually belonged to different genera. Among the most widely circulated was Tabasco pepper or *xocoxochitl* (*Pimenta officinalis* Lindt.) described by Hernández.[7]

One long chapter may be considered a study of the Solanaceae, since it describes separately, pointing out their distinguishing characteristics, two species of *Nicotiana:* picietl (*Nicotiana rustica* L.) and "quauh yetl seu picietl montana" (*N. tabacum* L., wild tobacco). The last group of Solanaceae is spread over two chapters treating the species of Datura, one of which is stramonium (*Datura stramonium* L.). This plant was unknown in antiquity, but the traditional theory, based partly on a conflation of it with the *métel* (*Datura metel* L.), placed it on the shores of the Caspian Sea and had it coming into Europe during the early Middle Ages; however, between the wars first Safford and then Wein cleared up this confusion once and for all when they concluded that the stramonium is of Mexican origin and that it was introduced to Europe by way of Spain in about 1577.[8] This accords with the appearance of stramonium in the first of Hernández's two chapters, under its Náhuatl name, "tlapatl."

Yet, in the hundreds of chapters of the *Natural History* that treat species identified as Compositae, there are hardly any groups as important as those we have just described. The one chapter we might just mention is on "cempoalxochitl seu foliorum viginti flores," which discusses five species of *Tagetes* and one of *Zinnia*, the "pinks of the Indies."

As one might expect, one of the longest and most detailed chapters in Hernández's work is devoted to corn (*Zea mays* L.). The same is true of his discussion of "cacahoa quahuitl seu arbor cacahoatl," which deals with four types of cacao. "Cacahoa quahuitl," according to Miranda et al., corresponds to the varieties of *Theobroma cacao* L., and two of the others to the Mexican species of that genus: *Theobroma angustifolium* D.C. and *Theobroma color* H. & B. However, according to Sauer, the most commonly held view is that all cultivated cacao trees belong to the same species.[9]

Of course, a large part of the most outstanding contributions of the *Natural History* will not be found in taxonomic categories. But to those that we have mentioned already we may add those chapters relating to "epazotl" or "pazote" (*Chenopodium ambrosiodes* L.). The absence of any grouping of these chapters together does not prevent Hernández from making continual comparisons between the Mexican plants and similar ones native to Europe. For example, in addition to "epazotl" he treats three species of *Chenopodium*, each in a separate "book." He says that two of these are "species of wild armuelle," that is, like the *Chenopodium album* L. The third, he says, is similar to "our biengranada" (*Chenopodium botrys* L.).[10]

From a general perspective, it is interesting to note that Hernández describes practically every botanical species and

genus that N. I. Valivov, the great biologist and researcher of the origin and geographic distribution of cultivated plants, considered to be from Mexico and Central America.[11]

European Scientific Interest in Hernández's Work at the End of the Sixteenth Century

The importance of Hernández's expedition to New Spain is witnessed by the interest taken in his work by scientists from several European countries at the end of the sixteenth century. Their interest alone caused texts of Hernández to be published and disseminated during the early years of the next century and so encouraged the widespread welcome accorded the various editions of his work.

Spanish scientific interest in Hernández is well illustrated by three of Spain's foremost scientists, all of whom have been mentioned many times in these essays: the engineer and architect Juan de Herrera, the physician Francisco Valles, and the naturalist José Acosta. We have already mentioned Herrera's active role in early attempts to get Recchi's selection published. Valles was among the most important and influential physicians in Renaissance Europe, whose many books went through numerous editions all over the Continent. In one of them, first published in 1587, the year of Hernández's death, Valles spoke in general terms of the expedition to New Spain in connection with a discussion of royal gardens.[12] When Acosta mentioned the expedition in the second edition of his *Historia natural y moral de las Indias* (1590), he was much more explicit and detailed:

> Doctor *Francis Hernandes* hath made a goodly worke upon this subject, of *Indian* plants, liquors, and other phisicall things, by the Kings expresse commission and commaundement, causing all the plants at the *Indies* to be lively painted, which they say are above a thousand two hundred; and that the worke cost above three score thousand ducats: out of which worke the Doctor *Nardus Anthonius* an Italian Physitian hath made a curious extract, sending him to the foresaid bookes, that desires more exactly to knowe the plants at the *Indies*, especially for physicke.[13]

Acosta was much like Valles in scientific stature and influence. His summary of Hernández's activities in New Spain was the most widely disseminated of all the early notices, reprinted in twenty-five editions outside Spain and translated into German, French, English, Italian, Dutch, and Latin. In addition, the whole of Acosta's *Natural History* was plagiarized by Theodore de Brij, whose famous compilation suppressed the name of the author and presented Acosta's words as his own.

Contemporary interest in Hernández outside Spain falls roughly into two schools, headed by Ulisse Aldrovandi in Italy and Clusius in the Low Countries. The importance granted to American natural history in Italian scientific circles began soon after 1492, with the translation of the works by Peter Martyr, Fernández de Oviedo, Cieza de León, Francisco López de Gómara, Agustín de Zárate, and José Acosta. That interest never waned as these works were all repeatedly reprinted and absorbed by other naturalists throughout the sixteenth century.[14]

Aldrovandi stands out among Italians interested in American botany and materia medica, not only because of his far-reaching network of contacts but also because of his prominent role in the development of European studies in the field. His library and some of his surviving papers reflect his detailed knowledge of Spanish contributions to the subject. With the mediation of the Medici, Aldrovandi even attempted to get Philip II to arrange his travel to the West Indies. The most compelling evidence of his interest in the work of Hernández lies in the continual requests for information about Hernández scattered all over his personal correspondence. For example, on April 1, 1586, Aldrovandi wrote to Francesco de Medici, who, under the patronage of Philippo Segha, bishop of Piacenza, had been papal nuncio in Madrid when Hernández had returned from New Spain in 1577. Aldrovandi said he had heard that "in the court of King Philip [there was] a truly regal book with paintings of various plants and animals and other new things from the Indies," and he urged de Medici to appeal to his ambassador in Spain to help him obtain a copy.[15] It did not take Aldrovandi long to learn that Recchi had returned to Naples in 1589, and in no time he was writing to Giambattista della Porta requesting information about Hernández, which he did again twice in 1590.[16] Toward the end of 1595, Aldrovandi began his correspondence with Fabio Colonna,

who before becoming a member of the Accademia de Lincei (in 1603) was already well acquainted with the work of Hernández.[17] As we shall show, Colonna was in fact the first to publish any scientific information taken from Hernández. Later, Aldrovandi would enter into correspondence with Johannes Eck, a founding member of the Lincei and one of the people who traveled to Madrid with the specific intention of gaining access to the Hernández originals.[18]

It is well known that Clusius's *Rariorum aliquot stirpium per Hispanias observatarum historia* (1576) was the most important publication of the whole century on the flora of the Iberian Peninsula. Clusius gathered his materials on his travels around Spain in the 1560s, establishing in the meantime a number of important contacts with several Spanish naturalists. This was the beginning of a scientific collaboration that was to last for decades. Clusius had already translated Monardes into Latin and written commentaries on his work, as well as on García da Orta and Christopher Acosta, making all three of them accessible elsewhere in Europe. The main influence on Clusius's work on Iberian flora was Juan Plaza, predecessor of Pomar as holder of the chair of simples at the University of Valencia. Plaza's authority was provided by Guillaume Rondelet, who had taught Clusius at Montpellier. Clusius's book incorporated Plaza's observations on American as well as Mediterranean plants: the aguacate or avocado (*Persea americana* Mill.) and the *Agave atrovirens* Karw. In 1596 Clusius came into contact with the great naturalist Simon de Tovar, whose botanical garden in Seville was the first in Europe to have its own annual catalog of plants, the *Index horti Tovarici*. The catalogs were distributed to Tovar's correspondents in different countries, including the Dutchmen Beren ten Broeke (Bernardus Paludanus) and Karel van Aremberg. Tovar sent them full and exact descriptions of American plants, which Clusius translated and published. Clusius also obtained New and Old World botanical material from Juan de Castañeda of Seville and Francisco Holbecq, who worked in the great garden at Aranjuez. In his *Exoticorum libri decem* (1605), published at the end of his life, Clusius assembled in one book not only the "exotic" natural history that he had translated from Monardes, da Orta, and Acosta but also information received from his correspondents, Spanish and otherwise.[19]

The earliest reference to Hernández in Clusius's correspondence appears in January 1585 in an answer to a query from Joachim Camerarius of Nuremberg about "a work concerning exotic simples painted by the mandate and at the expense of the king of Spain." He replies that he has never heard of it but that "if such a work were to be published and was good enough, in the judgment of our friends, I would gladly get down to work translating it."[20] From then on, Clusius demonstrated a growing interest in Hernández. Early in 1597, Camerarius returned to the topic, this time in connection with what Colonna had told Clusius about it. Clusius said that his "old friend," the great scholar Benito Arias Montano, had retired to a small village outside Seville and could no longer help. But, Clusius went on, some acquaintances in Naples had told della Porta, who passed the news on to him, that they had seen a selection from Hernández in the home of Recchi.[21] Midway through that year, Ferrante Imperato, a correspondent in Naples, told Clusius of Recchi's death, but that did not stop him asking for more information about Hernández, with which Imperato obliged him in another letter early the following year.[22] It made sense that Clusius should also remain in contact with his correspondents in Seville, as he did until shortly before his death. However, neither Tovar nor Castañeda had any connections with the court, and they knew nothing about Hernández's work.[23]

Editions of Hernández in the First Half of the Seventeenth Century

As we stated above, the first information taken from the work of Hernández was published by Fabio Colonna even before he joined the Accademia dei Lincei, the group that would later edit and publish Recchi's selection of Hernández. In *Phytobasanos* (1592) Colonna mentioned a plant that Hernández had described, the "tlapatl" (*Datura stramonium* L.). Calling it "solanum manicum" and saying his information about it came from Recchi, "a most erudite physician of Philip II," Colonna then alluded to Recchi's selection, "which will be published by royal decree as soon as possible, thanks to the generosity of the monarch, by his mandate and at his expense."[24]

The first text of Hernández to be published was the *Index medicamentorum*, in which a list of Mexican plants that had been studied according to their therapeutic use was arranged in the order of parts of the body "from head to foot," as was customary at the time. This index appeared in a Spanish translation as an appendix to an important and fascinating medical treatise by Juan Barrios in 1607.[25] Barrios gave the index its title, which precisely explains its origin, and yet hypotheses have come thick and fast about why it is included in Barrios's book at all, one theory even suggesting that it had nothing whatever to do with Hernández. Even such accomplished scholars as García Icazbalceta and Somolinos dismissed it because of its content.[26] Surprisingly, until our own recent study of this topic, no one seems to have noticed the similarity between the Spanish text of the index printed by Barrios and the corresponding Latin index that appears at least once, sometimes twice, in the majority of extant copies of the Lincei's edition of Hernández. In contrast to Barrios, who explicitly attributed the index to Hernández, the Rome edition gives the impression that the index was compiled by Francesco Stelluti, who merely keyed the page references to the new edition.[27]

The first edition of Recchi's selection was also published, like this index, in Mexico City, eight years after Barrios. As we know, this was the *Quatro libros de la naturaleza y virtudes de las plantas y animales . . . en la Nueva España,* a Spanish translation made by a lay Dominican, Francisco Ximénez, from Aragón, who cared for the sick at the hospital in Huaxtepec. Hernández had worked at the same hospital during his time in central New Spain. Ximénez had obtained a copy of Recchi's manuscript, signed by Francisco Valles, which we now know had belonged to Barrios.[28] Detailed comparison of the text of the *Quatro libros* with other editions and with the surviving manuscripts helps to solve a number of mysteries.[29] When it is compared with the Rome edition, the differences are few but significant and revealing in the printing history of the *Natural History*. On the one hand, Ximénez included additions and commentaries, some of which were based on his own experience at the hospital at Huaxtepec, on his knowledge of the local flora there (and elsewhere), and on other authors who had written on the plants of the Americas, especially Oviedo,

Cárdenas, and Monardes. On the other hand, Ximénez's text omitted chapters that do figure in the Rome edition, the most important of which is the first text ever to deal with the tomato.[30] By relying solely on the text of the *Quatro libros,* Sauer made the mistake of saying that "it has been remarked repeatedly that Hernández in his description of the plants of Mexico did not include the tomato."[31] Even a glance at the Rome edition and at Nieremberg's *Historia naturae* would have put that error right.

From the beginning of the seventeenth century, Federico Cesi and the other founder members of the Accademia dei Lincei became aware of Hernández's work by way of two principal routes. The first and more important was via Naples, beginning with Cesi's residence there in 1603. The second route passed through the Escorial and examination of the original Hernández manuscripts deposited there. That work included the research and collaboration of Cassiano dal Pozzo, Johannes Eck, and Johannes Schreck (who took the name Terrentius). The gestation of the Lincei's project of publishing Hernández—not to mention the vicissitudes of the printing and distribution and the few copies mysteriously dated 1628, 1630—is far too complicated a subject to discuss here, but we might take note of several facets of the history of this edition that shed light on the diffusion of Hernández.

As we have noted above, Recchi took with him to Naples his selection of Hernández's work and copies of the paintings taken from the originals. Recchi's copies of the paintings were exhibited quite frequently in local scientific circles as well as for interested naturalists who visited from farther afield. In 1610, fifteen years after Recchi's death, Cesi bought the selection of texts from Recchi's heir, the legal scholar Marco Antonio Petilio. Cesi acquired the right to use, but apparently did not buy, the illustrations. The text of the *Natural History* edited by the Lincei scholars was Recchi's selection and is quite familiar now. However, it has escaped any critical notice that the treatises on animals and minerals were reproduced directly from Hernández's originals.

Once the texts were in Cesi's hands, he charged Terrentius with the task of writing commentaries and annotations, a labor that occupied him from September 1610 until the end of the following year. He wrote commentaries on about 60 percent of the chapters dealing with plants and on a smaller percentage of the texts on animals and minerals. He also wrote brief notes on more than three hundred illustrations (all plants) that were among the copies obtained by Recchi but that he had not selected and so lacked any corresponding text. The illustrations and commentaries were printed as an appendix entitled "Aliarum Novae Hispaniae Plantarum Nardi Antonii Recchi imagenes, et nomina Ioannis Terrentii Lyncei notatione."[32] Without altering in any way the contents and structure of Recchi's selection, Terrentius limited himself to complementing the descriptions with brief notes taken from other authors who had dealt with exotic botany or materia medica. Close to two-thirds of his citations come directly from Monardes or from Clusius's Latin translation, and most of the remainder come from Oviedo, da Orta, and Acosta, with occasional isolated references to other naturalists. The only obvious exceptions to this bookish commentary are seven mentions of plants that Terrentius had had the chance to see in the collection of Hendrik de Raaf and a few others he had seen thanks to his Jesuit connections.

Just as Terrentius was getting started on his commentaries, Johannes Faber was beginning to work on the zoology. If Herrera's efforts constituted the first attempt at botanical iconography of Hernández, the second was under way now, and Faber was in charge of that, too. Sixty-eight wood engravings of plants were printed in Rome in 1613 under the title *Mexicanarum plantarum imagenes,* dedicated to the bishop of Bamberg, Faber's birthplace, no doubt in the hope of obtaining financial assistance for the full edition. Faber continued his work until 1628, when the zoological part of the Hernández text and Faber's commentary appeared in print as *Animalia mexicana descriptionibus scholiisque exposita,* with its own title page, which was retained when the work was subsequently incorporated in the complete Rome edition of Hernández. In the same year Fabio Colonna finished his work, too, having written two hundred commentaries on many of the plants studied by Hernández. Colonna's essays were much more extensive and elaborate than those written by Terrentius. Colonna's solid background in natural history enabled these commentaries to become the first assimilation of Hernández's contributions in botany and materia medica in the seventeenth century.[33]

In the *Historia naturae*, Juan Eusebio Nieremberg included a large number of Hernández texts, among them 160 chapters from the *Natural History*, as well as five illustrations. Nieremberg taught natural history at the Imperial College in Madrid, so he naturally used the Hernández manuscripts that were among the college's collections.[34] Nevertheless, he also consulted the volumes at the Escorial, at least those containing the illustrations. As Somolinos points out, the five plant illustrations, as well as some that depict animals, show the native Mexican characteristics of the original drawings made during the expedition.[35] They are quite distinct from the Europeanized copies commissioned by Recchi, which served as the model for the Rome edition. Consequently, Nieremberg's engraver, Christopher Jegher, must have copied them from the volumes at the Escorial.

With rare exceptions, the Hernández texts selected by Nieremberg correspond to the precise descriptions of botanical species that have been identified with certainty. His selection includes a high percentage of the most important contributions to botanical science made by Hernández. Some chapters are dedicated to *tunas* and *piteras*, china root and sarsaparilla, tomatoes, chilis, squashes, legumes, and "pinks of the Indies." Others deal with important edible plants and foodstuffs, such as corn, cacao, sweet potatoes, yucca (or manioc), and fruits such as cherimoya, granadilla, capolin, Mexican espino, and so on. Still others describe medicinal remedies (balsam of Tolu, resins, purgatives), drugs (tobacco and coca), plants of ornamental value, and so forth. Although at 160 the total number of chapters selected by Nieremberg is far smaller than Recchi's selection, still there are thirty-seven chapters in Nieremberg that were not in the *Quatro libros* or the Rome edition, and another five whose illustrations appeared without any text in the Rome edition. Nieremberg also contains chapters on the different types of tomato, which, as we mentioned above, were not in the *Quatro libros*, as well as one, on "charapu" (*Sapindus saponaria* L.), that was not printed in the Rome edition. Some of Hernández's most outstanding work is to be found in chapters known only by means of Nieremberg's selection. Among these are the chapters on American

squashes, pinto beans, sweet potatoes, and bitter potatoes (*Ipomoea hederifolia* L.), yucca, granadilla, espino (*Crataegus mexicana* Moc. & Sessé), purgatives such as *Rumex mexicana* Meissn. and *Hura poliandra* Baill., two species of Ficus—*Canna indica* L. and *Musa textilis* Née. We should note that Nieremberg's work is the only place where Hernández's chapter on Mexican mushrooms can be found. Nieremberg also reproduced three chapters that were printed in the *Quatro libros* and the Rome edition yet were excluded from the Madrid edition of 1790 and the *Obras completas* (1959), in addition to some twenty chapters on plants of the Philippines and the Far East, which since his time have never found their way into print.[36]

The Assimilation of Hernández's Contributions in Early Modern Botany and Materia Medica

The assimilation of the contributions of the *Natural History* in Europe begins with the work of Johannes de Laet, a director of the Dutch West India Company, who used Hernández's work at practically the same time that Fabio Colonna was finishing his commentaries for the Rome edition and a little more than ten years after the publication of Francisco Ximénez's translation of Recchi's selection. Until de Laet, the first scientific and medical books printed in America had made barely any impact in Europe, but de Laet, by contrast, rushed to obtain a copy of the *Quatro libros* as soon as he heard about it. He then took full advantage of it, relying on it extensively for information about Mexican plants, which he had begun to include in the first Dutch edition of his book on the New World (1625). Selections from the *Quatro libros* were first added in the second Dutch edition (1630), then more in the Latin edition (1633), which was translated into French (1640). De Laet's work was the first in a long sequence of works that cited, summarized, or reproduced Hernández, all of them subsequently drawing on Nieremberg's *Historia naturae* and, after 1651, the Rome edition of Recchi's selection. Among the works that thus assimilated Hernández were the leading pre-Linnaean studies of botany and materia medica, such as Robert Morison's *Plantarum historia universalis oxoniensis* (1699) and Joseph Pitton de Tournefort's *Institutiones rei herbariae* (1700).[37]

However, among the works that demonstrate the importance of Hernández's contributions, John Ray's *Historia plantarum* (1686–1704) holds a special place, not just because of its importance generally in the history of botany but rather because of the emphasis that Ray placed on Hernández in various editions, summaries, and citations. In the bibliographical note that precedes the whole text, Ray referred to the Rome edition and to the "annotations and additions" of Colonna, yet he made no mention of the comparable notes by Terrentius, nor did he list numerous other works that he actually used as sources for Hernández, foremost among them de Laet and Nieremberg.

Ray reproduced in his treatise thirty-three whole chapters and twenty extracts taken from Hernández.[38] The texts of the chapters appear in full, except for the detailed information about the "temperaments" of the plants that followed the Galenic theory of "qualities" and a few other accessory details. The extracts are of varying length, ranging from an almost complete chapter to a mere paragraph on a specific aspect of a plant. Some of these chapters and extracts are arranged in groups with independent headings: thus ten chapters describing types of maguey are included under the general title "Aloes Americanae quaedam species e Fr. Hernandez historia," and eight chapters and two fragments, all taken from de Laet and Nieremberg, appear together under the heading "Arbores exotici e Jo. de Laet Descriptione Indiae Occidentalis et Nierembergii hist. Exot."[39] Occasionally, Ray restricts himself to keeping the original categories used by Hernández, as he does with the eight "differentiae" of *nochtli*. Ray clearly used his three Hernández sources with great care in order to complete his information. For example, in the chapter on the *capolín*, Ray followed the text of the Rome edition exactly, but he added a final paragraph on the various types of *capolín* (*Xitoma capolin, Helo capolin, Totocapolin*), which had been omitted by Recchi but included by Nieremberg. Ray even preserved Nieremberg's erroneous spelling of the third type, which he called *Tolacapolin*. Another demonstrable case is the reference to the "maripenda seu balsamiferus arbor III," in which Ray notes that de Laet's description of the plant comes from Hernández.[40]

At the end of his work, Ray offers fifteen pages of very small print under the heading "Compendium historiae

plantarum mexicanarum Francisci Hernandez," that is, a summary of the Rome edition of Recchi's selection.[41] After giving some general information based on the "first" book, he goes on to include chapters from books 2 to 4 in the same order as the Rome edition. He then continues with information from books 5 through 8, but in alphabetical order. This last section contains a summary of all the chapters except those that Ray had reproduced in whole or in part in the main body of his text. The compendium lacks any introduction, but Ray does justify the inclusion of this section with two brief statements, which serve as a colophon. The first is especially interesting: "Perhaps some may wonder to see that several new species of herbs not mentioned by others can be found in this work. Yet the reader will stop wondering if he will pause to consider, with me, that Francisco Hernández is the only person whose work brings together and describes the medicinal herbs that grow throughout New Spain: and besides, recorded travels, or general histories of America, include either flowers on account of their beauty or fragrance, or shrubs, roots, and other parts that people use for food."[42] The second text explains Ray's difficulties as he tried to use "Ad historia plantarum Francisci Hernandez illustrandam," because he could not situate "many kinds of species, owing to their brief and imperfect descriptions" in their proper categories, and thus he had decided to summarize them and include the "compendium" in his own work. He ingenuously adds, "A certain friend, whose opinion I esteem greatly, has pointed out to me that some would consider my *Historia* to be imperfect, if it did not contain species which have been made known by Hernández for the first time."[43] In addition, of the references included in this "compendium" and those in the "index," Ray cited in his text thirty-five descriptions from Hernández on plants and groups of plants. It is hardly necessary to say that these citations are sometimes accompanied by brief summaries that correspond to the species, which he was able to categorize according to his own classification in the fragments and chapters he reproduced.

Because of Ray's extraordinary influence on the subsequent development of botany, we should give here a brief general account of his selections from Hernández. The chapters whose texts are reproduced correspond first to the two principal categories of the *Natural History,* that is, the *Agave* and similar genera and the survey of the *tunas.* The others include some of the most important of all Hernández's contributions, such as those on vanilla, the pimiento of Tabasco, the purgative and bitter *batatas* (*Ipomoea jalapa* Pursh and *I. heterophylla* Ort.), the *epazotl,* the *dondiego de noche* (*Mirabilis jalapa* L.), the *capolín* (*Prunus capulli* Cav.), the "tiger flower" or *oceloxóchitl* (*Tigridia pavonia* Kerr.), the *espino* (*Crataegus mexicana* Moc. and Sessé), the *ciruelos* (*Cyrtocarpa edulis* [Brandt.] Standl. and *Spondias purpurea* L.), two species of ficus, the "ciprés de pantanos" (*Taxodium mucronatum* Ten.), the "brasil" (*Bocconea arborea* Watts), and so on. He also reproduced other chapters on species that were already known from excellent and widely disseminated descriptions, such as the "balsam of Peru," whose text he combined with that of Monardes. In the chapters that Ray partially edited, we find two Hernández categories: the section concerning the "claveles de Indias" and the series of sections on china root and the American sarsaparillas. Alongside these appears another group of Hernández contributions of the highest quality on cacao, corn, and the "nopal de la grana de Indias" (*Nopalea cochinifera* [L.] Salm.-Dyck.), as well as those descriptions of the various species that produce medicinal resins, or the "lignum nephriticum," which was famous at the time and which Ray identified as the *coatli* (*Eysenhardtia polystachia* D.C.). Ray also reproduced fragmentary texts from Hernández on plants from the Far East—or some that were not exclusively American in origin—among them ginger and the coconut tree and some from the New World that had been well known since the time of Fernández de Oviedo, including the tropical pineapple. In the references in his text, Ray included Hernández's category of plants that produce "copal" (*Elaphrium* or *Bursera*), which he subsequently incorporated at greater length in his "compendium." Ray also succeeded in classifying other descriptions of plants: the *granadilla,* the *anón,* manioc, the purgative *Jatropha curcas* L., the "hule" tree (*Castilla elastica* Cerv.), the *floripondio* (*Datura arborea* L.), the *Cassia occidentalis,* and others. Of course, by no means did he exhaust all the information that came from the *Natural History* and had been published by

his time. He even rejected three important Hernández contributions, on tomatoes, chilis, and tobacco.[44]

It would be impossible in this essay to cover the assimilation of Hernández by every botanist of the period. Instead, we shall limit ourselves to one case, an important and fundamental text of a stature in the history of pharmacotherapy similar to that of Ray's work in the history of botany: Etienne François Geoffroy's *Tractatus de materia medica.* This work was first published in Latin in three quarto volumes in 1741, ten years after its author's death. The most complete edition was in French, in seven octavo volumes, and appeared in 1743, reprinted in 1757. The section on European vegetable materia medica, which Geoffroy was unable to finish, was completed in three other volumes in 1750. The section on exotic vegetable materia medica (volumes 2 to 4 of the French edition of 1743) is structured according to the parts of the plants that were used in therapeutics. It is organized in nine long chapters, subdivided into "articles" dedicated to a species or a group of common species.[45] Hernández materials are used in the sections on American plants, except those dealing with cinchona (the source of quinine) and ipecac, described later, and the chapter on sassafras, well known since Monardes. Descriptions taken from Hernández include native American names and their Latin translations, among them the china root; the *contrayerva* (that is, the passionflower *Passiflora normalis* L.); the *cyperus americanus* or *souchet d'Amérique* (*Cyperus articulatus* L.); the purgative "mechoacanna alba" (*Convulvulus mechoacan* Vand.), which, he recalls, was introduced into Europe by Monardes; the New World sarsaparillas; guaiacum; nephritic wood, which Geoffroy identifies, as Ray did, with Hernández's *coatli;* the *Cassia grandis* L.; vanilla; allspice (Jamaica pepper); cacao; balsam of Peru; balsam of Tolu; American liquidambar; the resins copal, *caranna,* American dragon's blood, and *tecomahaca;* and the nopal of the "cochinelle." Two species from the East Indies are included here, too: ginger and "cassia caryophyllata" or "caninga" (*Myrtus caryophyllata* L.).[46]

Geoffroy uses the contributions from Hernández as if they were written by a contemporary author. He does not just allude to them but nearly always quotes them in full. For example, in his discussion of the four types of American sarsaparillas described by Hernández, Geoffroy refers not only to those belonging to the genus *Smilax* but also to those of the *Sapindácea Serjania mexicana* (L.) Willd. He also gives a great deal of attention to the four types of cacao.[47] An example of this kind of treatment is his article on nephritic wood: "Tournefort has been unable to describe [its flowers] because he has seen only dried specimens. Hernández says that they are a pale yellow, and that they are small, long, and in the form of a spike; the calyxes are all one piece divided into five parts, similar to a small basket and covered with a fine reddish fur."[48] In some cases, Geoffroy uses Hernández's descriptions in order to compare them with other people's, for example at the start of the article on vanilla: "This herb is similar to a 'centinodia' [*correhuela*], as Hernández states, which climbs up trees and surrounds them"—which is actually a paraphrase of Hernández—and then he goes on to deal with the "vanilla of the Island of Santo Domingo," adding, "It is certain that the vanilla of Santo Domingo is no different from that of Mexico, which was described by Hernández, save for the color of the flowers and the aroma of the pods since the Mexican flower is black and its pod has a pleasant aroma."[49]

The Continuation of Hernández's Work during the Eighteenth Century: The Spanish Botanical Expeditions to the Americas, especially New Spain

In the same decade that the French editions of Geoffroy were published, the influence of Hernández's work entered a new phase, which lasted for two hundred years in the development of modern botany and materia medica. The process of assimilation of Hernández's works that had begun with Ray culminated with Geoffroy. Hernández's *Natural History* served as a new point of departure for a continuation of his work on American, especially Mexican, flora, in accordance with the newly established approaches and techniques of classification. The beginnings of this new phase should be situated in relation to the work of Linnaeus, of course, as well as to the men responsible for organizing scientific activity in Spain during the eighteenth century. One of those men was Peter Löfling, Linnaeus's favorite student.

Linnaeus had agreed with Secretary of State José de Carvajal to initiate a scientific mission to study American plants, and Löfling arrived in Madrid in October 1751 to take charge of it. Having first established himself in the scientific circles at the court, and at Cadiz, Löfling began to study various aspects of the natural history of the Iberian Peninsula. In 1754 he was appointed botanist for the expedition to the zone of Cumaná and the mouth of the Orinoco; the whole expedition was directed by José de Iturriaga. In close collaboration with a team of artists, Löfling worked in this territory until his premature death in 1756. The collected graphic materials of this expedition were sent to the Royal Botanical Garden in Madrid, which had been founded the previous year. In the meantime, his manuscript, known as *Plantae hispanicae* and *Flora cumanensis*, together with letters addressed to his teacher, was edited by Linnaeus himself in 1758. The letters, with an introduction by Linnaeus, were translated into Spanish by the noted legal scholar and naturalist Ignacio Jordán de Asso and published between 1801 and 1802. These letters constitute the principal source for our knowledge of the importance that Löfling and Linnaeus alike recognized in the work of Hernández. Further evidence of Linnaeus's interest can be found in his monographs, especially the article, published in the Swedish Academy of Science's *Handlingar* in 1755, in which he identifies Hernandez's *atzoatl* as *Mirabilis longiflora*.[50]

During the first few weeks of his stay in Madrid, Löfling wrote to Linnaeus that he was going to "see an old herbarium which had been deposited in the Royal Library of the Escorial, which he believed had been collected by Dr. Hernández." This scrap of information must have interested Linnaeus because, in his next letter, he replied, "What you tell me about Hernández's herbal would be an excellent thing, if the Escorial holds herbs from the Indies under his name, but since those which are there are plants from the country [that is, Spain], I rather think that such information must be wrong."[51] Halfway through 1753, when Löfling was planning his voyage to America, he related to Linnaeus the substance of his conversations with the Marqués of Grimaldi: "I had said that it would be advantageous to go to Mexico, where Hernández had been . . . and then the Marqués told me that he had been of the same mind, and that part of the Hernández manuscript should still be in the Library of the Escorial, and that the other part should be in the Imperial College of Madrid, or at least that something could be salvaged from there. . . . If I have the opportunity to go to Peru, I will not lose hope of going to Mexico."[52] In October that year, on the eve of his departure, Löfling communicated to his teacher his concern that among the indispensable books he still "lacked Margraw and Hernández," but he was "confident that [he] would not leave without them"; and, sure enough, in December, writing from the Port of Santa María, he wrote that he "had already bought the Hernández in Madrid at a reasonable price" and that he would attempt to illustrate it as best he could.[53] When he was in Cumaná, in April 1754, he wrote that he had already complied with Linnaeus's charge about a plant described by Hernández: "I have been successful in obtaining in Mexico the curious tree *Malpalkochith Qualhuith Hern.* which you asked me to find. . . . I have made four copies of what is contained in the Hernández text about this tree, so that I may send it to different parts."[54] Up to the last moment he harbored the illusion of going to Mexico and "illustrating" the work of Hernández: "I have a branch, a flower, and a fruit that I want to send you, in case I do not get the opportunity to go back to the country where it grows."[55]

During the first decade of its existence, the Royal Botanical Garden in Madrid and the scientific activity that took place there were organized on the basis of Tournefort's system. José Quer, who was "principal professor" and director of the garden, was a disciple of Tournefort. In 1772, the directorship passed to Casimiro Gómez Ortega, whose tenure lasted until 1801. For thirty years, while he implemented the new Linnaean system, one of the most important aspects of his activity was to promote and centralize the administration of the great Spanish botanical expeditions to the Americas. These expeditions were headed, in general, by naturalists who had studied in the school that functioned as a part of the Botanical Garden. The first of these was the Royal Botanical Expedition to the New Kingdom of Granada, led by José Celestino Mutis, who had received his scientific training in the early years of the garden. In 1764, four years after his arrival in New Granada, he sent to Charles III a document in which he declared himself a fol-

lower of Linnaeus and added that he wished to continue the work of Löfling. That same year he sent a specimen of quina de Loja to Linnaeus, thus initiating a correspondence between the two that lasted until the great Swede's death in 1778, though Mutis prolonged it by corresponding with various of Linnaeus's disciples. The expedition to New Granada was officially organized under Mutis's direction in 1782 and functioned with great intensity until shortly before Mutis died, in 1805. One of the primary reference texts for the expedition was to be the Rome edition of Hernández.[56] Gómez Ortega himself had the responsibility of finding a copy to send to Lima in 1777, when his former disciples Hipólito Ruiz and José Antonio Pavón had been named directors of the Royal Botanical Expedition to the Kingdoms of Peru and Chile.[57]

By far the greatest and most direct influence of Hernández's work can be seen quite clearly in the third of these great undertakings, the Royal Botanical Expedition to New Spain. At the end of the 1760s, Juan Bautista Muñoz, "principal cosmographer of the Indies," found in the library of the Imperial College in Madrid "draft manuscripts by Hernández, revised and corrected in his own hand, and consisting of five volumes." As soon as a decision was taken to publish these papers, Casimiro Gómez Ortega took on its editorship. This publication, as we know, was printed in three volumes, although five were originally projected. The whole publication, a Latin text of the section on plants from the *Natural History,* was published in Madrid in 1790, and is always known as the Madrid edition.[58] Copies of the illustrations of the plants, which scholars hoped to find in Mexico and Italy, never turned up. In addition, it was necessary to complete, rearrange, and update Hernández's descriptions, and it was in this context that the physician Martin de Sessé stepped in. Sessé had traveled to America in 1780 and finally settled in Mexico City, where he was living when, in May 1785, he was appointed commissioner of the Royal Botanical Garden in Madrid—this after maintaining correspondence with Gómez Ortega. Three months later, he wrote a document to the viceroy Bernardo de Gálvez, in which he noted that "there is no need to lay the foundations" of Mexican natural history, because that had been done "during the last century by Dr. Francisco Hernández by a royal commission," and he went on to offer "to continue the said work of Dr. Hernández in the same language [and] order in which it was written." He undertook "to travel to those regions where exotic research and analysis" of plants and other natural products might take him. In this document he also proposed the foundation of a botanical garden in Mexico City and a chair of botany to be associated with it.[59] With a favorable report on the part of Gómez Ortega, a royal edict dated March 13, 1787, decreed that "a botanical garden be established in that capital [Mexico] and that an expedition begin which is to travel through the provinces in order to make drawings, collect natural products, and illustrate and complete the writings of Dr. Francisco Hernández."[60] A week later Sessé was named director of the expedition with a title that justified the undertaking:

> For the benefit of my service and the good of my subjects, who, following my royal decree which is taking place in the kingdoms of Peru and Santa Fe [New Granada], I command that the natural products of the most fertile dominions of New Spain be examined, illustrated, and methodically described, not only for the important and general purpose of advancing the progress of the physical sciences, of clarifying the doubts and adulterations which are found in the fields of medicine, tincture, and other useful arts, and to increase commerce, but also for the special purpose of filling in, illustrating and perfecting, given the present state of the natural sciences, the written original work which Dr. Francisco Hernández, protomédico of Philip II, left behind as the fruit of an expedition of a similar nature and one which was funded by that monarch.[61]

From 1788 to 1802 the expedition covered the central territories of New Spain, continued into more or less adjacent areas, from California to Guatemala, to Nutka on the west coast of present-day Canada, and to the islands of Cuba and Puerto Rico. Members of the expedition studied and collected more than fifteen hundred botanical species, half of which were unknown at the time to European naturalists. In a considerable number of cases, they noted the native name given to the species by Hernández, and in some they included the binomial term in accordance with the Linnaean classification system.[62] However, the expedition predictably went beyond the scope and limits of Hernández's work, in

quality and quantity. Still, it was an authentic continuation, expansion, and updating of Hernández, who, from that moment, became a classic author.[63]

Conclusion

The survival of Hernández's work as a classic continued to depend fundamentally on people devoted to botany and materia medica. Here we can note the eponymic homage paid to Hernandez, who had already had the genus *Hernandia* named after him by Plumier in his *Nova plantarum americanorum genera* (1703). Plumier similarly named *Ximenia* in honor of Francisco Ximénez, whose edition of Hernández, the *Quatro libros,* had been "recommended by Johannes de Laet in numerous places in his work on the New World."[64] More than a century later A. P. de Candolle gave the name *Opuntia hernandezi* to a species of cactus in his *Podromus systematis naturalis regni vegetabilis* (1824–73), a fundamental source of systematic botany.[65] Hernandez has a definite presence in treatises on materia medica, such as Tschirch's great *Handbuch der Pharmakognosie* (1909–27), which includes a detailed and rigorous account of the Hernandez manuscripts and editions from the first half of the seventeenth century. Reutter, too, in his *Traité de matière végétale* repeated this information and affirmed the importance of Hernández's work.[66] Finally Janzen (1967) emphasized that the first printed description and illustration on the relationship between one plant and a hymenopteran was that of Hernández on the "horns" of the *hoitzmamaxalli* (*Acacia cornigera* L.) produced by the *Pseudomyrmex ferruginea* F. Smith.[67] On the other hand, historical studies have never reached the level of Hernández's importance, unless we except some Mexican and Italian studies of the Rome edition, whose international circulation and renown have remained inadequate.

NOTES

1. See J. M. López Piñero and J. Pardo Tomás, *La influencia de Francisco Hernández (1515–1587) en la constitución de la botánica y la materia médica modernas* (Valencia: Instituto de Estudios Documentales e Históricos sobre la Ciencia, 1996).
2. See *Codex Pomar* and López Piñero, "The Pomar Codex."

3. Archivo General de Simancas, Quitaciones de Corte, bundle 35, February 21, 1580.

4. *OC* 5:425.

5. "La nomenclatura de los vegetales," *Anales del Museo Nacional de México* 3 (1886): 145–64. Also, Efrén del Pozo, "La botánica indígena de México," *Estudios de cultura náhuatl* 5 (1965): 57–73; Bernard Ortiz de Montellano, "¿Una clasificación botánica entre los nahuas?" in *Estado actual del conocimiento en plantas medicinales mexicanas,* ed. X. Lozoya (Mexico City: Instituto Mexicano para el Estudio de las Plantas Medicinales, 1976), 27–49. And J. M. López Piñero, "Francisco Hernández: la primera expedición científica a América," in *Medicinas, drogas,* 197–315.

6. *Mexican Treasury,* MB (see list of abbreviations in that volume) 3.15.

7. See María José López Terrada, "Hernández and Spanish Painting," below.

8. Quoted by Paul Fournier, *Le livre des plantes médicinales et vénéneuses de France,* 3 vols. (Paris: P. Lechevalier, 1947–48), 3:455, summarized by P. Font Quer, *El Dioscórides renovado,* 8th ed. (1962; Barcelona: Labor, 1980), 597.

9. F. Miranda et al., *Francisco Hernández: Historia de las plantas de Nueva España* (Mexico City: Imprenta Universitaria, 1942–46) 3:908. C. O. Sauer, "Cultivated Plants of South and Central America," in *Handbook of South American Indians,* ed. J. Steward (New York: Cooper, 1963), 6:539.

10. For commentary on Hernández's taxonomic criteria, see our *Nuevos materiales,* esp. 48–57; our *Influencia* includes a detailed analysis of the question.

11. N. I. Valivov, *Origin and Geography of Cultivated Plants* (Cambridge: Cambridge University Press, 1992), 207–23.

12. Francisco Valles, *De iis quae scripta sunt physice in libros sacros sive de sacra philosophia,* 2d ed. (Lyon, 1592), 588. (The first edition was published in Lyon, 1587.) See J. M. López Piñero and F. Calero, *Las "Controversias" (1556) de Francisco Valles y la medicina renacentista* (Madrid: CSIC, 1988).

13. 1590 ed., p. 267; we quote from the first English edition, *The Naturall and Morall Historie of the East and West Indies* (London, 1604), bk. 4, chap. 29, p. 290. See J. M. López Piñero and M. L. López Terrada, "Las plantas en la *Historia natural y moral de las Indias* de Jose de Acosta," in *La influencia española en la introducción en Europa de las plantas americanas (1493–1623)* (Valencia: Instituto de Estudios Documentales e Históricos sobre la Ciencia, 1997), 126–35.

14. See J. Pardo Tomás, "Obras españolas sobre historia natural y materia médica americanas en la Italia del siglo XVI," *Asclepio* 43 (1991): 51–94.

15. "Le lettere di Ulisse Aldrovandi a Francesco I e Ferdinando II," ed. O. Mattirolo, *Memoria della Reale Accademia delle Scienze di Torino,* 2d ser., 54 (1904): 353–401.

16. See Giuseppe Gabrielli, *Contributi alla storia dell'Accademia dei Lincei* (Rome: Accademia Nazionale dei Lincei, 1989), 731–34.

17. Ibid., 1518.

18. Ibid., 1084–87.

19. F. W. T. Hunger, *Charles de l'Ecluse (Carolus Clusius) Nederlandsch Kruidkundige, 1526–1609* (The Hague: Nijhoff, 1927), and José M. López Piñero, *La "Historia medicinal de las cosas que se traen de nuestras Indias Occidentales" (1565–1574), de Nicolas Monardes* (Madrid: Ministerio de Sanidad y Consumo, 1989).

20. Clusius to Camerarius, Vienna, January 31, 1585, in Hunger, *Charles de l'Ecluse,* 2:404.

21. Hunger, *Charles de l'Ecluse,* 2:447–48.

22. Imperato to Clusius, Naples, August 8, 1597, in *Clarorum hispaniensium atque exteriorum epistolae,* ed. Ignacio Jordán de Asso (Saragossa: Typographia Regia, 1793), 101. Recchi had by this time been dead two years.

23. The letters of Tovar and Castañeda to Clusius appear in Jordán de Asso, *Clarorum hispaniensium,* 41–51, 53–69. For a detailed study of the descriptions and materials that Tovar and Castañeda sent to Clusius, see J. M. López Piñero and M. L. López Terrada, "Las plantas americanas en relacion de Clusius con los naturalistas españoles," in *La influencia española,* 66–103.

24. Fabio Colonna, *Phytobasanos sive plantarum aliquot historia* (Naples, 1592), 50. The second edition was published in Milan in 1744.

25. Juan Barrios, *Verdadera medicina, cirugía y astrología* (Mexico City, 1607). The appendix is separately, and erratically, foliated, fols. 59r–69v. Cf. *Mexican Treasury, Index medicamentorum,* for Barrios's translation of Hernández and for López's translation of a corresponding text.

26. J. García Icazbalceta, *Bibliografía mexicana del siglo XVI* (Mexico City: Fondo de Cultura Económica, 1954), 239; Somolinos, "Vida y obra," 404–5.

27. See our *Nuevos materiales,* 103–17.

28. Barrios said, probably in 1609, that he owned the manuscript signed by Valles. He is quoted in Antonio de Leon Pinelo, *Question moral si el chocolate quebranta el ayuno eclesiastico* (Madrid, 1636).

29. See the discussion by G. Gándara, "La obra de fray Francisco Ximénez comparada con la del doctor Francisco Hernández recompuesta por el Dr. Nardo Antonio Recco," *Memorias y revista de la Sociedad Científica Antonio Alzate* 39 (1921): 99–120.

30. See *Nuevos materiales,* 119–27.

31. Sauer, "Cultivated Plants," 521.

32. *T* 345–55.

33. *Nuevos materiales,* 133–43.

34. Book 14 of Nieremberg's *Historia naturae* contains 58 chapters from Hernández (pp. 294–334); book 15 contains another 102 (pp. 335–72). For a selection of these, translated into English, see *Mexican Treasury.*

35. "Sobre la iconografía botánica original de las obras de Hernández y su sustitución en las europeas," *Revista de la Sociedad Mexicana de Historia Natural* 15 (1954): 73–86.

36. *Nuevos materiales,* 129–32.

37. See Rafael Chabrán and Simon Varey, "Hernández in the Netherlands and England," below. In *La influencia* we discuss in detail the Hernández material incorporated in the works of Ray, Tournefort, and their European contemporaries.

38. John Ray, *Historia plantarum,* 3 vols. (London, 1686–1704), 196, 292, 343, 399, 655–57, 728–29, 1165, 1200–1201, 1249–50, 1314, 1330–33, 1356–59, 1397, 1463–65, 1507, 1540, 1647, 1670–71, 1685–86, 1757–59, 1771, 1789–93, 1804, 1846–48, 1856, 1884. The three volumes are continuously paginated.

39. Ibid., 1200–1201, 1789–94.

40. Ibid., 1550, 1759.

41. Ibid., 1929–43.

42. Ibid., 1943.

43. Ibid., 1943, and see the comments on Ray by Chabrán and Varey, "Hernández in the Netherlands and England," below.

44. *Nuevos materiales,* 145–53.

45. Étienne François Geoffroy, *Traité de la matière médicale . . . Traité des végétaux. Section I. Des médicamens exotiques,* 7 vols. (Paris, 1743).

46. Ibid., 2:59, 62, 84, 176, 229, 300, 392, 410; 3:152, 178, 206, 261, 386, 390, 401; 4:1, 34, 82, 103, 478.

47. Ibid., 2:229; 3:261.

48. Ibid., 2:412.

49. Ibid., 3:179.

50. Peter Löfling, "Observaciones de historia natural hechas en España y América," translated from the Swedish by Ignacio de Asso, *Anales de ciencias naturales* 3 (1801–2): 3:278–315; 4:155–91, 324–39; 5:82–104, 297–340. See Linnaeus, "Mirabilis longiflora," *K. Svenska Vetenskapakademie Handlingar* 16 (1755): 176–79.

51. Löfling, "Observaciones," 4:159, 163.

52. Ibid., 5:99–100.

53. Ibid., 5:316, 326. "Margraw" means Georg Marcgraf: for his selections from Hernández, see *Mexican Treasury*.

54. "Observaciones," 5:337. The tree is *macpalxochitl quahuitl,* or *Chiranthodendron pentadactylon* Larr.

55. Ibid., 5:337.

56. See A. F. Gredilla, *Biografía de José Celestino Mutis* (Madrid: Junta de Ampliación de Estudios, 1911), and E. Pérez Arbeláez, *José Celestino Mutis y la real expedición botánica del Nuevo Reino de Granada* (Bogotá: Autares, 1967).

57. Arthur Robert Steele, *Flowers for the King: The Expedition of Ruiz and Pavon and the "Flora of Peru"* (Durham, N.C.: Duke University Press, 1964), 59.

58. *Opera* (Madrid, 1790), and see Somolinos, "Vida y obra," 329–53, and Jesús Bustamante, "The *Natural History of New Spain,*" in *Mexican Treasury*.

59. Petition from Sessé to the viceroy Gálvez, Mexico City, August 10, 1785, in J. C. Arias Divito, *Las expediciones científicas españolas durante el siglo XVIII: Expedición Botánica de Nueva España* (Madrid: Cultura Hispánica, 1968), 337–38.

60. Royal decree, March 13, 1787, in Arias, *Expediciones,* 340–41.

61. Certificate issued to Sessé, March 20, 1787, in Arias, *Expediciones,* 341–42.

62. To take one representative example, the "coztomatl" of Hernández corresponds to *Physalis coztomatl* Moc. & Sessé ex Dunn. See J. Valdés and H. Flores, "Historia de las plantas de la Nueva España," *OC* 7:7–222.

63. However, in the first half of the nineteenth century, Hernández's findings were still being used in connection with specific American plants. An obvious case is the standard reference work of the period, F. V. Mérat and A. J. de Lens, *Dictionnaire universel de la matière médicale* (Paris: Baillère, 1829–47), for instance, on the subject of varieties of smilax (6:378).

64. C. Plumier, *Nova plantarum americanarum genera* (Paris, 1703), 6–7.

65. A. P. Candolle and A. L. P. de Candolle, ed. *Prodromus systematis naturalis regni vegetabilis* (Paris: Fortin, Treuttel & Wurtz-Masson, 1824–73), 3:474.

66. A. W. O. Tschirch, *Handbuch der Pharmakognosie* (Leipzig: Tauchnitz, 1909–27), vol. 1 part 1, 757–59. L. Reutter, *Traité de matière végétale* (Paris: Baillière, 1923), 13.

67. D. H. Janzen, "Interaction of the Bull's-horn Acacia (*Acacia cornigera* L.) with an Ant Inhabitant (*Pseudonmyrmex ferruginea* F. Smith) in Eastern Mexico," *University of Kansas Science Bulletin* 67 (1967): 315–58.

HERNÁNDEZ IN THE NETHERLANDS AND ENGLAND

RAFAEL CHABRÁN

SIMON VAREY

One of the most surprising developments in the dissemination of the work of Hernández was its appearance in the Netherlands in the 1630s and in England toward the end of the seventeenth century. We discuss the manuscript and printing history in the text volume, and although that aspect of the history is really inseparable from the movement of the plants themselves, we try to avoid repeating ourselves as we attempt in this essay to show how Hernández was used as an authority in the places in northern Europe where botanical and medical research made use of plants that are native to Mexico.

The connection between Hernández and the Low Countries originated with the Botanical Garden at the University of Leiden. Toward the end of his life Clusius showed an interest in Hernández and a willingness to translate him, but he seems not to have gone any further than that. After Dirk Cluyt's great catalog of the plants cultivated at Leiden (1594), Peter Paaw's updated revision (1601) adds considerably to the sum of our knowledge of Leiden's holdings (including aloe, five species of asphodel, balsam, three varieties of calendula, *Datura indorum,* and dozens of varieties of ranunculus).[1] A further revised catalog appeared in 1668,

and when the accomplished Paul Hermann was supervisor of the Leiden garden, he produced yet another catalog that is just as important.[2] Hermann's authorities include Fabio Colonna's essay in the Rome edition of Hernández, and although his list does not name Recchi, it does include Hernández by name, without a date. He obviously used the Rome edition, as anyone would expect by 1687, for by then the Rome edition had become the editio princeps of Hernández. Hermann's principal authorities for nomenclature are Jean Bauhin and Robert Morison.

In addition to affording us occasional insights into the transportation of plants between countries, Hermann's catalog is most valuable in general for what it says about Leiden and the advanced state of northern European botanical studies. Extremely useful, too, for what it says about Hernández, the catalog provides evidence that at least thirty Mexican plants were being cultivated in Leiden in Hermann's time and that Hernández was the principal authority, sometimes the only one, who described them. Of course, in an indirect way, this was another means of disseminating the work of Hernández, not by way of reprinting or editing his texts but by using them as the scientific base for identification, weaving him into the fabric of everyday study. The same procedure had begun in Paris, where a specimen of *Datura stramonium* is said to have come from Hernández himself, as early as 1601.[3] By 1613 the bishop's garden at Eichstätt certainly grew a few Mexican plants, such as tobacco, *Papaver spinosum,* and *Opuntia ficus-indica,* though whether or not anyone there had read any Hernández manuscripts at the time is unknown.[4] The same sort of thing would happen, as we shall see later, in England.

Hermann relied on Hernández and others for six entries in his catalog.[5] Two more could not be definitely identified by reference to Hernández, but for fourteen species and their multiple varieties, Hernández was Hermann's sole authority. Hermann's use of Hernández illustrates the status of Hernández and the Rome edition in the Netherlands in the later seventeenth century. Hermann shows that at Leiden the *Thesaurus* was being used as an encyclopedic reference work should be used. Mexican plants are still cultivated at Leiden's Hortus Botanicus: four varieties of *Agave,* two of *Beaucarnea, Nolina longifolia,* and many varieties of *Passiflora* are all on public view today. Without Hernández, Europeans would not have known what the specimens were. Without Johannes de Laet, they would not have known very much about the geography of the Americas.[6]

As we explain in some detail in our text volume, de Laet was instrumental in publishing Hernández texts, but as far as we know he had little or nothing to do with the distribution of seeds or specimens. The same is true of Georg Marcgraf, whose work on Brazilian natural history was posthumously decoded and edited by de Laet in 1648. Willem Piso did send specimens back to Leiden from Brazil, which may have been transplanted in the University Botanical Garden.[7]

We should also take notice here, if only briefly, of the Groningen family of Munting, in particular the work of Abraham Munting, who is described in our text volume and whose citations of Hernández appear among our texts. But it is not only for citations of the Hernández texts that Munting matters to us. He also tells us occasionally how he came by a particular plant: for example, a specimen of *Arundo americana striata,* "of which my father, Hendrick Munting, was sent the first specimen from Paris in the year 1640, by Mr. Robin, who had himself obtained it from the Caribbean

Islands. All the other examples that can now be found in the Netherlands came from this one specimen."[8] Clearly, Munting came across other Mexican plants, not necessarily associated with Hernández at all, among the more surprising being the datura (in Dutch) or stramonium (Latin) or "nux metella" as well as the more familiar opuntia. Further evidence that the acquisition of specimens was unglamorous and haphazard is that Munting got his specimen of the opuntia, or *Indiaanse doornappel* (Indian thorn apple, *Pomum spinosum opuntiatum*) from a ship's captain, Henrik Barendsz, in 1654.[9] Just as Clusius once bought a handful of beans from a French ship's captain returning from Brazil, Hermann (and others) no doubt received specimens in these unspectacular ways, too.[10]

The Muntings were "moderns," as the designs of the engraved plates of the *Naauwkeurige Beschrijving* demonstrate. Compared with most of their contemporaries in the Netherlands, they were internationally minded pioneers of new scientific systems of taxonomy and nomenclature.[11] Abraham Munting's citations from Hernández in 1696 do not quite mark the end of Dutch interest in Hernández, but it is the last time that Hernández appeared in print in the Netherlands until late in the eighteenth century, when Arnout Vosmaer included a description of the bison, based on the Rome edition of Hernández, in his *Natuurkundige Beschrijving eener uitmuntende verzameling van zeldzame gedierten, bestaande in Oost- en Westindische viervoetige dieren, vogelen en slangen* (Amsterdam, 1766–72). Each animal in this delightfully personal book of exotic quadrupeds, birds, and snakes has its own dated title page and pagination: the bison is dated 1772, and there Vosmaer cites Hernández ("Hist. Mex. p. 587 & Hist. Nov. Hisp. p. 10") as his authority.[12] For his description of a rattlesnake (1768) Vosmaer cites Marcgraf, Piso, and Nieremberg, which in fact means that he was referring to Hernández.

———

English interest in Hernández, like the Dutch, has remained an entirely unexplored subject until now. We have discovered manuscript evidence of considerable English interest in Hernández, as well as printed English translations of some 150 selections from the *Natural History of New Spain* that have remained for the most part unnoticed since their first publication, between 1659 and 1752. These texts are represented in our text volume.

As we explain in our text volume, Robert Lovell's *Pambotanologia* (1659) listed ninety-five Mexican drugs, all taken directly from Hernández. Lovell's book appears to have had little or no impact in its field, in the sense that it attracted virtually no contemporary comment (not even dismissal), so that it is hard to speak of a contribution by Lovell to any genuine dissemination of knowledge about the medicinal plants of New Spain. Yet Lovell's work warranted a second edition, which is not a mere reissue but a new book whose whole text was reset: a publisher would not go to that trouble and expense for a title that was not selling. The extremely slim bibliographic evidence therefore suggests that the audience for Lovell's book was most likely popular, not academic. That in turn suggests that drugs made from East and West Indian plants were perhaps not such exotic rarities as we might suppose.

If Lovell had any colleagues at Oxford, even any friends with similar interests, we have found no evidence of them. Lovell seems to have worked in isolation. The Oxford University Botanical Garden may well have owned the relevant texts of Hernández that enabled Lovell to do his own research, but we have not been able to determine this. The Oxford garden certainly did cultivate a significant number of Mexican plants, and its leading botanists knew the Rome edition of Hernández, which was easy to obtain in the mid-seventeenth century, unlike the *Quatro libros*. The garden's first and second catalogs of plants offer ample proof, although, as always, identification of specific plants is problematic. Jacob Bobart the elder's anonymous *Catalogus plantarum horti botanici Oxoniensis* (Oxford, 1648) and its revision by his son, Jacob Bobart the younger, Philip Stephens, and William Brown, *Catalogus horti botanici Oxoniensis* (Oxford, 1658), listed sixteen hundred plants, including hundreds of exotics in alphabetical order of their Latin names, with English equivalents, which makes tracing plants by their Náhuatl names difficult, but they do include Hernández as an authority. Both editions of the Oxford catalog demonstrate that Mexican plants were being cultivated at Oxford, but unlike Paul Hermann's equivalent work at Leiden, they do not tell us specifically how much use they

made of Hernández, or any other source for that matter.[13] Stephens and Brown added an English translation of their Latin preface, in which they defiantly declare:

> We chearfully undertook this work being moved by the solicitations of students in Physick & lovers of plants... being confident it will not be only an ornament but of use also to the true Physitian.
>
> But if any one be puffed up with a vain perswasion of his own abilities, and shall think because he hath the title of Doctor he may be as idle as he please, and slight the study of Simples let him (if he will take so much paines) read the life of *Fernelius*, and the Epistles of *Bauhine*, *Lobell*, *Mathiolus*, and *Fuchsius* that he may know that we have reason to be of another mind. (190)

Thus, at least we know that they felt there was a growing rift between medicine and botany in England. That was 1658. By the end of the seventeenth century, as we shall see, there was, if anything, a closer relationship between the two.

Two much better known Britons, contemporary with Lovell, were also working with the texts of Hernández: Robert Morison and John Ray. Morison's scheme of classification was based on a clear, and indeed pioneering, concept of genus, species, and family. In his major posthumous work, the *Plantarum historiae universalis oxoniensis*,[14] Morison listed Hernández and Recchi, "who composed [plural] the Mexican history," as well as Acosta, Monardes, Marcgráf, Piso, da Orta, Laguna, Fragoso, and Amatus as his Iberian authorities.[15] His list of assistants and authorities, especially northern Europeans, is enormous. Morison's use of Hernández is mainly as an identification authority, along with many others. He seldom quotes Hernández (or Recchi), and if he does, it is usually a brief citation designed to show the physical characteristics of a plant.

A personality in sharp contrast to the vainglorious Morison was one of England's finest botanists, a truly generous man of principle, and one of the most formidable intellects of his time: John Ray, whose first botanical work, his table of plants, had promptly been attacked in print by Morison.[16] Although Ray never visited Spain, one of his companions on the early tour to the Low Countries and Italy did. The ornithologist and ichthyographer Francis Willughby wrote a brief account of his travels in the Iberian Peninsula.[17] Willughby's narrative is largely unrevealing of anything that might cast light on Hernández, but references to Mexican birds and Hernández's identifications of them scattered throughout Ray's correspondence with Willughby and Hans Sloane show that the men in Ray's circle habitually used Hernández as a source of reference.

In the *Historia plantarum*, which appeared in two volumes (London, 1686–88, with a reissue of volume 2 in 1693) and a supplement (London, 1704), Ray's purpose was to produce a rational, ordered classification. Hernández is one of dozens of authorities to appear throughout volumes 1 and 2. De Laet and Nieremberg are much in evidence as well. In volume 3 (pp. 1929–35) appears Ray's appendix, entitled "Compendium historiae plantarum mexicanorum Francisci Hernandez," consisting of a terse summary of the Rome edition, book by book, chapter by chapter, which is followed by an index in alphabetical order of all the remaining Mexican plants from the Rome edition. As Ray himself says in a note between these two sections, the summary of books 2–4 of the Rome edition consists of trees and shrubs in the order in which they appear, and the remaining plants, all herbs, are arranged alphabetically. That alphabetical arrangement suits Ray's concept of classification, while the entire appendix devoted to Hernández is the only one of its kind devoted to anyone. There is no doubt that Ray accorded Hernández a kind of special treatment, or a special place, in the botanical classification that he was seeking to establish. Not everything in the appendix appears scattered through the text proper of Ray's *Historia plantarum*, however. In the main body of the text, the plants whose descriptions are attributed to Hernández tend to be those that were more familiar by this time in northern Europe. We have no recorded evidence of Ray's criteria for exclusion of any plant from the text proper, though one of his two paragraphs at the end of the appendix makes his attitude to the sheer novelty and uniqueness of the work of Hernández quite clear: "Perhaps some may wonder to see that several new species of herbs not mentioned by others can be found in this work. Yet the reader will stop wondering if he will pause to consider, with me, that Francisco Hernández is the only person whose work brings together and describes the medicinal herbs that grow throughout New Spain: and besides, recorded travels, or general histories of America, include either flowers on account of their beauty or fragrance, or shrubs, roots, and other parts that people use for food."[18]

In the appendix itself, the summaries of books 2–4 give alternative names, very brief botanical features, and the basic therapeutic application, all in two or three lines, usually. There is no mention of the kind of terrain where any of these plants grow or any mention of their humoral nature. The alphabetical index of herbs pays less attention generally to applications, sometimes omitting them altogether, and thus appears on the whole to be of more use and more interest to the pure botanist, the gardener, or collector rather than the physician.

The appendix concludes with Ray's judgment of Hernández, in which he acknowledges that some of the descriptions are obscure because they are so short and obviously imperfect, and then mentions the advice of a trusted friend, probably Sloane, who suggested that Ray's work would be considered defective if it lacked those species newly brought to light by Hernández. Ray decided to incorporate them in this summary form, rather than attempt to edit imperfect texts. In some cases Piso and Marcgraf are the recognized authorities on American plants. Ultimately, Ray's is a statement of recognition that there is still a vast amount of work to be done identifying American plants and that if Hernández was unable (sometimes) to cast any light on specific plants, then Ray was certainly not about to volunteer to do a better job.

While Ray was seeking to organize the chaotic and inchoate science of botany, the proximate cause of early English interest in Hernández, de Laet, Nieremberg, Cárdenas, Colmenero, and Acosta is easy to ascertain: Jamaica. In 1655, desiring to compete with Spanish colonizing efforts in the Caribbean, and probably just as eager to busy giddy minds with foreign quarrels, Oliver Cromwell initiated the quasi-military fiasco in which inadequately armed English troops were outnumbered in guerrilla warfare for four years before finally taking control of the island of Jamaica. The immediate political benefit to Cromwell himself never materialized, because he died in 1658, but the benefit to sugar and cocoa merchants was, for the next thirteen years, immense. In 1671, close to the time that the Escorial was ablaze, a hurricane swept through the island of Jamaica, wiping out most of the cacao "walks," as the plantations were known. Those that were replanted did not mature until well into the eighteenth century.[19]

Jamaica also became a haven for British botanists, entomologists, and natural historians, who began to explore the island's rich resources. Once a steady supply of cacao began to come to England, chocolate began to be manufactured and consumed on a commercial scale, and those scientists began to read the work of Spanish physicians, naturalists, scientists, and travelers, who had encountered many Jamaican species elsewhere in New Spain, especially Mexico. Two early works on chocolate in English date from this period: those by John Chamberlayne and Henry Stubbe (discussed and represented in our text volume). For this reason, as well as uncomplicated intellectual curiosity, the work of Hernández became one of the obvious places in which to look for information about Jamaican plants that were common to Mexico.

The Natural History of Jamaica, published in two lavish volumes in 1707 and 1725, remains a treasury of valuable information to this day. Its author, Sir Hans Sloane, has a rather ill-deserved place in the history of medicine as an entrepreneur and facilitator, partly because he was not a prolific writer and is thus seen as an underachiever who did not fulfill his promise. This is a slight to Sloane's learning, which is amply demonstrated on every page of his work on Jamaica. His modern reputation also undervalues his extraordinary role at the center of his own circle of affinity in London. Just by being at the center of such a circle, Sloane advanced the twin causes of botany and medicine, because he was able to distribute information and opinions to correspondents in all parts of the British Isles, as well as to others elsewhere in Europe. He not only exchanged specimens but also cheerfully sought out and bought books for friends and acquaintances who had difficulty tracking down rare titles; he was also a great giver of presentation copies of his own books.[20]

Dr. Richard Richardson, a physician in Yorkshire, asked Sloane to locate rare books for him: among the few books that Sloane did *not* buy was Stubbe's *Indian Nectar,* which he said in 1731 was "not to be found."[21] Richardson also wanted a copy of Colonna's *Phytobasanos,* which Sloane did succeed in finding for him, saying, "Fabius Columna I could not get till a week ago; it is not a fair copy, but the book is one of the scarcest in Botany."[22] As he painstakingly compiled the *Natural History of Jamaica,* Sloane, a gifted linguist, translated from the recognized Spanish sources and from Nieremberg, de Laet, Piso, and Marcgraf where relevant, and he incorporated forty-eight extracts from Hernández, together with comments on the accuracy or inaccuracy of the illustrations or the descriptions. A selection of these appears in our text volume. With healthy and pragmatic skepticism, volume 1 (1707) and volume 2 (1725) of Sloane's *Natural History of Jamaica* made available in English significant portions of Hernández of most interest to English botanists, physicians, apothecaries, settlers, merchants, and consumers. Like the brief excerpts cited and translated by Stubbe, Sloane's more substantial translations have eluded the attention of Hernández scholars despite the renown of Sloane's work and its dissemination all over Europe.

Sloane had already begun to amass the largest single collection of medical and botanical materials that perhaps any individual has ever attempted to create—but then, he was a multimillionaire.[23] He was also as generous in searching for specimens as he was in looking for books for people who could not gain easy access to suppliers.

———

Although the long-term therapeutic use and value of plants from the Americas may have faded during the nineteenth century, their impact on European pharmacopoeia was immense both when Hernández was writing and, little more than a century later, when Sloane was reading him. Every day the English could read about the commodities produced by Jamaica for consumption in England: cacao, indigo, cotton, sugar, and

> DRUGS, which this Island produces in great abundance, as, *Guiacum, China-roots, Sarsaparilla, Cassia-Fistula, Tamerinds, Vinello's* [i.e., vanilla] and *Achiots* or *Anetto,* which is like to prove a good Commodity. There are also divers sorts of
> GUMS and *Roots* wherewith experienced Planters cure divers Wounds, Ulcers, and other Maladies; as, *Aloes, Benjamin,* and the like: And by the report of an intelligent *Physician,* who made it his business to enquire and

search after such things, there is likewise *Cyperas, Contrayerva, Adjunctum nigrum, Cucumis agrestis, Sumach, Acacia, Mistleto*, with many other *Drugs, Balsams* and *Gums*, whose Names and Virtues are not known or remembred. However the Planters begin every year to be better and better acquainted with their Nature and Use, and endeavour to encrease them in order to their supplying *England* with them.[24]

Without English interest in Jamaica at the dawn of the early modern period, the medical botany of the Spanish Renaissance in Mexico would probably never have made any inroads at all into England. At the levels of diplomacy and warfare, colonial expansion and imperial ambition, politics made this particular kind of cultural import (hardly an interaction, as England returned little to either Mexico or Spain at the time) a reality.[25]

Hernández was not alone, of course, in making his particular botanical and medical knowledge available to Europe, even if it was not eventually made available in the way he had wanted to organize it, but he was nonetheless the presiding authority, though again not the only one, on the medicinal plants of Mexico. Monardes was still considered important, but Hernández can be seen profitably in the context of the other Spanish medical writers working and writing in Mexico at much the same time. The work of such men as Agustín Farfán and Alonso López de Hinojosos did not overlap much with that of Hernández, but instead of accompanying his studies in their fitful dissemination across northern Europe, the work of these two was almost totally neglected and remained unknown to all but the devoted specialist.[26] The obvious reason for neglect was pragmatic. Stressing the practical aspects of his botanical survey, Sloane anticipated his critics:

It may be objected, that 'tis to no purpose to any in these Parts of the World [i.e., England], to look after such Herbs, &c. because we never see them; I answer, that many of them and their several Parts have been brought over, and are used in Medicines every day, and more may, to the great Advantage of Physicians and Patients, were People inquisitive enough to look after them. The Plants themselves have been likewise brought over, planted, and throve very well at Moyra, in Ireland, by the Direction of Sir Arthur Rawdon; as also by the Order of the Right Reverend Dr. Henry Compton, Bishop of London, at Fulham; at Chelsea by Mr. Doudy; and Enfield by the Reverend Dr. Robert Uvedale; and in the Botanic Gardens of Amsterdam, Leyden, Leipsic, Upsal, &c. but especially at Badminton in Glocester-shire, where they are not only rais'd some few handfuls high, but come to Perfection, flower and produce their ripe Fruits, even to my Admiration; and that, by the Direction of her Grace the Duchess of Beaufort, who at her leisure Hours, from her more serious Affairs, has taken the pleasure to command the raising of Plants in her Garden, where, by means of Stoves and Infirmaries, many of them have come to greater Perfection, than in any Part of Europe.[27]

We shall introduce Compton, Doody, Uvedale, and the Duchess of Beaufort shortly. Although it may come as a surprise to see American plants being cultivated by three botanists in and around London, it should be more striking that Sloane omitted Oxford from the list of places where botanical gardens had been established. Stubbe and Chamberlayne, both Oxford men, do not make an appearance in Sloane's work, either (and Barrios qualifies for only one line).[28] Stubbe, Chamberlayne, and Sloane (who was the youngest of the three) appear to have had nothing in common and to have known nothing of one another's work.[29] With the obvious exception of cacao, nothing from Hernández selected by Sloane is to be found in the work of Stubbe or Chamberlayne. Except for tobacco, there is no passage in Lovell that is duplicated in Sloane, and he does not mention cacao, so that between 1659 and 1725 these four writers, quite independent of one another, produced more than 150 selections from Hernández in English, with almost no overlap. Sloane's omission of Colmenero, Chamberlayne, and Stubbe from the text proper of the *Natural History of Jamaica* seems to confirm that there was no continuous tradition at Oxford, or at any rate none of which Sloane cared to be cognizant.[30]

Sloane rarely specified the particular plants grown by the people he names in the preface to volume 2, though other sources confirm that this is the beginning of general evidence of possibly the most unexpected legacy of Francisco Hernández. Some of the Mexican plants he described were being cultivated in the inhospitable climate of northern Europe about 150 years after he wrote his great work. We would not wish to claim that Hernández was somehow responsible for their cultivation anywhere but Spain, where, according to a stubbornly persistent myth, Hernández was supposed to have introduced tobacco in 1559 (he did nothing of the sort).[31] But the fact that Sloane was so interested in the work of Hernández tells us conveniently what some scattered sources also record, that drugs derived from Mexican plants were being manufactured, on the scale of a cottage industry (there being no other kind) in England in the early modern period.[32]

The reason that the drugs made from plants that grow in distant places were desirable at all is clear from a loaded commentary by the greatest of Anglo-Irish politicians and orators, Edmund Burke, as he looked back on the Renaissance as "an extraordinary coincidence of events at the time that the discovery of America made one of the principal; the invention of printing, the making of gunpowder, the improvement of navigation, the revival of ancient learning, and the reformation; all of these conspired to change the face of Europe entirely."[33] When Burke came to generalize about Mexican medical practice, he declared:

> Their physicians generally treat [patients], in whatever disorder, in the same way. That is, they first enclose them in a narrow cabbin, in the midst of which is a stone red hot; on this they throw water until the patient is well soaked with the warm vapour, and his own sweat; then they hurry him from the bagnio, and plunge him suddenly into the next river. This is repeated as often as they judge necessary; and by this method, extraordinary cures are sometimes performed. But it frequently happens too, that this rude method kills the patient in the very operation, especially in the new disorders brought to them from Europe; and it is partly owing to this manner of proceeding, that the small pox has proved so much more fatal to them than to us. It must not be denied that they have the use of some specifics of wonderful efficacy; the power of which they however attribute to the magical ceremonies with which they are constantly administered. And it is remarkable, that purely by an application of herbs they frequently cure wounds, that with us refuse to yield to the most judicious methods.[34]

The rational British had found that there were "alternative" medicines, starting probably with tobacco. Of course, tobacco had not come to England from Mexico, but William Coles wrote in 1657 that tobacco had been successfully cultivated in Gloucestershire and that the only reason it was no longer grown there was the bureaucracy of taxation. Tobacco might be smoked for pleasure, but one would never know it from Coles's solemn (yet typical) description of the application of the green juice of the leaves as a cure for fresh wounds and old sores. And as early as 1657, Coles knew the Náhuatl word for tobacco, *picietl,* which barely suggests that tobacco smoked in England was not all best-quality Virginia.[35] Guaiacum, ginger, china root, and sarsaparilla were among the other common plants used for medicines in England, as Johannes Renodaeus and his English translator, Richard Tomlinson, noted, lumping them all together as cures for the French pox under the general heading "Exotical Calefactives."[36] A commercially manufactured drink called sarsaparilla (later, sasparilla) with only the vaguest medicinal claims attached to it was probably not made from the root described by Hernández, nor, presumably, was its purpose the same when it was on offer to small children in "one of those pungent herb shops" in Manchester in the 1920s remembered by Anthony Burgess.[37] If sarsaparilla provides a false continuity to the twentieth century, the same cannot be said of tobacco, ginger, chili, cacao, and a host of other plants, which have remained in northern European cultures, long after they ceased to be considered drugs. Their impact is not on pharmacopoeia but on food, both of which, we should remember, are more likely to be considered two aspects of the same thing in Michoacán than they are in Middlesex.

———

Several other English people, including those named by Sloane, were involved with the cultivation of Mexican plants. Space forbids a full exploration of them all, so we must be content with a summary.

A now obscure amateur botanist, James Newton (1639–1718), left at his death an unfinished manuscript of a book published by his son as *The Complete Herbal* in 1752. Newton's book contains, as an appendix, *Enchyridion Universale Plantarum: or, An Universal and Complete History of Plants, with Their Icons, in a Manual,* with several extracts from Hernández (which appear in our text volume). It was probably this Newton who was looking for a copy of the Rome edition of Hernández in the 1680s. On August 7, 1685, an English student named George London wrote a letter from the Netherlands addressed jointly to "Dr. Plukenet, Dr. Newton, Mr. Doodie." London had been viewing plants and buying books. He found a copy of Piso for only eight guilders, and for Newton he bought a copy of Munting, adding—remarkably—"for Rechiis, here is not one to be had."[38] It was in 1698 that Newton read a hilarious paper to the Royal Society on the effects of overindulgence in the roots of the horned poppy, but he was not in public view much longer.[39] Newton was quietly cultivating exotics, though how many of them were Mexican we cannot say.

There is no doubting that some Mexican plants had become popular, if not yet altogether fashionable, in England by the early eighteenth century. A professional gardener and commercial florist in London, Thomas Fairchild, wrote of "aloes and torch-thistles" as "yet little known in *London*," although he mentions that "many sorts of Aloes . . . do very well in *London*."[40] Fairchild had much to say about the success of a grower named Jobber who had cultivated numerous species of aloe in London, and Fairchild recommended them as ornamental plants that "add an extraordinary Gaiety" to a room if they are placed on a mantelpiece.[41]

Samuel Doody (1656–1706), mentioned by Sloane as one of the Englishmen who grew American exotics, was a botanist who took over his father's apothecary business in London in 1696. Doody was "memorable for having been the first who extended the *cryptogamous* class."[42] He was appointed head of the Chelsea Physic Garden (discussed below) in 1693 and elected a fellow of the Royal Society in 1695. There is a manuscript list, which seems to be in his hand, of American plants extracted from Ray's *Historia,* and although he turns up in the correspondence of this whole English circle, we know very little more about him.[43]

James Petiver (1663–1718) was a botanist, entomologist, and apothecary. A fellow of the Royal Society from 1695 and quite distinguished in his day, Petiver was a good friend of Ray's and Sloane's. In fact, when Petiver went to the Netherlands in 1711, it was because he had been charged by Sloane with the task of buying Paul Hermann's museum.[44] Petiver's role in English work with connections to Hernández occurs mostly in his capacity as apothecary, because he was always on the lookout for new ingredients to incorporate in his medications, and as a result of these interests he owned a formidable library.[45] Petiver was the author of several works, including the very rare *Hortus Peruvianus Medicinalis: or, The South-Sea Herbal* (London, 1715), which is quoted in our text volume. As we explain in the text volume, Petiver's annotations of the 1658 Piso/Marcgraf and particularly of Nieremberg's *Historia naturae* reveal his interest in Hernández, in the service of his efforts to make and market drugs.

The garden at Badminton in Gloucestershire, in the west of England, is a place that still attracts tourists and amateur botanists. In Sloane's time, the Duchess of Beaufort (d. 1714) assembled a collection of exotic plants that was simply extraordinary: Sloane said her collection of West Indian plants was the best outside the West Indies.[46] The duchess kept an annual catalog of plants, which Sloane later acquired—of course—but despite Sloane's implication when mentioning her name in his *Jamaica,* she seems not to have relied on Hernández much for identification.[47]

Henry Compton (1632–1713) was a major player in England's religious and theological (which meant political) controversies in the 1680s. In 1686 he retired to his garden at Fulham (southwest London), where he cultivated exotics. He himself did not write any published account of his plants, but Petiver later owned a manuscript that he called "Codex Comptoniensis," which has disappeared. According to Richard Pulteney, "Compton obtained most of his rare plants from correspondents in North America."[48] Ray mentions fifteen specimens of Compton's, and in 1751 Sir William Watson described another thirty-three in an address to the Royal Society.[49]

Robert Uvedale (1642–1722) was well known in his own day as the headmaster of the Grammar School at Enfield, north of London.[50] It is not for his abilities as a schoolteacher but as the creator of a botanical garden there that he is known today, if he is known at all, among specialists in the history of botany.[51] A brief note on Uvedale's garden, dated January 26, 1691, described his priorities: "Dr. *Uvedale of Enfield* is a great lover of plants, and having an extraordinary art in managing them, is become master of the greatest and choicest collection of exotic greens that is perhaps any where in this land. His greens take up six or seven houses or roomsteads. . . . But, to speak of his garden in the whole, it does not lie fine to please the eye, his delight and care lying more in the ordering particular plants, than in the pleasing view and form of his garden."[52]

Uvedale certainly knew the other men in Ray's circle: from the fairly extensive surviving correspondence with Sloane we know that the author presented him with a copy of *The Natural History of Jamaica*,[53] and we know, too, that Uvedale corresponded with Petiver. In January 1699 Uvedale sent a package of 215 minerals and therapeutic plants, all from Siam, to Petiver and Sloane, a practice he would repeat from time to time.[54] Uvedale was in correspondence in this way with several botanists and doctors, including the Duchess of Beaufort, Leonard Plukenet, William Sherard, Caspar Commelin, Hermann, Tournefort, and Magnol on isolated occasions, and Peter Hotton, Ray's "singular friend" who was professor of botany at Leiden.[55] Thus Uvedale's garden at Enfield became well stocked with exotics from all over the world, particularly from India, China, and the West Indies. Uvedale is most interesting for being a part of that European circle of botanists and medical men who so generously shared their knowledge and their specimens with one another; he is also important as one who collected and distributed "a few West Indians [that is, plants] from the Continent."[56] At some time he sent to Richard Richardson six varieties of aloe (though they may have been African rather than American), an opuntia, and a yucca.

Fortunately, Uvedale's fourteen-volume herbarium has survived, like many of his contemporaries', and also like most of them, his was acquired by Sloane. Among the plants preserved in it are many that apparently came from Virginia and at least two that, at the time, could not have done so: the *Solanum mexicanum flore magno* C. B. and *Nasturtium indicum maximum odoratum scandens* (*Tropaeleum majus* ?L).[57] He also had a specimen of *Papaver spinosum*, which is native to Mexico.[58]

Leonard Plukenet (1642–1706) owned a garden in Westminster and a farm in Hertfordshire and set out ambitiously to compile one continuous description (in as many volumes as he needed) of plants from all over the world. He

succeeded in publishing enough botanical works to get himself appointed by Queen Mary as "Queen's botanist," which meant, in practice, superintendent of the royal gardens at Hampton Court. Even though he could be a quarrelsome man, and he later sharply criticized some of the entries in Sloane's *Catalogus*, Plukenet nonetheless was an able botanist who assisted Ray in arranging volume 2 of the *Historia plantarum*, in which Ray referred to him as "a learned man, whose knowledge of plants is second to none."[59] Among Plukenet's many books, the *Phytographia*, with its baffling organization, is the one that shows, in a minor key, his acquaintance with Hernández. The cumulative evidence of all these botanists, whether professional or amateur, is that they needed Hernández as their authority on Mexican plants.

———

At the center of the Chelsea Physic Garden in southwest London stands a statue of the greatest benefactor in the institution's history. It is no surprise that the benefactor was Sir Hans Sloane. The garden was founded by the Society of Apothecaries in 1673, at a time when, according to one amiable historian of the place, the average Londoner's knowledge of botany was less than that of a caveman.[60] In London, the apothecaries, who prepared remedies from spices, leaves, and roots, were separate from the grocers, who imported, stocked, and sold those ingredients. Further, the apothecaries were serenely convinced that physicians knew nothing about drugs—at least, this was later said on their behalf by a member of the House of Lords during a debate.[61] This meant war. It also meant, a little surprisingly, that the Chelsea garden was devoted to the study of botany rather than medicine. But when the Society of Apothecaries ran into financial difficulties in 1721, Sloane, who had recently bought the manor of Chelsea, bailed it out by leasing to the society the land that included the garden at the low annual rent of £5, on condition that the society should give samples of its medicinal plants to the Chelsea Hospital. In other words, whatever his immediate and pragmatic motive may have been, Sloane shifted the emphasis of the garden from botany to medicine.

The effect of this shift can be seen in two published lists. The more important of them is the catalog of the medicinal ingredients stored in the Hall of the Society of Apothecaries, that is, ready to be prepared and dispensed as drugs. It includes scores of American, particularly Mexican, ingredients. The other published work that casts a little light on the activities at Chelsea, though less revealing than this list, is the later catalog of the society's library, which shows, in the somewhat fragmented form in which it has come down to us since the vicissitudes of the nineteenth century, that botany and medicine had indeed become blended into virtually one science and that American plants were likely to be as familiar as any other exotics to the scientists at Chelsea.

The evidence suggests that American and Mexican plants could be studied by the Society of Apothecaries without direct reference to Hernández, yet all the significant works that made use of Hernández during the corresponding period, from de Laet to Sloane, were there in the society's library. This foreshadowed a pattern that would develop everywhere, for Hernández had in fact begun to be absorbed into English writing about American plants and into English study of them on the ground in all probability.

As in the Netherlands, so too in England, Hernández's encyclopedic work was used in piecemeal fashion by people with particular interests in certain parts of it. The desultory appearances of Hernández's writings in northern Europe demonstrate the apparent paradox of the Renaissance doctor's work becoming absorbed in a world trying to adapt to recognizably "modern" changes. Yet it is not so paradoxical really: Spanish and English colonizing efforts in the Caribbean and Mexico, mutually hostile and competitive, meant that the colonizers gradually acquired a common stock of knowledge, which brought their cultures closer together intellectually without generating or requiring any concomitant political, economic, or diplomatic bond. That Hernández had not been superseded by anyone, Spanish or otherwise, may mean no more than that Renaissance botanical classification took longer than most other branches of intellectual pursuit to be redefined and reorganized: it was, after all, still waiting for Linnaeus.

Ultimately, Hernández did not disappear from English horizons, for the appearance of the Madrid edition in 1790 meant at least that English libraries could make a new purchase, which, with the notable exception of the British

Museum, they did. Major scientific, botanical, and national collections in Britain all owned either the Madrid edition or the Rome edition, or both, by about 1825, as their published catalogs witness. Gradually, Hernández's name drops out of printed English discourse, but his words remain, sometimes attributed to his anthologizers, sometimes not. One picturesque example occurs in a footnote to Erasmus Darwin's extraordinary poem *The Botanick Garden*: "Mancinella. l. 188. Hippomane. With the milky juice of this tree the Indians poison their arrows; the dew-drops which fall from it are so caustic as to blister the skin, and produce dangerous ulcers; whence many have found their death by sleeping under its shade."[62] These words will be familiar to anyone who knows Sloane: "They are most pernicious to People lying in their Shade, their whole Bodies swell, their Eyes and Eyelids being most estreamly so, as if they had been burnt, if by Chance any of the Dew touch the Flesh, it burns wherever it falls, as if it was *Aqua Fortis*. . . . The Indians poison their Arrows with this Fruit . . . *Xim*."[63] Darwin's is not an exact transcription by any means, but it is good evidence of how the Hernández text as printed by Ximénez in the *Quatro libros* has been condensed, edited, and paraphrased yet still retains its core. Even in a note to an eccentric poem on botany, Hernández was still able to make an anonymous appearance in England, and even in anonymity, he was at the forefront of an adventitious movement that took Mexican plants, or their exact equivalents from North American territories, to England. When we ourselves were even younger than we are now, a British author, Alexander Nelson, was compiling a standard textbook on medical botany. In various parts of it he lists and describes the medicinal plants that were in use in the British pharmacy at the time of writing, 1951. The point of Nelson's book is to indicate the botanical ingredients of pharmaceuticals that were commonly manufactured in Britain at midcentury, not, in the main, as simples but in compounds. Some of those ingredients might still raise a few British eyebrows: pineapple, tomatoes, avocado, coconut oil, papaya, and so forth. But many will be quite familiar to anyone who has studied Hernández: *Datura stramonium* (for asthma), sarsaparilla, canela (Mexican cinnamon), sassafras, numerous aloes, copals, and balsams (including balsam of Tolu), guaiacum, cassia fistula, cacao, peppers, and euphorbias.[64] Nelson was a pragmatist, not a historian, so he was not concerned with identifying Hernández or anybody else as his authority, but really, by then, Hernández did not need to be cited as an authority any more, because his descriptions were the basis of observation and application; in short, Hernández provided all that anyone needed on Mexican medical botany, and his authority had passed into the unquestionable authority of tradition.

NOTES

1. Peter Paaw, *Hortus publicus Academiae Lugduno-Batavae* (Leiden, 1601). The British Library copy (988 e 10) was owned by eighteenth-century England's premier gardener, Philip Miller, and later by Sir Joseph Banks. The moving force behind the institution of Kew Gardens, Banks owned nearly all the seventeenth-century botanical works we discuss in this essay. José M. López Piñero and José Pardo Tomás discuss Clusius in "Contribution of Hernández," above. Clusius's posthumous *Histoire des drogues, espiceries, et de certains medicamens simples, qui naissent e's Indes & en l'Amérique* (Lyon, 1619) draws on Monardes, da Orta, Christopher Acosta, and López de Gomara, but never Hernández.

2. Florentius Schuyl, *Catalogus plantarum horti academici Lugduno Batavi* (Leiden, 1668); Hermann, *Horti Academici Lugduno-Batavi catalogus* (Leiden, 1687).

3. Pierre Delaveau, *Histoire et renouveau des plantes médicinales* (Paris: A. Michel, 1982), 138–39. Delaveau says that the datura was quickly cultivated "dans tous les jardins botaniques," which presumably means those in France. "On le signale," he adds, "à Blois dans le jardin de Gaston d'Orléans, en 1653." French gardens certainly did grow American plants: Guy de la Brosse listed at least four dozen in his *Description du Iardin Royal des plantes medicinales* (Paris, 1636). In connection with large numbers of exotic plants (Blois claimed to have twenty-three hundred), Antoine Schnapper warns that "these figures must be treated with caution, for the distinction between species and variety was still vague" ("Gardens and Plant Collections in France and Italy in the Seventeenth Century," *The Architecture of Western Gardens: A Design History from the Renaissance to the Present Day*, ed. Monique Mosser and Georges Teyssot [Cambridge: MIT Press, 1991], 175).

4. See Nicolas Barker, *Hortus Eystettensis: The Bishop's Garden and Besler's Magnificent Book* (London: British Library, 1994), plates 55, 69, 72, 73.

5. The "others" named here include Christopher Acosta, Jan Huygen van Linschoten, Jacob Bondt, Willem Piso, and Jean and Caspar Bauhin, the foremost classification authorities of the day.

6. For de Laet, see our introductory essay, "The Hernández Texts," in *Mexican Treasury*.

7. The best account of this Brazilian expedition is P. J. P. Whitehead and M. Boeseman, *A Portrait of Dutch Seventeenth Century Brazil: Animals, Plants, and People by the Artists of Johan Maurits of Nassau* (Amsterdam, North-Holland Publishing Co., 1989).

8. Abraham Munting, *Naauwkeurige Beschrijving der Aardgewassen* (Utrecht, 1696), 367. Hindrick (or Hendrick) Munting compiled the *Hortus, et Universae Materiae Medicae Gazophylacium* (Groningen, 1646).

9. Munting, *Naauwkeurige Beschrijving*, 541–42, 573, 575.

10. F. W. T. Hunger, *Charles de l'Ecluse (Carolus Clusius) Nederlandsch Kruidkundige, 1526–1609* (The Hague: Nijhoff, 1927), 142, and Johannes Theunisz, *Carolus Clusius, het merkwaardige leven van een pionier der wetenschap* (Amsterdam: Kampen, 1939), 77. Apparently Clusius obtained some notes and information from the captain and promptly incorporated them at the last moment in the second edition of his Latin translation of Monardes. James Petiver, whom we shall meet later, established an extensive network of acquaintances "amongst seafaring men," in order to acquire specimens (Edward Edwards, *Lives of the Founders of the British Museum* [London: Trübner, 1870], 301).

11. Probably more typical of its time was Jan van Beverwijk's *Schat der Ongesontheyt, ofte Genees-konste van de Sieckten* (Dordrecht, 1649), whose second part is an eclectic mix of classical and contemporary authors, all enlisted in support of the curative properties of native Dutch plants. It is a scholarly book, though not in any sense pathbreaking, and it does give French and Latin (and, very occasionally, Spanish) names of plants in addition to the Dutch.

12. The references are to the Rome edition, specifically to Faber's commentary in the scholia (587) and to the separately paginated *Historia animalium* (10).

13. We should emphasize that many of the plants that are "Mexican" are widespread in the Americas and by no means unique to Mexico. Hence, William Coys (whose garden at Stubbers in Essex had a large number of Spanish plants, incidentally) is credited with being the first person to cultivate the yucca in England, which flowered in 1604, but, like his other "American novelties," his specimen came from Virginia, not Mexico. See R. T. Gunther, *Early British Botanists and Their Gardens* (Oxford: Clarendon Press, 1922), 17–18, 312–13. Coys is virtually unknown today.

14. Robert Morison, *Plantarum historiæ universalis oxoniensis*, 2 vols. (Oxford, 1680–99). These were termed parts 2 and 3. Part 1 was apparently never published.

15. Ibid., pt. 3, preface, n.p., sig c, verso, and c2 recto. Jacob Bobart the younger added a preface (1698) to part 3, in which he named some thirty contemporaries (English and Dutch, mainly) who had made significant contributions in botany, chemistry, pharmacy, and anatomy.

16. Ray's table was printed in John Wilkins, *Essay towards a Real Character, and a Philosophical Language* (London, 1668).

17. John Ray, *Observations Topogaphical, Moral, & Physiological; made in a Journey through part of the Low-Countries, Germany, Italy, and France . . . Whereunto is added A brief Account of Francis Willughby Esq; his Voyage through a great part of Spain* (London, 1673). Willughby's narrative is at pp. 463–99.

18. John Ray, *Historia plantarum*, 3 vols. (London, 1686–1704), 1943.

19. Edward Long, *The History of Jamaica*, 3 vols. (London, 1774) 3:695.

20. One such is the copy of the *Natural History of Jamaica* now at the Henry E. Huntington Library, San Marino, Calif. Sloane gave this one to Abbé Bignon, who obtained another copy for the library of Cardinal Dubois, in time to put it up for auction—which is odd, because Sloane's second volume was published in 1725, and Dubois's library was sold (and Sloane's two volumes listed in the sale catalog) in 1723.

21. Sloane to Richardson, April 24, 1731, in *Illustrations of the Literary History of the Eighteenth Century*, ed. John Nichols, vol. 1 (London: Nichols, Son & Bentley, 1817), 286. Richardson was himself a decent amateur scholar and author of *De cultu hortorum* (London, 1699).

22. Ibid.

23. See Arthur MacGregor, ed., *Sir Hans Sloane: Collector, Scientist, Antiquary, Founding Father of the British Museum* (London: British Library, 1994), especially the editor's essay, "The Life, Character, and Career of Sir Hans Sloane," 11–44. For J. B. Palmer's useful notes on Sloane, see <http://www.gpl.net/users/bradley/sloane.html>.

24. *The Present State of His Majesties Isles and Territories in America* (London, 1687), 16.

25. Spain certainly discouraged any trade between British Jamaica merchants and Spanish America. The Treaty of Madrid (1670) explicitly forbade English and Spanish merchants to trade with any possession of the other in the "Indies." The War of the Spanish Succession changed this picture somewhat. See Curtis P. Nettels, "England and the Spanish-American Trade, 1680–1715," *Journal of Modern History* 3 (1931), repr., 14.

26. Agustín Farfán, *Tractado breve de anathomia y chirugia, y de algunas enfermedades que mas communmente suelen hauer en esta Nueva España* (Mexico City, 1579); Alonso López de Hinojosos, *Suma y recopilacion de chirugia con un arte para sangrar muy util y provechosa* (Mexico City, 1578). These two are extremely rare books: even facsimile reprints are rare and the works themselves little studied. This situation will be corrected by a new series, "Latino Medical Classics," which will be published, under our editorship, by the Center for the Study of Latino Health and Culture at UCLA.

27. Hans Sloane, *Natural History of Jamaica,* 2 vols. (London, 1707–25), vol. 1, pref., no pag.

28. Barrios appears briefly in Sloane's Royal Society paper, "A Description of the Pimienta or Jamaica Pepper-Tree, and of the Tree that Bears the Cortex Winteranus," *Philosophical Transactions* 16, no. 191 (December 1687): 462–68. In a fascinating case for textual bibliographers, the transmission of this printed text when Sloane revised it for incorporation in his *Jamaica* meant that Barrios was finally omitted altogether.

29. Sloane was only sixteen when Stubbe drowned (aged forty-four) in 1676, but he came to know Chamberlayne (1666–1723) well enough to correspond with him between 1700 and 1721. Sloane himself was born in 1660 and lived to be ninety-three.

30. Sloane did, however, acquire Stubbe's library catalog (and possibly his library). The catalog is now British Library, MS Sloane 35.

31. This myth should surely have been laid to rest by Sarah Augusta Dickson, *Panacea or Precious Bane: Tobacco in Sixteenth-Century Literature* (New York: New York Public Library, 1954), 80, yet the myth still shows up from time to time. In his brief Dutch translation of Monardes on tobacco, Nicolaes van der Woudt emphasized L'Obel's point that tobacco came to Portugal, France, England, and the Netherlands, in that order (*Beschrijvinge van het heerlijcke ende vermaede kruydt waasende in de West Indien aldaer ghenaemt Picielt* [Rotterdam, n.d. (c. 1600?)], no fol.).

32. The eccentric Philip Wharton thought that "larger Quantities might be made of [Jamaican] Cocoa, Tobacco, Anatta; more Gums might be gathered, and probably Drugs discovered," adding that medicinal trees could easily be "transplanted from the Continent and other Territories; but I am sorry to say Things of this kind are scarce ever thought on" (*Whartoniana: or, Miscellanies in Verse and Prose. By the Wharton Family, and Several other Persons of Distinction,* 2 vols. [London, 1727], 2:11–12).

33. *An Account of the European Settlements in America,* 2d ed., 2 vols. (London, 1758), 1:3.

34. Ibid., 1:174–75. Burke is describing the *temaxcalli,* the steam bath mentioned several times by Hernández in the *Antiquities.*

35. *Adam in Eden: or, Natures Paradise* (London, 1657), 150–51 (erroneously paginated for 200–201). All the same, Coles knew his Monardes.

36. *A Medical Dispensatory, Containing the Whole Body of Physick* (London, 1657), 288–89.

37. Anthony Burgess, *Little Wilson and Big God* (London: Heinemann, 1987), 9.

38. British Library, MS Sloane 4062, fol. 214.

39. For the paper, see *Philosophical Transactions* 20 (1698): 263–64.

40. Thomas Fairchild, *The City Gardener* (London, 1722), 62, 65. Fairchild deserves credit for creating the first recorded artificial hybrid. In addition to numerous contemporary comments (mostly laudatory) about him, there is a brief account of Fairchild by Conway Zirkle, "Some Forgotten Records of Hybridization and Sex in Plants, 1716–1739," *Journal of Heredity* 23 (1932): 435–37, reprinted in *Cotton Mather and American Science and Medicine: With Studies and Documents Concerning the Introduction of Inoculation or Variolation,* ed. Bernard Cohen, 2 vols. (New York: Arno, 1980).

41. Fairchild, *City Gardener,* 65.

42. Richard Pulteney, *Historical and Biographical Sketches of the Progress of Botany in England,* 2 vols. (London, 1790), 1:284. Doody's commonplace book survives, British Library, MS Sloane 3361.

43. The list is British Library, MS Sloane 2022, fols. 1–21.

44. Information about Petiver comes from his own voluminous papers, scattered now throughout the Sloane MSS at the British Library, and from the DNB. There is a good biographical account of him by Raymond Phineas Stearns, "James Petiver: Promoter of Natural Science, c. 1663–1718," *Proceedings of the American Antiquarian Society* 62 (1952): 243–365, and some further information about him in P. J. P. Whitehead, "The Biography of Georg Marcgraf (1610–1643/4) by His Brother Christian, translated by James Petiver," *Journal of the Society for the Bibliography of Natural History* 9 (1979): 301–14. Petiver's extensive herbarium was acquired by Sloane and is now in the Natural History Museum in London. One of Petiver's correspondents was Joan Salvador i Riera (1683–1725), whose father, Jaume, knew John Ray. For details, see Ángel M. Romo, "Un herbario prelinneano en el Institut Botànic de Barcelona: El herbario Salvador (Finales del siglo XVII y principios del XVIII)," <http://flora.uv.es/herbarios/salvador.htm>.

45. His library catalog is now British Library, MS Sloane 3367.

46. Sloane to Richard Richardson, May 13, 1703, in Nichols, *Illustrations* 1:273.

47. Her 1699 catalog, for instance, lists *Aloe americana* (four varieties), ananas, benjamin or balsam tree, capsicum, ficus from Barbados, corn, guaiacum, mandragora, pepper tree, sassafras, *Solanum mexicanun,* and tamarind. Her references are to "Plantini Plantarum," Plukenet, Munting, Tournefort, *Hortus Eystettensis,* Parkinson, and Ogilby's America, but not to Hernández. British Library, MS Sloane 525, fols. 5r, 8r, 9r, 15r, 17r, 22r, 26r, 30r, 31r, 33r. See Gordon D. Rowley, "The Duchess of Beaufort's Succulent Plants," *Bradleya* 5 (1987): 1–16.

48. Pulteney, *Sketches,* 2:105–7, 302.

49. *Philosophical Transactions* 47 (1751): 241–47.

50. The best account of Uvedale that we can find is a slight paper by J. G. L. Burnby and A. E. Robinson, *And They Blew Exceeding Fine: Robert Uvedale, 1642–1722,* Edmonton Hundred Historical Society, Occasional Papers (new ser.), no. 32 ([Enfield, Middlesex]: Edmonton Hundred Historical Society, 1976).

51. See *Reliquiae Hearnianae: The Remains of Thomas Hearne,* ed. Philip Bliss, 2d ed. (London, 1869), 3:37. The Reverend John

Laurence told Charles Evelyn in 1717 that he hoped to find some-one better than himself to write a book on gardening, and "I would have perswaded Mr. *Uvedal* of *Enfield,* or Mr. *Lloyd,* Rector of *Covent-Garden,* to undertake that very Thing you now attempt," but they both declined. That very thing became *The Lady's Recreation: or, the Third and Last Part of the Art of Gardening Improv'd* (London, 1717), in which Evelyn printed some of Laurence's letters (this quotation at 197). Edward Lloyd was one of the people acknowledged for his learning by Robert Morison.

52. The description, signed J. Gibson, was printed in *Archaeologia* 12 (1794): 188.

53. British Library, MS Sloane 4040, fol. 345.

54. Ibid., 4067, fol. 177.

55. Ray to Sloane, January 7, 1705, ibid., 4039, reprinted in *The Correspondence of John Ray,* ed. Edwin Lankester (London: Ray Society, 1848), 459. As often, Lankester got the year wrong, apparently not recognizing that March 25, the Feast of the Annunciation, was New Year's Day in the British Isles until the reform of the calendar in 1752.

56. August 6, 1701, in Nichols, *Illustrations,* 3:328.

57. London, Natural History Museum, Sloane collection, vol. 305, fol. 115, and vol. 306, fol. 105. Very useful summary information can be found in *The Sloane Herbarium,* ed. J. E. Dandy (London: British Museum, 1958).

58. Sloane collection, vol. 309, fol. 105.

59. Ray, *Historia plantarum,* pref, n.p., sig. A2f, recto. Stearns, "James Petiver," 254, calls Plukenet "lofty but unpopular."

60. F. Dawtrey Drewitt, *The Romance of the Apothecaries' Garden at Chelsea,* 3d ed. (Cambridge: Cambridge University Press, 1928), 3.

61. See Arthur MacGregor, "The Life, Character, and Career of Sir Hans Sloane," in *Sir Hans Sloane,* 17.

62. Erasmus Darwin, *The Botanick Garden* (London, 1825), pt. 2, *Loves of the Plants,* canto 3, line 188, note. Erasmus Darwin, grandfather of Charles, has attracted praise and ridicule for his verses. See Desmond King-Hele, ed., *The Essential Writings of Erasmus Darwin* (London, 1968), 11, and on the poem itself, 132; and Lester S. King, *The Medical World of the Eighteenth Century* (Chicago: University of Chicago Press, 1958), 220.

63. Sloane, *Natural History of Jamaica,* 2:5.

64. Alexander Nelson, *Medical Botany* (Edinburgh: Livingstone, 1951), 243–471.

HERNÁNDEZ AND SPANISH PAINTING IN THE SEVENTEENTH CENTURY

MARÍA JOSÉ LÓPEZ TERRADA

Recent developments in research on Francisco Hernández and his work—as the essays in this volume testify—have radically altered our understanding of the great naturalist, not just in strictly biographical ways or even only in analyses of his works but especially in the influence he had in diverse scientific and cultural fields. In this essay I propose to build on the most recent research by exploring the influence of Hernández's work in one specific area in the history of art: plants in Spanish baroque painting. More specifically still, my objective is to offer a representative selection of Spanish pictorial works of the period that depict plants described by Hernández in his *Natural History of New Spain*. As other essays in this volume show, many of those plants first became known in Europe by way of the selections published in the Rome edition of Hernández (1651) and those included by Juan Eusebio Nieremberg in his *Historia naturae* (1635).

In my selection of painters and paintings I endeavor to reflect the genre painters who specialized in still life and flower studies just as much as the mainstream dominated by the great figures of Spain's Golden Age. Hence, side by side with works by the famous, Juan Sánchez Cotán (1560–1627),

Francisco de Zurbarán (1598–1664), Diego Velázquez (1599–1660), and Bartolomé Esteban Murillo (1617–82), are works by the relatively little known Madrid painters Juan van der Hamen y León (1596–1631), Juan de Arellano (1614–76) and his pupil Bartolomé Pérez (1634–98), and the Valencian Tomás Hiepes (c. 1600–1670).

In addition to offering some basic description, this essay seeks to set out a preliminary approach to the ways in which New World plants described by Hernández were absorbed in the traditions and patterns of symbolism in Spanish painting.[1] This involves a process parallel to that in which numerous American medicinal and alimentary plants were tried out, some used as substitutes or put to the same use as their European equivalents.[2]

One fundamental question that must be addressed is how Spanish painters gained access to the text or illustrations of Hernández's work. There are essentially four ways: (1) First and most obvious is direct use of published editions of Hernández. The case of Murillo is a good example because, thanks to the publication of his library catalog by his son Gaspar, we know that among numerous titles on American plants, he owned the works of Fernández de

Oviedo, López de Gómara, and Monardes, as well as the Rome edition of Hernández.[3] It has been noted that a good proportion of this collection did not actually belong to Murillo but to his son, who inherited it from his uncle, José de Veitía y Linage, king's councillor and private secretary. This part of the library was included in the catalog anyway and, incidentally, contained two books in English, on the Casa de la Contratación in Seville, "the first governmental institution for the promotion of technology," in Ursula Lamb's expression.[4] In any case it seems undeniable that the painter knew the work of Hernández, either firsthand or from his brother-in-law. (2) The artists could also consult the unpublished pictures from the expedition of Hernández, whose originals were kept at the Escorial until the fire in 1671,[5] or they could look at copies destined for the Rome edition of Recchi's selection, some of which were gathered in collections such as the *Codex Pomar*, which Philip II presented to Jaime Honorato Pomar, professor of medical botany at the University of Valencia. Although these copies are considered in Europe to be derived from the Florentine school of Ligozzi, they clearly contain two styles: the Amerindian, which is also reflected in the engravings illustrating Nieremberg's selection, copied directly from the Escorial originals, and the European Renaissance style that corresponds to the illustrations in the Rome edition.[6] (3) The artists could paint the plants from life, since many varieties had begun to be cultivated in Spain by this time, mainly in the environs of the court in Madrid, as well as in Seville and Valencia. (4) Last, they must have made the most of personal contacts in the places where there were people taking an active interest in the work of Hernández, such as these three major Spanish cities. In this connection it is curious that two Spaniards with strong Flemish connections should have resided in Madrid at exactly the same time: Juan Eusebio Nieremberg and Juan van der Hamen y León. At the same time Valencia had a prestigious chair of "herbs," which was attached to a botanical garden and was connected with the court through Pomar, his predecessor Juan Planza, and his successor Melchor de Villena. The leading figure in medical botany in sixteenth-century Valencia, Planza maintained close professional contact with Clusius, who spoke highly of him in his letters and elsewhere and reproduced materi-

als that Planza had sent him. In some cases these were plants that are typical of the area around Valencia, such as *Pancratium maritimum* L., and in others, plants from the Americas, such as agaves, which came to be known all over central Europe, via Clusius, as *filiagulla,* or "needle and thread."[7]

In this study I am mainly concerned with eleven plants associated with Hernández: pimento, tomato, and chayote among the alimentary; bouvardia, American marigold, damask rose, nasturtium, tuberose (lily of the Indies), *dondiego de noche* (*Mirabilis jalap*), passionflower, and sunflower, all of which are used mainly as ornamentals.

The pimento (*Capsicum annuum* L. and related varieties) was among the earliest plants to be imported from the Americas, where the Spanish found that it was commonly consumed. Spurred by their desire to find spices, the first Europeans to arrive in the Antilles identified the piquant variety of this plant with Asian pepper, which was then one of the principal spices and one of the most expensive.[8] (This explains Columbus's entry in his diary for January 15, 1493.)[9] After that the process of diffusion to Europe began, and in this particular case it was extremely rapid. In 1535 Fernández de Oviedo, like the authors of earlier texts, recognized the importance of this plant in the native diet, but he added that it had already begun to be accepted as a foodstuff by Europeans living there as well. Thanks to Oviedo we also know that commercial networks were established very early on to import the pimento into Europe, where it quickly became a prized spice.[10] In this way the pimento, especially the hottest species and varieties, was commercialized, consumed, and adopted in European cuisines in place of Asian pepper. Furthermore, its adaptability enabled it to be cultivated easily in Spain, from where it soon spread all around the Mediterranean and to eastern Europe. Evidence of this is the Hungarian pepper known as paprika, which has become a central element in Hungarian culture, to the point where legends are associated with its cultivation and use and a major character in folklore in the seventeenth century, Jancsi Paprika, is named after it. European botanical writings in the sixteenth century confirm these early patterns of distribution, since this plant appears, with illustrations, in the first editions of the works of those "German fathers of botany," Fuchs and Bock, in 1542 and 1552.[11]

It is clear from contemporary sources in the sixteenth and seventeenth centuries that this American plant was among the commonest vegetables and flavorings in the Spanish diet. For example, Monardes says that the "Peper that thei dooe bryng from the Indias . . . is knowen in all Spaine, for there is no Gardeine, nor Orcharde, but that it hath plentie thereof in it."[12] The main interest was still in the hottest varieties, because "in all maner of meates and Potages . . . it hath a better taste then the common Peper hath." The only difference, said Monardes, is that "that costeth many Ducattes: the other doeth coste no more but to sowe it."[13] On the contrary, the work of Hernández shows many more differences than that, in his detailed analysis of the distinct species and varieties of pimento.[14]

This same desire to say that there was little difference between the American plant and any other type, like the high value attached to it as a foodstuff, was expressed years later by Sebastián de Covarrubias in his *Tesoro de la lengua* and even turns up in literature. In *The Country Wedding Party* (*Boda y acompañamiento del campo*), Quevedo says:

All bluster and noise
All bragging and boasting,
Here comes Sir Pepper
Dressed fit for a roasting.

while the refrain, "Garlic, salt, and chili; the rest is nothing," suggests that pimento had arrived as a flavoring and a sauce.

All of this explains the early appearance of pimento in Spanish seventeenth-century painting. For example, a still life from the school of Sánchez Cotán (Madrid, private collection) dated about 1615–25 depicts pimentos next to an American pumpkin, bunches of grapes, peaches, a lily, and a basket of figs. In the *Food of the Angels* (*Cocina de los ángeles*) by Murillo (fig. 1), the pimento appears amid common vegetables used in the Spanish cuisine of the day. Velázquez, too, included pimentos in several of his best-known works, such as the *Old Woman Frying Eggs* (*Vieja friendo huevos*) (Edinburgh, National Gallery of Scotland) and *Christ in Martha's House* (*Cristo en casa de Marta*) (fig. 2), both of which have been interpreted as symbolic.[15] Juan van der Hamen y León seems to have given the pimento a special meaning, perhaps an allusion to fertility, when he put it among the fruits and vegetables in his mythological painting of *Vertumnus and Pomona* (fig. 3).

Alongside the pimento, the tomato (*Lycopersicum esculentum* Mill.) was the other major contribution that the New World gave to European food. However, unlike so many other American plants, this one has never been the object of rigorous study, and unfortunately even present-day guides to culinary plants continue to offer eccentric, if not downright sloppy, explanations of its origin and diffusion in Europe.[16] We must therefore welcome studies in the history of science that reconstruct the route of the tomato from its places of origin. Prominent among them is the work of José M. López Piñero, who has done more than merely make known the importance of Hernández's contributions on this subject to the history of science; he has gone on to collate scattered information about its introduction to Europe, using previously neglected sources.[17] All the evidence suggests that the tomato came into Spain by about the middle of the sixteenth century, in spite of the absence of any earlier reference to it by any of the earliest travelers, chroniclers, and naturalists. The earliest mention of the plant appears in the commentaries of Mattioli on Dioscorides, first published in 1544 and reissued several times. In his notes to the chapter on the mandrake, Mattioli includes a short note on the "malum insanum"—the eggplant, or *Solanum melongena* L.—and goes on to mention the "pomo d'oro" (love apple) or "mala aurea" (golden apple), to which he devotes two lines and a half, saying that the fruits are sometimes yellow, sometimes red. Gesner, too, briefly mentions "malum aureum" or "pomum amoris" in *De hortis Germaniae liber* (1561), noting that the fruit could be yellow, red, or white and adding that there are some who think this fruit is the eggplant. Laguna, for example, thought so, saying in his translation of Dioscorides that he considered "verengenas," "mala insana," and "poma amoris" synonymous.[18]

Nevertheless, during the second half of the sixteenth century and the first half of the seventeenth, some authors used the terms *malum aureum, pomum aureum, pomum amoris,* and their translations, mainly in Italian, German, Dutch, French, and English, to designate a vague group of American "solanos" that could be identified with species of the genus *Physalis* and also *Lycopersicum esculentum*. The

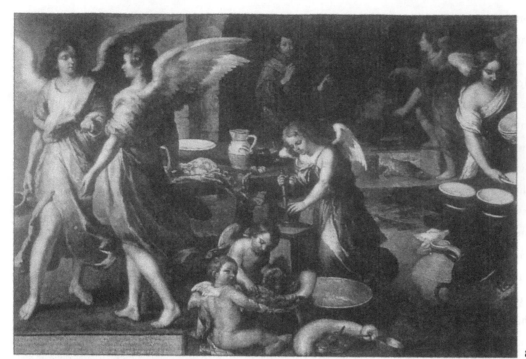

a

1a
Bartolomé Estaban
Murillo,
Food of the Angels
(*Cocina de los ángeles*)
(1646), oil on canvas,
180 × 450 cm.
Paris, Musée du Louvre.

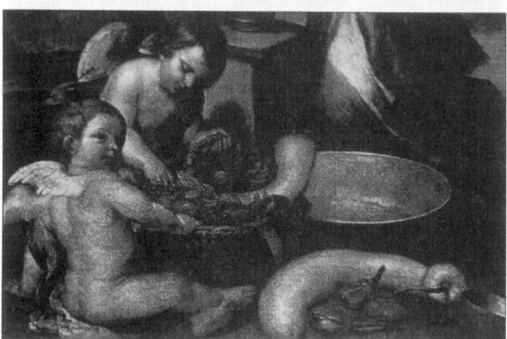

b

1b
Murillo,
Food of the Angels detail.

two exceptions that stand out are illustrations in the botanical treatises of L'Obel (1576) and Dodoens (1583), which unmistakably refer to *Lycopersicum esculentum,* with the image from L'Obel going on to be crudely copied in the *Herbario nuovo* (1585) of Durante. The Náhuatl word *tomatl* turns up in this period only in the commentary on Pliny by the Italian Guilandini (1572), who speaks of the "tumatl Americanorum," and in two Spanish works, one by Acosta (1590), who says that in America "they use also *Tomates,*

which are cold and very wholesome . . . the which gives a good taste to sauce, and they are good to eat," and the other by Gregorio de los Ríos (1592), who speaks of "pomates" being cultivated in Spanish gardens.[19]

In contrast to this panoply of inaccurate or fragmentary information, Hernández's treatment was a typically systematic review of "the species of solano" known in the New World as "tomatl." He describes the "xitomame," the species we recognize today as the tomato, as well as a series of

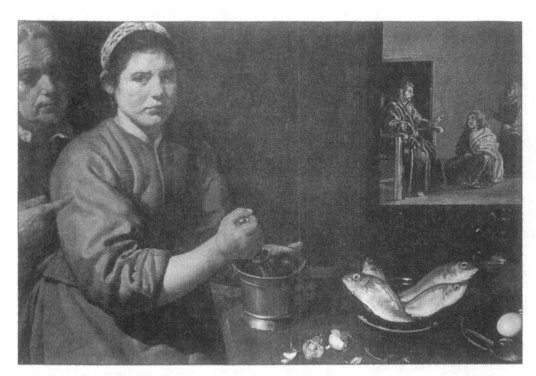

2
Diego Velázquez,
*Christ in Martha's House
(Cristo en casa de Marta)*
(1618), oil on canvas,
60 × 103.5 cm.
London, National Gallery.

"tomames," which correspond to other species of *Physalis*.[20] He also notes that "European pharmacists who are familiar with any of these fruits have named them 'love apples.'" Apart from the intrinsic interest in his descriptions and botanical conceptions, Hernández brought together all the information he could find about the main uses of the tomato, especially in cooking. Cultivation of the tomato and its use in salads and sauces were well established in Spain during the seventeenth century, yet in central and northern Europe it did not assume its everyday place in the kitchen until the end of the nineteenth century and the beginning of the twentieth.[21]

This assimilation of the tomato accounts for its appearance in seventeenth-century Spanish painting and literature and its corresponding absence in northern European art. The widespread diffusion and regular consumption of tomatoes and chili peppers in Spain at the end of the seventeenth century are reflected in lines of verse such as these by Anastasio Pantaleón (1580–1629)—"Innocent blood flows / red as a tomato, / red as a pepper"—or in a traditional Spanish saying: "Tomatoes and chilis, like good friends, always go together."[22] In the same way, as I have already indicated, Murillo puts them among typical foodstuffs in his *Food of the Angels* (fig. 1). Nonetheless, it is possible to find earlier examples. One of the earliest representations of a tomato in

an oil painting is in *Frutero con dulces* by Juan van der Hamen y León, painted about 1623 and now in the collection of the Bank of Spain in Madrid. Three years later, the same artist depicted it again among the fruits and vegetables in his *Vertumnus and Pomona* (fig. 3), next to other American species, such as the pimento or squash, possibly as an allusion to fertility.

The chayote (*Sechium edule* Sw.) is also depicted early on in Spanish painting. The problem of the origin and distribution of the squashes of the New and Old Worlds has never been satisfactorily resolved despite all the scholarly attention paid to the subject. The generally accepted conclusion is that the *Cucurbita*, *Sicana*, *Sechium*, and *Cyclatera* were American in origin and that the European *Lagenaria* was transplanted to America at an early date.[23] Hernández, who took up this subject in his study of the different types of American squash, devoted one chapter to the "*chayotl* or plant that bears prickly fruit."[24] Jordan and Cherry pointed out that the appearance of this species in *Still Life with Game* (*Bodegón con piezas de caza*) by Sánchez Cotán (fig. 4) is one of the earliest examples of New World fruits in a European still life.[25]

The bouvardia (*Bouvardia longiflora* L.) is an American plant now very widespread in gardening. The scientific name of the genus honors Charles Bouvard (c. 1572–1658), physician to Louis XIII of France and superintendent of the Jardin

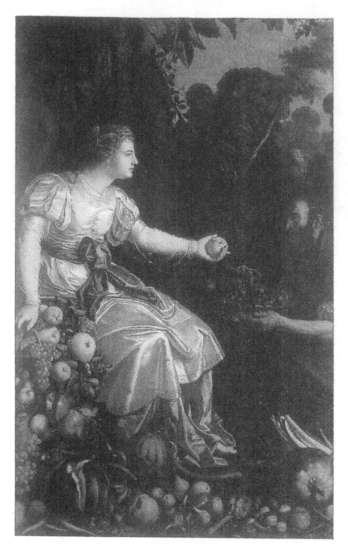

3
Juan van der Hamen y León,
Vertumnus and Pomona (1626), oil on canvas,
229 × 149 cm. Madrid, Banco de España.

du Roi.[26] But the plant was not yet known by this name. Hernández described it using its Náhuatl name, *tlacoxóchitl*, which means "flower staff," which is the way Murillo depicted it in *The Two Trinities (Las dos Trinidades)* (fig. 5), where it represents the staff of Saint Joseph next to another Mexican flower, the *Tagetes erecta* L., or marigold of the Indies.[27]

As I mentioned above, the incorporation of new American plants into religious painting, especially in contexts in which an iconography already existed, poses problems of interpretation. To take a specific example, the subject of the Two Trinities arose with the Counter-Reformation at the end of the sixteenth century and established a parallel between

the Holy Trinity, with Father, Son, and Holy Ghost in Heaven, and a terrestrial trinity, in which the Son is a link with the earth, accompanied by Mary and Joseph, his earthly parents. The Holy Family became a way of affirming the humanity of Jesus and at the same time a way of attaching more importance to Mary and Joseph, who then began to become popular cult figures.

In Murillo's work, the bouvardia appears next to flowers that were traditionally associated with Saint Joseph and had clear symbolic connotations, such as the rose and the lily. Murillo may have painted this species with nothing more in mind than to display its spectacular flowers, but that he chose a plant known as the flower staff to represent the staff of Saint Joseph probably means something more. Perhaps the bouvardia shared the religious connotations of the crucifix, but it is just as plausible that, like so many other American plants, it took over the traditional symbolism of a European species. It is interesting to note in this context that Murillo frequently used jasmine in depictions of Saint Joseph's staff. But then the representation of jasmine as a flower with four petals was quite frequent in contemporary religious painting, perhaps in an attempt to make a religious reading even clearer. This is how it is represented, for example, by Sánchez Cotán in his *Mystic Wedding of Saint Catherine (Desposorios místicos de Santa Catalina)*, at the Museum of Fine Arts in Granada. When Murillo put the "flower staff" in Joseph's hands, he may have been thinking of the likeness between the white flowers of the American plant and those of jasmine, which they resemble except that they are larger and have four petals.

Several species of the *Tagetes*, whose name seems to come from the Etruscan god Tages, son of Jupiter, came into Spain through the main gate of gardening.[28] The principal ones were the *damasquina*, or Moroccan carnation (*Tagetes patula*), and the marigold, or flower of death (*Tagetes erecta*).[29] During the sixteenth and seventeenth centuries, these species were known in Spain by the catchall name of "carnations of the Indies," differentiated almost exclusively by size and raised fundamentally as ornamentals. Acosta testifies to the high regard that they enjoyed at the time, stressing that these American flowers "which they call pinks of the Indies, the which are like to a fine orange tawny vel-

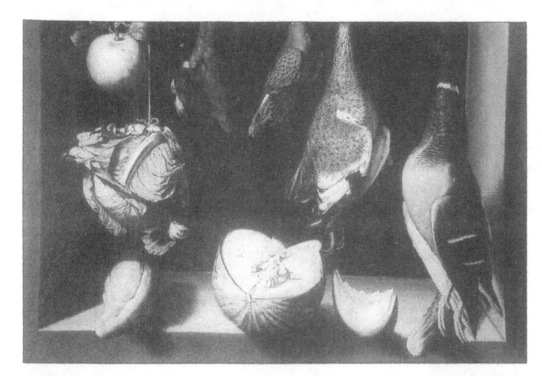

4
Sánchez Cotán,
*Still Life with Game
(Bodegón con piezas
de caza)* (c. 1600),
oil on canvas,
67.8 × 88.7 cm.
The Art Institute
of Chicago.

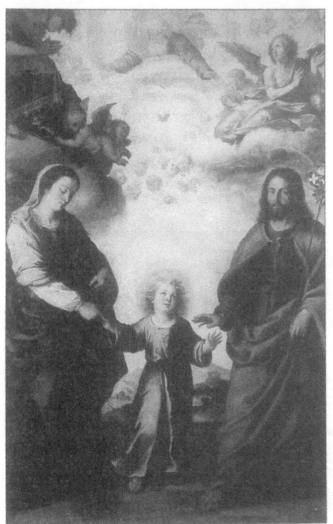

a

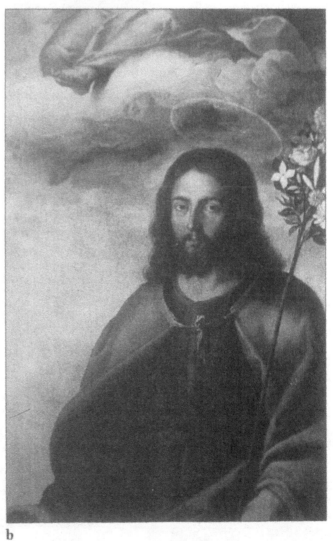

b

5 a, Bartolomé Estaban Murillo, *The Two Trinities, or Holy Family (Las dos Trinidades o la Sagrada Familia)* (c. 1640),
oil on canvas, 222 × 162 cm. Stockholm, National Museum; **b,** Murillo, *The Two Trinities* detail.

vet, or a violet; those have no scent of any account, but onely faire to the eye."[30] However, Francisco Hernández was the first to describe the different varieties and their properties, accompanied eventually by eight woodcuts in the Rome edition.[31] In his chapter on "cempoalxóchitl or flower with twenty leaves," he says: "Seven main varieties can be found of the flower known among the Mexicans as cempoalxóchitl, because it has so many leaves, and which the Spanish call carnation of the Indies, and which the ancients used to call, wrongly as some say, otona and flower of Jupiter, although there are here in New Spain other varieties that are distinguished by their flowers, their names, and their size."[32] Further on he adds: "I have seen all of these varieties growing in all sorts of places and different seasons; they have flourished in Spain, especially in warm places, and they have given their bright flowers to foreign countries, too."[33]

The early dissemination of these American species and their value as ornamental plants meant that they appeared in floral paintings all over Europe from the first half of the seventeenth century. Juan van der Hamen y León's *Still Life with Fruit Basket and Bunches of Grapes (Bodegón con frutero y racimos de uvas)* (1622; fig. 6) is one of the earliest examples of European still life to depict the *Tagetes patula*, or *damasquina*. Sam Segal shows that this species was also represented in Dutch flower paintings contemporary with Juan de Arellano or Tomás Hiepes; the latter included it frequently in his compositions (fig. 7).[34] Segal also emphasizes the symbolism that the various types of Tagetes had at the time, since, like other New World plants, these had taken over the symbolic role previously assigned to European plants. Generally speaking, they seem to have assumed the rich religious connotations of the carnation, and for that reason they appear in some flower paintings as symbols of Christ.[35] The *cempoalxóchitl* (known in Spain as the *clavelón*), or flower of death, similarly acquired much of the significance previously attached to the marigold, on account of its large golden flowers, to the point where it was even used as a substitute.[36] Because the sunflower turns to face the sun, a metaphor for heaven, it was used mainly as a symbol for those who closely follow the teachings of Christ.[37] The characteristics of the sunflower and the marigold illustrated this concept much more clearly than the European counterparts that they replaced. All these connotations, combined with their early appearance in Spanish gardens, explain their appearance in Spanish religious paintings such as the *Holy Family* of Zurbarán (fig. 8) and another by Murillo (fig. 5).

The species *Tropaeolum majus* L. was the most widely cultivated of the nasturtiums for the beauty of its yellow or

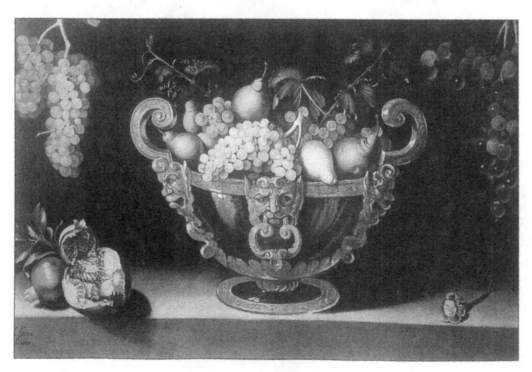

6
Juan van der Hamen y León,
Still Life with Fruit Basket and Bunches of Grapes (Bodegón con frutero y racimos de uvas)
(1622), oil on canvas, 59 × 93.3 cm.
Madrid, private collection.

Hernández also gave his attention to this plant, which he called the nasturtium of Peru, and referred not just to the way it was used as an ornamental that "adorns and beautifies the gardens, espaliers, windows, and courtyards of houses, being planted in clay flowerpots," but also to its use "in a salad, for they are very appetizing, so that afterwards the main dishes taste even better."[40] Use of the nasturtium as a religious symbol, albeit not a very precise one, in seventeenth-century flower painting has been mentioned in several studies and is explained fully by Hernández, who describes the nasturtium:

> The flowers are of an extraordinary, showy yellow color shading to red, as are those of the columbine or linaria, or those of the osiris. On their undersides these have a twisted little stem, which terminates on the upper side in seven sepals, of which two are bigger than the rest and two others [are] smaller than the remaining three. All have certain visible red lines, very similar to the wounds of Our Lord Christ as they are usually painted upon crucifixes. The other three remain in the middle of the aforementioned ones. These have three markings in the shape of a crown of thorns.[41]

Given the diffusion of the work of Hernández to so many parts of Europe, it is probably because of him that the nasturtium became, like the passionflower, a specific symbol of Christ.

Segal's study shows that these American species were represented in Dutch painting of the seventeenth century, appearing, for example, in the works of Elias van den Broeck (1659–1708) and Jan van Huysum (1682–1749). In Segal's view, both species had been recently introduced into northern Europe when they began to appear in paintings there, and they were represented with a clear symbolic meaning.[42] The appearance of this species in Italian and Spanish still life and flower paintings, like those of Mario Nuzzi or Arellano (fig. 9), began very early but illustrates at the same time its rapid dissemination all over seventeenth-century Europe, where it became fashionable and highly regarded as an ornamental plant.

The *Polianthes tuberosa* L., known variously as the tuberose, oriental hyacinth, and rod of Jesse, is another of the Hernández plants that was quickly established in gar-

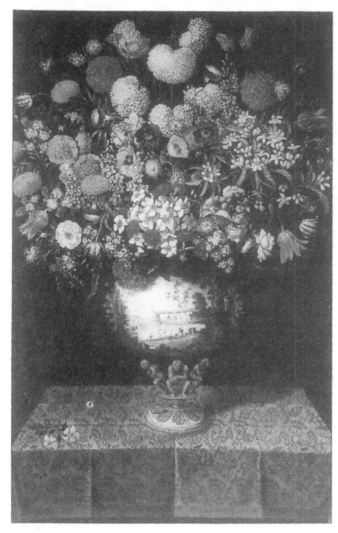

7

Tomás Hiepes, *Still Life with Flowers (Florero)* (1664), oil on canvas, 148 × 96 cm. Principado de Asturias, Pedro Masaveu Collection, Museo de Bellas Artes de Asturias.

orange flowers. The first to describe this plant, which from the end of the seventeenth century was also introduced in European materia medica under the various names of *berros, mastuerzo,* or *de los capuchinos,* was Monardes in 1590. He calls them "flowers of blood" and explains that he obtained them from "a seed brought over to me from Peru, more for its beauty than for any medicinal virtue."[38] He goes on to describe the species exactly and writes of its use as an ornamental plant. The literature of the period similarly shows that the nasturtium was an early import to Spanish gardens. In a passage from *El peregrino en su Patria (The Pilgrim in His Homeland),* Lópe de Vega says: "The brave young man gathered rosebays, sedges, and nasturtiums, which the freshness of a stream absorbed."[39]

dening. Hernández called it *omioxochitl*, or stoneflower, considering it "a species of narcissus unknown in the Old World."[43] Then he explained that the white flowers were used to make bouquets and perfumes and that they have "an aroma like that of the lilies of our country, hence they are sometimes called lilies of the Indies."

The fact that in Spain at the time the tuberose was known as lily of the Indies and that early-nineteenth-century gardening treatises would go on to call it the rod of Jesse would certainly suggest a religious connotation.[44] Such symbolism could be derived from the features of the flower, with its white color, clearly an allusion to purity, or the

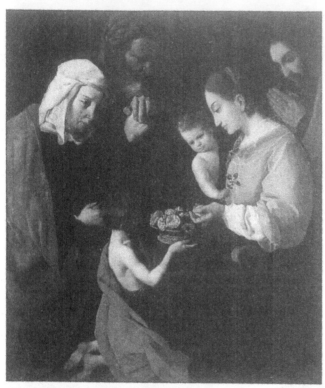

a

8a
Francisco de Zurbarán,
Holy Family
(*Sagrada Familia*)
(c. 1625–30),
oil on canvas,
126 × 128 cm.
Madrid, private collection.

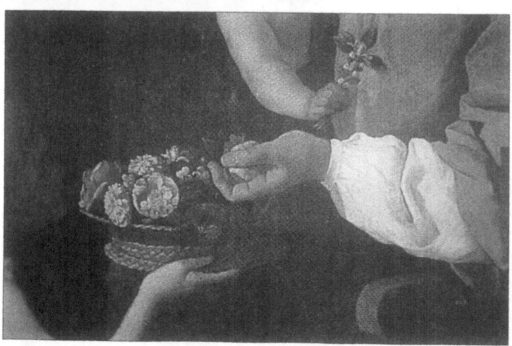

8b
Zurbarán,
Holy Family detail.

b

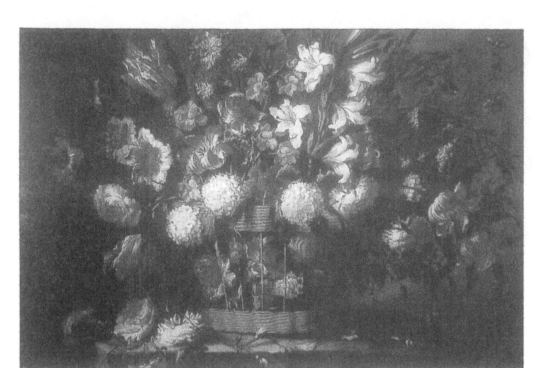

9
Juan de Arellano,
Basket of Flowers
(*Cesto de flores*)
(c. 1670–75),
oil on canvas, 84 × 105 cm.
Madrid, Museo del Prado.

sweetness of its aroma, commonly identified with virtue.[45] But it is also possible that, as with other American plants, it was identified with an Old World species with a long symbolic tradition, such as, in this case, the lily or the biblical rose.[46] On the other hand, the intense aroma of these flowers perhaps turned them into a clear symbol of smell, whose allegorical representation, always taken from floral attributes, was commonplace in seventeenth-century painting.[47]

The single flowers of the lily in the form of a funnel, intensely white and with six open petals, were represented early on in Spanish painting, as witnessed by the flower paintings of Hiepes (fig. 10) and Arellano (fig. 11). By contrast, this species is very hard to find in floral compositions anywhere else in Europe, at least in the seventeenth century. It is especially rare in the north, where the colder climate made reproduction of the plant difficult, which is why it was imported there so much later.[48] The Neapolitan flower paintings are a separate case, since the lily was commonly represented throughout the second half of the seventeenth century in works by Andrea Belvedere, Giuseppe Reco, and Paolo Porpona.[49] A good example is Belvedere's *Vase of Flowers* (*Jarrón de flores*) at the Prado, Madrid. The representation of this American plant in a painting by an Italian artist could be directly attributable to Spanish influence, as suggested

by Pérez Sánchez, who has also noted the possibility that Belvedere painted this work during his stay in Madrid at the end of the century, when the lily had become commonplace in Spanish gardens.[50] However, one must remember that the work of Hernández was well known by this time in Italy and that many American species spread quickly around Italian gardens.

The *Mirabilis jalapa* (*dondiego de noche* in Spanish) is a species native to Mexico that takes its botanical name from the Latin *mirabilis*, "wonderful," because a single plant could bear flowers of different colors. It is now called *dondiego,* Don Juan, or *bella de noche,* because its flowers open at nightfall and remain open until sunrise. Its extraordinary characteristics explain the name *admirabilis* or marvelous (*maravilla*), as it was known in the seventeenth and eighteenth centuries, when it became highly valued as an ornamental plant.[51] Hernández, who referred to this plant as *tlaquilin,* emphasized its long flowers of different colors and noted that "it grows in various places in Mexico, where it is cultivated in gardens as an ornamental and for its flowers."[52]

The commentaries that Clusius devoted to the *Mirabilis jalapa* in 1583 testify not only to its diffusion as an ornamental plant in Europe at the time but also to the confusing

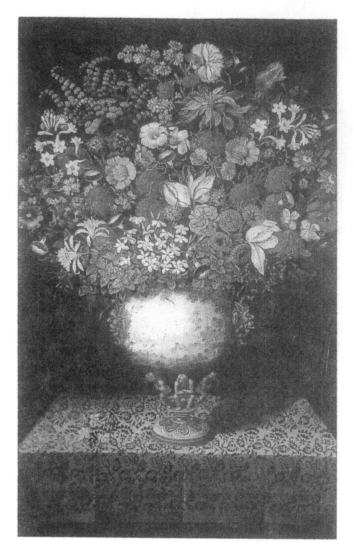

10
Tomás Hiepes, *Still Life with Flowers (Florero)* (1664),
oil on canvas, 149 × 98 cm. Principado de Asturias, Pedro
Masaveu Collection, Museo de Bellas Artes de Asturias.

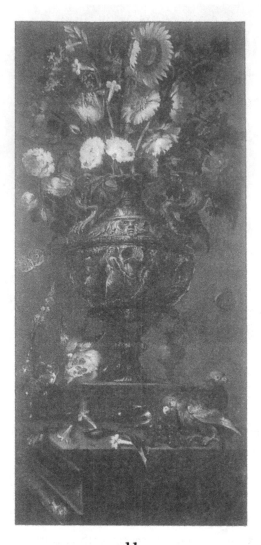

11
Juan de Arellano, *Still Life with Flowers, Birds, and Fruit
(Florero con pájaros y frutas)* (1647), oil on canvas.
Madrid, private collection.

diversity of the names it was given: "The seed was originally sent by the Spanish under the name of Marvel of Peru because of the amazing variety of the flowers and, later, under that of blusher. In Italy it was called Mexican jasmine, or jasmine of the Indies, on account of the sweet fragrance of the flowers. The Flemish call it *Solanum odoriferum* because of the leaves' similarity to those of the *Solanum* and the flowers' aroma. The Peruvians, from whom the Spanish took their name for it in the first place, call it, I believe, *Hachal indi,* in their native language. Viennese ladies of the night, who have a great liking for it, know it as *Gescheket Indianische Blumen,* that is, multicolored Indian flowers."[53]

As was the case with the nasturtium, the lily, the sunflower, or the *claveles de Indias,* the *dondiego de noche* was another American species that was common in Spanish gardens when it was adopted by painters of the period.[54] Its appearance in seventeenth-century flower paintings could be a response just to its popularity as an ornamental. However, the unique characteristics of its flowers, as interpreted by the baroque symbolists, give this plant a clear symbolic significance, which suggests that its appearance in the paintings was more than merely decorative.

Being a nocturnal flower, the *dondiego de noche* was likened to a modest and humble man, "who never shows the splendor of his wit to the eyes of others, nor seeks to display it in the theater of the world."[55] It seems, furthermore, that this characteristic caused this American species to be identified with the *selinotropo* mentioned by Piero Valeriano and Cesare Ripa, that is, the plant that follows the course of the moon. For these two authors, the *selinotropo* has the same significance as the sunflower, since both flowers symbolize unity, harmony, and the Platonic correspondences between earthly and heavenly things.[56]

This religious reading could fit the flower painting by Hiepes belonging to the Masaveu collection (fig. 10), in which the *dondiego de noche* is shown among such obviously symbolic species as the passionflower, *agnocasto,* jasmine, amaranth or tulip, and many others.

Picinelli found another emblem devoted to this flower, significantly called Spanish wonder (*miraculum hispanicum*), with the motto "Appearance is useless." In this emblem the property of the flower, that "it does not show its virtue on the outside," is related to the contemporary concept that worldly glory was worthless.[57] In this form, without necessarily excluding its religious connotations, the *dondiego de noche,* like the rest of the species represented and, in general, many flower paintings of the period, could carry an allegorical significance related to the theme of *vanitas,* or worldly vanity, commonplace in seventeenth-century Spain.

The passionflower was one of the most spectacular of the plants brought to Spain from the Americas in the seventeenth century. The best-known variety and the earliest to be disseminated was *Passiflora caerulea* L., which can be seen today in arbors, on walls, and in gardens everywhere in Europe. One of the first descriptions of this plant was by Hernández, who called it "the herb that the Spanish call 'granadilla.'"[58] We know from Monardes, who expounded not just on the fruit but also on the rest of the plant, that it was already being cultivated in Seville by 1580.[59] Ten years later, Acosta emphasized its main property: "The flower of Granadilla is held for an admirable thing, and they say it hath in it the markes of the Passion, and that therein they note the nailes, the pillar, the whips, and crowne of thornes, and the woundes, wherein they are not altogether without reason, and yet to finde out and observe these things, it

requires some pietie to cause beleefe: but it is very exquisite and faire to the eye."[60]

In 1605, this plant was sent to Pope Paul V and grown in Rome. It was then that Simón Palasca wrote a detailed description of the appearance of those parts of the flower associated with Christ's Passion. Its long interior leaves arranged in a circle were compared to the crown of thorns, its five stamens with the five wounds, and its three *styli* with the nails.[61] This interpretation was revised and enlarged in later treatises that saw, for instance, the five wounds in the five red markings of the corolla, the *stilus* as the scourge or the pillar where Christ was flagellated, and in the stamens the shape of the hammer and tongs or of the sponge soaked with wormwood and gall.[62]

The use of the passionflower as a symbol of the Passion spread all over Europe at the beginning of the seventeenth century. It seems that in both France and Italy the flower was venerated because it supposedly portrayed the instruments of Christ's martyrdom and the cross itself.[63] One of the earliest illustrations of the flower in the Low Countries appeared in a supplement to Theodore de Brij's *Florilegium* (1614), with the name of "passionflower, or granadilla." The symbolic associations must have spread quickly in northern Europe, because in 1629 they were condemned by the Protestants: "Some superstitious Jesuits design to make people believe that the flower of this plant displays all the signs of the passion of our Savior . . . but this is just another of their lucrative lies . . . which they use to instruct the commonfolk."[64]

Picinelli cited several examples of seventeenth-century emblems using this flower, "which miraculously reveals many of the instruments of Christ's passion," and proposed that it was an image of the torment of all the martyrs, not just of Christ. He also cited several contemporary literary references to support this symbolic interpretation of the passionflower, such as these lines by Giuseppe Baptista:

> The grieving of Venus is incarnate in the anemone,
> So too is the passion of Christ revealed in a flower. . . .
> As the flowers of the earth incorporate torments,
> So to God sufferings are made manifest in flowers.[65]

This symbolism lies behind the appearance of the passionflower in the garland of flowers surrounding Saint Anthony with the Child, in a painting by the chief pupil of Arellano, Bartolomé Pérez, at the Prado (fig. 12). Pérez, like Hiepes (fig. 10), also represented the passionflower in several flower paintings, very likely with the same religious implications.

Segal has noted the use of the passionflower as a religious symbol in several works by Daniel Seghers, who portrayed different varieties in the compositions he completed while in Rome (1625–27) and again twenty-five years later when he was working in Antwerp. Similarly, in the second half of the century, Hieronimus Galle and Elias van der Broeck included the passionflower alongside other recent American imports such as the sunflower.[66] However, this gaudy flower was generally not much depicted in seventeenth-century flower paintings, possibly because at the time it was not as easy to grow or propagate as it is now. A century later, the passionflower's symbolism had become entrenched in Spanish culture, when Antonio Palomino said, "It is well known in this realm today by the name of Passion Flower, containing as it does all the signs of the Passion."[67]

The sunflower (*Helianthus annuus* L.) is a clear example of the problems that common names still cause to this day in natural history. *Girasol, tornasol,* and *heliotropo* were all Spanish terms for Old World plants.[68] In America, these names were given almost immediately to the *Helianthus,* a native species that was transported to Europe and became widespread there during the sixteenth century.

The first reference to *girasol* in the European sources appears in Fernández de Oviedo's *Sumario de la natural y general ystoria de las Indias* (1526), although it is not certain that he was referring to *Helianthus annuus.*[69] Some forty years later, Fragoso called attention to the plant's characteristic of turning to face the sun, mentioning no fewer than seven popular names.[70] Monardes's passing allusion to the sunflower as "a herb of unusual size . . . with a strange flower" shows that by 1580 it had begun to be cultivated in Spain and had acclimatized well, mainly in gardens.[71] Hernández also refers to this plant, as the great Peruvian *chimacatl,* also called the sunflower, and in his detailed description he notes its curative properties and culinary uses.[72]

In the baroque period, *girasol* signified both the European heliotrope and the American sunflower. Emblematists differentiated the two formally but not very clearly and used both of them to organize concepts around its basic property of turning toward the sun.[73] Laguna eloquently expresses the importance of the heliotrope for people of the sixteenth century:

> The heliotrope is admirable and imitable in her nature, for she receives such frequent gifts from the sun, unique

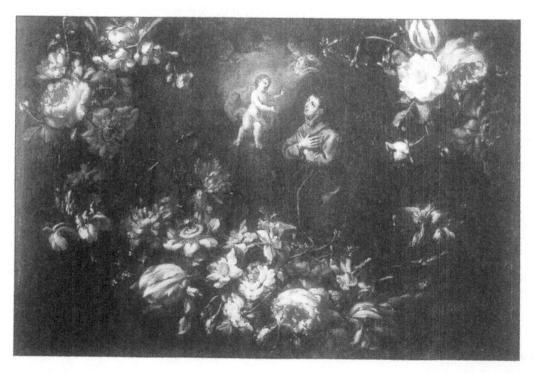

12
Bartolomé Pérez,
*Garland of Flowers
with Saint Anthony
and the Baby Jesus
(Guirnalda de flores con
San Antonio y el Niño Jesús)*
(c. 1689), oil on canvas,
65 × 84 cm.
Madrid, Museo del Prado.

in her being and her growth, forgets herself as she follows him, declaring with her stems, with her leaves, and with her flowers, no common desire but an intense love, full of a gratitude so remarkable that whichever part inclines toward the refulgent planet, the stems stand up straight, and at night they shrink like a grieving widow. From this we judge that this plant serves us not merely as salutary medicine, but also as the accurate timepiece that regulates the orderly progress of our daily life, as its punctual movements measure the day and, dividing it into equal portions, indicate the passing of each hour.[74]

Much more spectacular in size and in its corolla's resemblance to the sun, the American sunflower embodied more of these properties than its little European cousin, which it soon, and not surprisingly, replaced. A poem by José de Litala expresses that property of measuring the hours of the day but uses the sunflower as a metaphor for the poet's love of his mistress:

> In the Indies that fragrant flower is made
> That trails the sun's parched steps in order
> And from these hot paths espies the verdure,
> Mark'd by the orient, of the cooling shade.
> Its leaves unfailing mark chronology:
> Every hour of this diurnal round.
> In winds or calm this timepiece of the ground
> Functions in silent astrology.
> So likewise I, your Siren of beauty,
> The flower that your eyebeams do desire,
> Count the hours in my prison of duty.[75]

The sunflower was used emblematically with amorous connotations, for instance, by Otto Vaenius in an emblem with the motto "Wherever you are, I turn," in which the plant has become the supreme example of submission and servitude.[76] This symbolism may explain its presence in the Putti in a *Cartouche with a Garland* (*Amorcillos en una cartela y guirnalda de flores*) by Antonio Ponce (about 1650, Madrid, private collection) and the *Tribute to Flora* (*Ofrenda a Flora*) by Juan van der Hamen y León (fig. 13). Julián Gállego interprets this latter painting not just as a mythological work but, probably, as a floral poem dedicated to a woman, in which roses allude to love, the sunflower to fidelity, and so on.[77]

Use of the heliotrope as a symbol of love goes back a long way. Since antiquity it has been associated with the

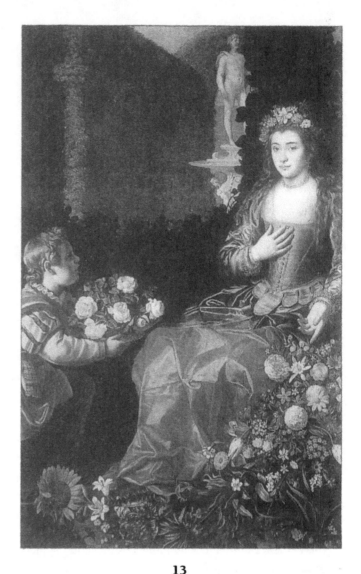

13
Juan van der Hamen y León,
Tribute to Flora (Ofrenda a Flora) (1627), oil on canvas,
216 × 140 cm. Madrid, Museo del Prado.

myth of Clytie and Leucothoe. In Ovid's *Metamorphoses*, book 4, the nymph Clytie is loved by Apollo until he turns his attention to her twin sister, Leucothoe. Clytie's jealousy causes the death of her sister, who is buried alive by her father (the traditional punishment of a Vestal Virgin found guilty of unchastity). Despite Apollo's efforts to revive her, the weight of the earth is too much for Leucothoe, who is gradually consumed until she is metamorphosed into the flower that always turns her face toward the sun. In the seventeenth century, the sunflower sometimes replaced the heliotrope in versions of this myth. Philotheus transformed Ovid's myth of Clytie and Leucothoe into a Christian version, in which love becomes the Christian's love of God.[78]

This religious meaning is predominant in our period. In a large number of emblems, the sunflower appears as the flower that follows the sun's course across the sky, metaphorically following Christ or God and thus inviting a comparison with people who follow divine teachings attentively and carefully. Camerarius devoted an emblem to the sunflower, which he called *Chrysanthemum peruvianum* "because it was recently imported from Peru," and said, "As the sun's rays make these flowers turn, so direct my heart, O Christ, with goodness." In the explanatory text, Camerarius exhorts people to imitate the behavior of the sunflower and direct their gaze to heaven, above the fragile, material world.[79]

Picinelli found several examples of the sunflower as an image of obeisance and of the love of God entirely free of worldly affection. Moreover, the concepts of fidelity and constancy are in perfect accord with the characteristics of this plant, as a good number of emblems suggest.[80] The sunflower as religious symbol also turns up in contemporary Spanish literature, such as a poem by Leonor de Cueva y Silva, on "the beauty and variety of spring flowers":

> You show us that the sunflower is divine,
> Following the stars of the celestial sun,
> And we mere mortals call this flower a rose.[81]

All this evidence points to a symbolic intention in the pictorial representation of the sunflower during the seventeenth century. Its religious connotations explain its appearance in Arellano's garland of flowers surrounding an allegory of vanity by Francisco Camilo (1646, Valencia, private collection). Segal has noted its similar symbolic use in Dutch flower painting, in which it appeared frequently at midcentury.[82] One of his most interesting examples is a work by Jan Davisz de Heem, now at the Bode Museum, Berlin, which is remarkably similar to the *Still Life with Flowers, Birds, and Fruit (Florero con pájaros y frutas)* by Arellano (fig. 11). Detailed analysis of contemporary symbolic sources leads Segal to conclude that Heem used the flowers and fruits as attributes of Christ and the Redemption. In this work, like that of Arellano, a sunflower appears in the upper part of the canvas, "where it has a clear symbolic function as a divine flower," an open pomegranate, "which could be an allusion to the church and its mem-

bers," and birds and butterflies, "which symbolize the redeemed soul."[83]

On the other hand, the work of Arellano bears a great resemblance to the engravings of Adrian Collaert, Claes Jansz Visscher, and Elías Verhulst, all of which were executed about 1615 and reissued many times and disseminated all over Europe. These images were accompanied by biblical references, such as this text from Isaiah 40:6–8:

> The voice said, Cry. And he said, What shall I cry? All flesh is grass, and all the goodliness thereof is as the flower of the field:
> The grass withereth, the flower fadeth: because the spirit of the Lord bloweth upon it: surely the people is grass.
> The grass withereth, the flower fadeth: but the word of our God shall stand for ever.

These are verses that the flower painters took it upon themselves to illustrate. Several elements of this work, such as the baroque vase, the arrangement of the flowers, butterflies, and shells, and in particular the bird pecking at cherries, all seem to have been taken directly from these earlier engravings.[84] Nor should we forget that, in this period, originality was extremely rare and such use of engravings by the artists as a source of inspiration for their own iconography and compositions was common practice.[85] These considerations suggest that Juan de Arellano was using a symbolic language common to European culture in the seventeenth century.

The paintings discussed here are representative of their artists, their genre, and their time. They also clearly demonstrate the earliest depictions of American plants in Spanish painting. Francisco Hernández was the ultimate authority on these plants—and sometimes on their symbolism—and the Rome edition provided the artists with images that they could copy. In any case, we may say now that Hernández made his mark in art as well as science.

NOTES

1. See María José López Terrada, "El mundo vegetal en la pintura española del siglo XVII: Aproximación a su estudio" (M.A. thesis, University of Valencia, 1995), and María José López Terrada, "Tradición y cambio en la pintura valenciana de flores en la tran-

sición de la Ilustración al Romanticismo" (Ph.D. diss., University of Valencia, 1995).

2. On these aspects of New World plants, see *Medicinas, drogas.*

3. Santiago de Montoto, "La biblioteca de Murillo," *Bibliografía hispánica* 6 (1946): 467–70.

4. "Veitía y Linage, José de," in José María López Piñero et al., *Diccionario histórico de la ciencia moderna en España* (Barcelona: Península, 1983), 2:402–3. On Veitía, see also Santiago de Montoto, "Don José de Veitía y Linaje y su libro 'Norte de la Contratación de las Indias,'" *Boletín del Centro de Estudios Americanistas* 4 (1921): 1–27.

5. See Jesús Bustamante, "The *Natural History of New Spain,*" in *Mexican Treasury.*

6. See especially *Códice Pomar* and *Nuevos materiales.*

7. José María López Piñero, *Clásicos médicos valencianos del siglo XVI* (Valencia: Conselleria de Sanitat i Consum, 1990), 48–49.

8. The identification of the American plant pimento with the *pimenta* (*Piper nigrum* L.) caused untold linguistic confusion. American peppers introduced in Europe were frequently called "Indian pepper," "Spanish pepper," or "piper presilianum" (*Medicinas, drogas,* 61). In the eighteenth century, the Royal Spanish Academy's *Diccionario de la lengua castellana* (Madrid, 1726–39), 3:273, maintained that the pepper belonged to the genus *Piperitis.* However, there are two distinct families. The *Piper nigrum,* from which we get both black and white pepper, is a climbing plant that grows mainly in India; the *Capsicum* is a genus of plants native to tropical America and the West Indies, with a great many varieties, not all of them piquant, and many hybrids and intermediates.

9. José Pardo Tomás and María Luz López Terrada, *Las primeras noticias sobre plantas americanas en las relaciones de viajes y crónicas de Indias (1493–1553)* (Valencia: Instituto de Estudios Documentales e Históricos sobre la Ciencia, 1993), 172–74, 259, explain that the term *axí* or *ají* used by Columbus is a Taino word that corresponds to *chilli* in Náhuatl, from which we get the term *chili* in common use today. But it was more common to find earlier authors speaking of "Pimento of the Indies."

10. Gonzálo Fernández de Oviedo, *La historia general de las Yndias* (Seville, 1535), fol. 75r.

11. Pardo and López Terrada, *Primeras noticias,* 174.

12. Nicolás Monardes, *Joyfull Newes out of the Newe Founde Worlde,* trans. John Frampton, 2 vols. (1577; London: Constable, 1925), 1:47; idem, *Historia medicinal* (Seville, 1580), fol. 19r.

13. Monardes, *Joyfull Newes,* 1:48.

14. See *Mexican Treasury,* "Five Special Texts."

15. See commentary by Julián Gállego in the Prado's Velázquez exhibition catalog (Madrid: Ministerio de Cultura, 1990), 62–67, 74–79.

16. For example, Jan Kybal, *Plantas aromáticas y culinarias* (Madrid: Susaeta, 1993), 122, says that the tomato was not eaten until the nineteenth century because Mattioli had called it *mala insana* and because scientific textbooks kept insisting that it was poisonous. But the most ridiculous explanation is that of John Seymour, *Los placeres del huerto* (Madrid: Mondadori, 1987), 74, who does not name his sources: the first seeds of the tomato to come to Europe, he says, were not sown in Spain but in Morocco, which explains the name *pomo de mori* (Moors' apple) given to it in Italy and subsequently distorted as *pomo d'oro.*

17. *Medicinas, drogas,* 222–24. I am indebted to this work for all my information, including early sources, and I summarize it in the succeeding paragraphs. See also José M. López Piñero and José Pardo Tomás, "Contribution of Hernández," above.

18. P. A. Mattioli, *Commentarii in sex libros Pedacii Dioscoridis Anazarbei de materia medica* (Venice, 1565); Conrad Gesner, *De hortis Germaniae liber,* in V. Cordus, *Annotationes in Pedacii Dioscoridis Anazarbei de materia medica libros quinque* (Strasbourg, 1561), 236–301; Pedacio Dioscorides Anazarbeo, *Acerca de la materia medicinal y de los venenos mortiferos,* trans. and ed. Andrés Laguna (Antwerp, 1555).

19. M. Guilandini, *Papyrus, hoc est, Commentarius in tria C. Plinii majoris de papyro capita* (Venice, 1572); José Acosta, *Naturall and Morall Historie of the Indies,* trans. Edward Grimestone (London, 1604), bk. 4, chap. 20, p. 266; Gregorio de los Ríos, *Agricultura de jardines, que trata de la manera que se han de criar, governar, y conservar las plantas* (Madrid, 1592; facsimile ed., Madrid: CSIC and Ayuntamiento de Madrid, 1991), fol. 59.

20. López Piñero, *Medicinas, drogas,* 224, notes that in Mexico today a good deal of the Náhuatl terminology recorded by Hernández is still in use. *Jitomate* designates basically the species that Europe recognizes as the tomato (*Lycopersicum esculentum*), while with the exception of a few places in northern Mexico, *tomame* refers to various species of the genus *Physalis* and other, related genera.

21. According to Pío Font Quer, *Plantas medicinales: El Dioscórides renovado,* 8th ed. (Barcelona: Labor, 1980), 588, cultivation of the tomato in northern Europe in the eighteenth century was an amusement for the curious, who grew it as a decorative houseplant. As late as the mid-nineteenth century, in the great French reference work on materia medica, Mérat and Lens noted *pomme d'amour* and *tomate* as interchangeable common names of *Lycopersicum esculentum,* which they considered "a plant grown in gardens for its fruit, usually a beautiful red color," though they did go on to mention its consumption as a foodstuff and its cultivation in Spain. F. V. Mérat and A. J. Lens, *Dictionnaire universel de matière médicale,* 7 vols. (Paris: J. B. Ballière, Méguignon-Marcis, Gabon, 1829–47).

22. Anastasio Pantaleón de Ribera, *Obras completas.* Rom. 20, quoted in the Royal Spanish Academy *Diccionario,* 3:295.

23. *Medicinas, drogas,* 225–26, and Pardo and López Terrada, *Primeras noticias,* 270–71.

24. *Mexican Treasury,* "The Low Countries, 1630–1648," Juan Eusebio Nieremberg, N 14.33.

25. William B. Jordan and Peter Cherry, *Spanish Still Life: From Velázquez to Goya* (London: National Gallery, 1995), 30.

26. Francesco Bianchini and Azzurra Carrara, *Guía de plantas y flores,* 10th ed. (Barcelona: Grijalbo, 1975), 66.

27. For Hernández's use of the plant's Náhuatl name, see *Mexican Treasury,* "England, 1659–1825," "Seven English Authors."

28. On *Tagetes* deriving from Tages, see Bianchini and Carrara, *Guía,* 248. Tages was endowed with great wisdom and possessed extraordinary powers of prophecy; once written down, his words became the basis of the sacred Etruscan prophetic texts (Pierre Grimal, *Diccionario de mitología griega y romana,* 5th ed. [Barcelona: Paidós, 1991], 489).

29. Font Quer, *Plantas medicinales,* 799.

30. Acosta, *Naturall and Morall Historie,* 4.27.

31. See *Mexican Treasury,* QL 2.1.29; for a more thorough analysis of this chapter, see *Medicinas, drogas,* 220.

32. Among the authorities who identified the American plant with otona was Laguna, for whom the species "that produces beautiful orange colored leaves, called carnation of the Indies, which does not grow except in gardens, I take to be the true othona" (*Pedacio Dioscorides Anazarbeo acerca de la materia medica y de los venenos mortiferos* [Antwerp, 1555], 3.122). At 2.173 he had already noted

that "some moderns want the othona to be the common plant, whose flower is known as carnation of the Indies."

33. *Mexican Treasury, QL* 2.1.29.

34. Sam Segal, *Flowers and Nature: Netherlandish Flower Painting of Four Centuries* (The Hague: SDU, 1990), 197–98. This species appears, for instance, in the flower paintings of Gillis van Caninxloo the younger, or Anthony Claesz. On the plants represented by Tomás Hiepes and Juan de Arellano, see María José López Terrada, "La flora mediterránea y exótica en la obra de Tomás Yepes (ca. 1600–1674)," in *Actas del XI Congreso del Comité Español de Historia del Arte: El Mediterráneo y el Arte Español* (Valencia, 1998), 175–79, and idem, "Las plantas ornamentales en la obra de Juan de Arellano," in *Juan de Arellano (1614–1676),* ed. Alfonso Emilio Pérez Sánchez (Madrid: Caja Madrid, 1998), 79–111.

35. Ibid., 176. This similarity had already been noted in the Royal Spanish Academy's *Diccionario,* 1:375–76 ("this orange or yellow flower is like the carnation in every respect"). That the same name was given to both species at the time is good proof of the identification of the two.

36. Similarities between this marigold and the genus *Tagetes* have caused errors of identification. For example, Jordan and Cherry, *Spanish Still Life,* 122, analyzing *Still Life with Grapevine, Marigolds, and Fruit* by Hiepes in the Plácido Arango collection, Madrid, describe as "a robust African marigold plant" a potted *Tagetes erecta.*

37. An emblem in Claude Paradin, *Devises héroïques* (Lyon, 1551), with the motto "Non inferiora sequutus" carries this sense and was later adopted and modified by Camerarius in his emblem of the sunflower.

38. Monardes, *Historia medicinal,* facsimile ed., fol. 84v. As López Piñero explains in his introduction to the facsimile of the 1590 edition, Monardes mentions many American plants, almost all of them medicinal (57–58). The only exceptions are the *cuantas xaboneras,* used as a soap substitute, and the nasturtium, which interested Monardes mainly because of its beautiful flowers.

39. Bk. 5, cited in Royal Spanish Academy, *Diccionario,* 2:509. Sebastián de Covarrubias Horozco, *Tesoro de la lengua castellana o española,* ed. Martín de Riquer (1611; Barcelona, S. A. Horta, 1943), 793, also calls the nasturtium "mastranto."

40. *Mexican Treasury, QL* 2.1.35.

41. Ibid.

42. Segal, *Flowers and Nature,* 231. Unaware of the Spanish sources, Segal maintains that the nasturtium was not introduced into Europe until the seventeenth century, and he claims that the earliest mention of it is in 1684 (*A Prosperous Past: The Sumptuous Still Life in the Netherlands, 1600–1700* [The Hague: SDU, 1988], 104, 215).

43. *Mexican Treasury,* "England, 1659–1825," "Seven English Authors" (Lovell). The lily belongs to the amarillidaceae, like the narcissus and pancratium.

44. Claudio Boutelou, *Tratado de las flores, en el que se explica el método de cultivar las que sirven para adorno de los jardines* (Madrid: Imprenta de Villalpando, 1804), 93.

45. Mirella Levi D'Ancona, *The Garden of the Renaissance: Botanical Symbolism in Italian Painting* (Florence: Leo S. Olfschy, 1977), 148–51, on the general symbolism of flowers.

46. The lily mentioned in the Bible has been identified as the *Nardostachys jatamansi* D. See Juan Gualberto Talegón, *Flora Bíblico-poética o Historia de las principales plantas que aparecen en la Sagrada Escritura* (Madrid: Widow and Son of D. E. Aguado, 1871), 486–92, who picked up its symbolism not only from the Bible but also from the classics. The identification of *Polianthes tuberosa* L. with the biblical rose was customary in the nineteenth century.

The Royal Spanish Academy's *Diccionario,* 595, adds to its description of the rose this meaning: "The aromatic balm made from the leaves of the rose and its thorns, like that used by Mary Magdalene to wash the feet of Christ."

47. Segal, *Flowers and Nature,* 25.

48. According to Boutelou, *Tratado,* 99, at the beginning of the nineteenth century the lily was exported from Italy or southern France to northern Europe, including England, where it was highly prized.

49. In *Still Life with Black Servant (Bodegón con criado negro)* by Giuseppe Recco (1679), now in the ducal palace of Medinaceli, Seville, lilies are depicted next to anemones and tulips in a vase.

50. Alfonso Emilio Pérez Sánchez, *Pintura española de bodegones y floreros: De 1600 a Goya* (Madrid: Ministerio de Cultura, 1983), 127, fig. 100. On the work of Belvedere, see also *Pintura napolitana: De Caravaggio a Giordano,* exhibition catalog, Palace of Villahermosa (Madrid, 1985), 84–89.

51. Pío Font Quer, *Botánica pintoresca* (Barcelona: Ramón Sopena, 1978), 432.

52. *Mexican Treasury, T* 8.29. The plant that Hernández described as "second atzoyatl" (*T* 5.47) has been identified as a variety of the *Mirabilis.*

53. Clusius, *Rariorum aliquot stirpium, per Pannoniam, Austriam, et vicinas quasdam provincias observatarum historia* (Antwerp, 1583), 401. On this theme, see José María López Piñero and María Luz López Terrada, *La influencia española en la introducción en Europa de las plantas americanas (1493–1623)* (Valencia: Instituto de Estudios Documentales e Históricos sobre la Ciencia, 1997), 82–84.

54. Ríos, *Agricultura,* fol. 251.

55. Filippo Picinelli, *Mundus symbolicus* (Cologne, 1694), XI, 15, no. 165, facs. ed. (New York: Garland, 1976).

56. Giovanni Piero Valeriano Bolzani, *Hieroglyphica, sive de Sacis Aegyptorum aliarumque gentium literis commentarii* (Basle, 1556), fol. 423v; Cesare Ripa, *Iconologia* (Rome, 1593), facs. ed. (Madrid: Akal, 1987), 2.234.

57. Picinelli, *Mundus,* XI, 15, no. 166.

58. *Mexican Treasury, M* 22.35.

59. Monardes, *Historia medicinal,* fol. 89. López Piñero, 55–56, says these "granadillas" appear to correspond to the *Passiflora edulis* Sims., or another, similar variety of the same species.

60. Acosta, *Naturall and Morall Historie,* 4.27.

61. S. Parlasca, *Il fiore della Granadiglia avero della passione di Nostro Signore Giesu Christo* (Bologna, 1609), quoted by Segal, *Flowers and Nature,* 223. According to Linda Kuscar, *Una flor para tí* (Madrid: Mondibérica, 1986), 73–74, it was the Augustinian fray Manuel de Villegas who brought the first dried specimen to Rome from Mexico and sent it to fray Giacomo Bosio, who was so impressed by it that he wrote a treatise on the Crucifixion that contains the earliest description of the plant later known as the passionflower. As usual, earlier Spanish sources have gone unnoticed.

62. See, for example, Royal Spanish Academy's *Diccionario,* 3:154. [Our editorial distinction is not merely pedantic: the history of *stylus* and *stilus* is carefully outlined by William T. Stearn, *Botanical Latin: History, Grammar, Syntax, Terminology, and Vocabulary* (London: Nelson, 1966), 42.—Ed.]

63. Angelo de Gubernatis, *La mythologie des plantes ou les légendes du règne végétal* (Paris, 1876–82), 2:282.

64. Segal, *Flowers and Nature,* 223. The quotation is from John Parkinson, *A Garden of Pleasant Flowers: (Paradisi in Sole, Paradisus Terrestris)* (1629; facs. repr. London: Dover, 1991), 393.

65. Picinelli, *Mundus,* 11.8. It is interesting that Baptista should make a connection between the flower that symbolizes the Passion of Christ and the anemone, the flower that represents Venus's grief for the dead Adonis.

66. Segal, *Flowers and Nature,* 222–23, 231.

67. Antonio Palomino, *El Museo pictórico y la escala óptica: El Parnaso español pintoresco laureado* (Madrid, 1715–24), 2, chap. 2.

68. Covarrubias, *Tesoro,* 641, 968.

69. Fernández de Oviedo, *Historia,* fol. 96. See Pardo and López Terrada, *Primeras noticias,* 286.

70. In Spanish: *flor del sol, gigantea, sol de las Indias, corona real, copa de Júpiter, trompeta de amor,* and *rosa de Jérico.* See Juan Fragoso, *Discurso de las cosas aromáticas, árboles, y frutales, y de otras muchas medicinal simples que se traen de la India Oriental, y sirven al uso de la medicina* (Madrid, 1572), fols. 25r–27v. See José Luis Fresquet Febrer, in *Medicinas, drogas,* 359–60.

71. Monardes, *Historia medicinal,* fol. 89v. Ríos, *Agricultura,* fol. 250, also describes this as a garden plant, calling it *gigantea* "because it grows much," and *flor del sol* "because it follows the sun."

72. *Mexican Treasury,* T 7.15. This evidence is clearly unknown to Kuscar, who declares that "as if by accident, some seeds of this plant came to Spain on board a ship in 1562, and grew in the royal gardens of Madrid . . . but it was a long time before the Spanish took any account of the nutritional properties that were so well known to the natives of America" (*Flor para ti,* 69–70).

73. Rafael García Mahíques, "Flora emblematica: Aproximación descriptiva del código icónico" (Ph.D. diss., University of Valencia, 1991), 243–63, brings together the different meanings attached by the emblematists to these two varieties.

74. Andrés Laguna, *Pedacio Dioscorides,* 4.193, Laguna's commentary on the lesser heliotrope (*Chrozophora tinctoria* Juss.).

75. "In the image of a flower, the clock of the Indies, resides her love" (José de Litala y Castelvi, *De cima del monte Parnaso español* [1672], fol. 128).

76. Vaenius, *Amorum emblemata* (Antwerp, 1608), no. 38. Santiago Sebastián López notes that the same theme can be found in Paradín and Scève ("Lectura critica de los *Amorum emblemata* de Otto Vaenius," *Boletín del Museo e Instituto "Camón Aznar"* 21 [1985]: 5–112). See also Mario Praz, *Studies in Seventeenth-Century Imagery,* 2d ed. (Rome: Edizioni di Storia e Letteratura, 1975), 109, noting Ramon Lull's *Libro del amigo y del amado.*

77. Julián Gallego, *Visión y símbolos en la pintura española del Siglo de Oro,* 3d ed. (Madrid: Cátedra, 1991), 200.

78. Philotheus [pseud. Karl Ludwig], *Philothei Symbola Christiana* (Frankfurt, 1677), 63.125–26, cited by García Mahíques, "Flora emblemática," 258.

79. Camerarius, *Symbolorum et Emblematum* (Mainz, 1668), 1.49, pp. 98–99. Other examples with similar meaning include Gabriel Rollenhagen, *Selectorum emblematum* (Cologne, 1613), 2.51, and Zacharias Heyns, *Emblemata* (Rotterdam, 1625), 41, who shows the sunflower facing the sun's rays accompanied by the text "Christi, actio imitatio nostra" and John 8:12: "I am the light of the world: he that followeth me shall not walk in darkness, but shall have the light of life." And see Segal, *Flowers and Nature,* 220–21.

80. Picinelli, *Mundus,* 11.10; García Mahíques, "Flora emblemática," 262–63.

81. This property of the sunflower is also sometimes ridiculed in Spanish literature, as, for instance, in one of Góngora's sonnets ("Round faces and sunflowers follow my fancy") cited in Royal Spanish Academy, *Diccionario,* 2:102.

82. Representation of the sunflower in Spanish painting is earlier, one of the earliest examples being *Dessert Still Life with a Vase of Flowers, a Clock, and a Dog (Florero y Bodegón con perro)* by van der Hamen, now at the Prado (no. 4158), dating from 1625–30 (reproduced in Jordan and Cherry, *Spanish Still Life,* 46).

83. Segal, *Flowers and Nature,* 35–36, 219.

84. See illustration 19a in ibid., 168.

85. Alfonso E. Pérez Sánchez, "Murillo y sus fuentes," in *De pintura y pintores: La configuración de los modelos visuales en la pintura española* (Madrid: Alianza, 1993), 129–46; Segal, *Flowers and Nature,* 40.

GLOBALIZING THE *NATURAL HISTORY*

JAIME VILCHIS

In August 1570, when Francisco Hernández, physician to the royal household, set out from Seville for New Spain, the first scientific expedition financed by a European monarch was under way. Hernández took with him all the cultural baggage of his era, much like the alchemist Paracelsus, who sought the philosopher's stone, not as the key to the elements but as the key to men's souls.[1] He took with him the concept of man as microcosm, all his concepts colored by the ethical systems of the neo-Stoics and the quirky northern European sect the "Family of Love."

Like a modern Prometheus, Hernández harbored a utopian desire to construct and order cities in the New World. In the utopian communities that were supposed to ensue, indigenous forces in combination with Christian Nicodemian thought would seek to return religion to primitive communities so that their members might dream of the immanence of a definitive kingdom of peace. Those whose religious views and visions of new horizons were at odds with those of the official church prompted a characteristic sixteenth-century "unbelief," which has been discussed lucidly by Lucien Febvre and by Leszek Kolakowski, who refer to this type of believer during the seventeenth century

as a "Christian without a church."[2] All these ideas and beliefs competed with Hernández's dual roles as chief medical officer in New Spain and experimental naturalist. In the seven years of his activity in New Spain, Hernández was able to create a magnificent summa that described the nature and the people of the New World. His tireless traveling and methods of producing a natural and moral history brought together and transcended a half century of historical chronicles and "discovery" literature, written between the Spanish conquest and the early phases of colonization.

Like Juan de Valdez and Fernando de Rojas, Hernández was born in La Puebla de Montalbán, near Toledo. Like Rojas (c. 1475–1541), the author of *La Celestina,* but of a different generation, Hernández saw his work suffer many trials in the composition and editing of the volumes he wrote in New Spain.[3] We know that he wrote two other works, the comparative index of plants and the treatise on the customs and laws of the natives of New Spain. The majority of his manuscripts were read but not published,[4] but they would be "globalized" much like Rojas's tragic comedy of Calisto and Melibella—with the important difference that Hernández never saw so much as a single letter of his encyclopedic work in print. By "globalization" I mean the global diffusion of modernity both through ideas and through conceptual tools. I emphasize three constituent parts in this process of "globalization": (1) the reception of something perceived as new and its diffusion within a given traditional context; (2) appropriation: the regionalization and translation of the cultural tradition and the critical production of these new ideas based on consensus; and (3) the re-creation of these ideas in the form of new contributions (brought about by nationalism and networks of transmission or patronage).[5]

As we know, the manuscripts had to wait until the second half of the twentieth century (1960) before the Madrid edition of 1790 began to appear in a Spanish translation, when the team of scholars led by Germán Somolinos d'Ardois started to publish the *Obras completas*. Despite the acknowledged importance of this collection, the attempt to establish a definitive Hernández canon remains today a laudable but unattainable objective. As Jesús Bustamante has observed, all the original manuscripts would have to be brought together, including some that have not been found yet, before anyone could even dream of assembling Hernández's complete works.[6] Recently Bustamante has revealed the existence of Hernández's translation of Pseudo-Dionysus, in a manuscript at the Biblioteca Nacional in Madrid. This translation will surely shed new light on perceptions of Hernández and will enhance our understanding of his work.[7] My purpose in this essay is to indicate the changing perceptions and interpretations of Hernández's work brought about by two centuries of reading and reception. As others in these two volumes point out, the publication history of Hernández's texts is a story of many vicissitudes, so that the reception of "the work" has always been subject to the historical contingency of interpretation of a shifting text. Reception has also varied because of the intellectual stature of the author, who was able simultaneously to participate in and resist the beginnings and development of modernity. I propose to delineate the diverse ways in which readers and authors received Hernández's thought, in particular by emphasizing the institutional and discursive necessities of his *Natural History of New Spain*.[8]

At the beginning of the seventeenth century, the Escorial librarian, fray José de Sigüenza, wrote a laudatory memoir of Hernández, a recollection of scholarly deduction and diligent experimentation generated by his empathy with the man and his work. Sigüenza wrote it only after a detailed examination of Hernández's writings, in which he detected the work of a theologian "whose profession was to observe what God had created for man's medicine."[9]

The fact that a biblical scholar such as Sigüenza, who belonged to the philological circle of Arias Montano, had recognized the religious tenor of Hernández's *Natural History* is significant. Within the context of Hebraic exegesis, and given Arias Montano's central role in the production of the Polyglot Bible (the *Biblia regia*), the idea that New World nature could be considered "the medicine of salvation" signified, metaphorically, the essential character of the new Jerusalem.[10] Revelation 22:1–2 relates how "in the middle of the street of the city" grows a tree of life whose "leaves serve as medicine to the people of the world," for the health of all people, as Daniel had prophesied. This biblical imagery, not surprisingly, inspired Hernández, as witnessed by his allusions to "the Garden of the Hesperides" in his poem to Arias Montano. The imagery turns up in the cabalist worldview, in which it is associated with "The Tree of the Ten Sephiroth," first planted by God and an image of divine health, whose innate wisdom generates creative forces that multiply.[11] For Hernández the Western paradise, "Hesperia occidua," is translated into the gardens and heights of New Spain, a new motherland with abundant resources, which flourishes with the assistance of inspiration and the aid of Christ. This image was held in especially high regard by *conversos,* for whom the Tree of Life was a metaphor for the Trinity.

Gregorio López (1542–96), a converso and hermit who at one time lived among the Chichimecas, is another example of a European who saw the Tree of Life planted in the new and exceptionally fertile Hesperides.[12] In 1583 he wrote a commentary on the Apocalypse, in which he described the outstanding characteristics of the New Jerusalem:

> The Tree of Life is Wisdom, which resides in the Father and which is one part of the River, and in the Son, which is the other part; the Holy Spirit is the River, so that these three together are Wisdom. The twelve fruits are the fruits

of the Holy Spirit, fruits which are enjoyed by those who are on a pilgrimage. . . . Each month the tree bears fruit which signifies the abundance of the motherland because the land which gives fruit twelve times a year must be fertile, and for this reason David said: I have eaten my fill once your glory was shown to me. It is said that this tree brings good health to all people. The leaves signify the humanity of Christ, which brings eternal health, and it is for this reason that he brought this name when he became a man. He was called Jesus, which means Savior or Health, and there will be no evil things in this land because all will be good in this City.[13]

Fray Jerónimo in his encomiastic gloss on Hernández also echoes the view of the noted court physician and royal councillor Dr. Francisco Valles, a close friend of Hernández's and one who knew his work well—well enough to have had a hand in the transmission of the manuscript of the *Quatro libros*. In *De sacra philosophia* Valles speaks of the physician and the pharmacist as "the ministers of nature and teachers of all people." According to Ecclesiastes 38, all health comes from God. Physicians and pharmacists—with the assistance of emperors—should seek medicine in "all kinds of exotic plants," which means nature that is already known and nature that is as yet undiscovered. The task itself will eventually lead to God.

Sigüenza, who had read the Hernández manuscripts in the library at the Escorial, not only gives Hernández's work the intertextual character I have sketched above but also—mindful that Philip II governed, from the Escorial, the first global empire—likens the work to that of Aristotle for Alexander the Great (as Hernández himself had done).[14] This was how Sigüenza, the wise monk and one of the best writers of the sixteenth century (according to Miguel de Unamuno and Menéndez y Pelayo), displayed the same heightened awareness and sense of purpose that Hernández felt about his expedition, in the face of obstruction from royal functionaries.

Let us leave Sigüenza and the Escorial and move to New Spain and the hospital at Huaxtepec, about sixty miles from Mexico City. It was at Huaxtepec that the Dominican lay brother Francisco Ximénez read the manuscript selection of the *Natural History of New Spain* that had been prepared by Recchi. Hernández had been to this hospital, and Gre-

gorio López had convalesced there when he was ill with "tabardete."[15] Both Hernández and López had written a major part of their works on materia medica within the walls and gardens of this hospital. The hospital was founded in 1569 by Bernardino Alvarez, and, as Carlos Zolla has indicated, it "was a point of confluence for prehispanic herbal medicine and Spanish colonial medicine."[16] In native codices as well as in the historical chronicles and geographical surveys, we can find evidence of the importance of the gardens of Huaxtepec and of the solace and respite they offered the Mexican kings, such as Moctezuma and Netzahualcoyotl.

Gardens served as a metaphor and an important element in the Nahua worldview. Gardens symbolized Tlalocan, or paradise, the final resting place for warriors, sacrificial victims, the shipwrecked, and others who could not arrive in other regions of the complicated Aztec universe.[17] Jeanette F. Peterson makes use of these aspects of Nahua philosophy when she turns to the Augustinian convent of Malinalco, about thirty-seven miles southwest of Mexico City. Peterson develops her idea of "convergence" to support her thesis that "converging gardens" were central to the beginning of the "process of interculturalization" or "translation" as the garden becomes a conflation of Tlalocan, the pre-Columbian paradise, and Christian Europe's garden of Eden.[18]

I wish to emphasize two points intimately linked to the development of this symbolic and eschatological cultural complex. The first is obvious. When Hernández arrived in Mexico in 1571, he established his residence for a time in Cuernavaca, the home base from which he set out for Ocuilán and Malinalco at the time when the Creole frescoes were being designed in the convent of Malinalco. A native glyph of the period shows a friar receiving and greeting a physician, perhaps Hernández himself. Hernández normally stayed in monasteries during his botanical expeditions in New Spain.[19] The second point is that Hernández included in the *Antiquities* a description of the homeland of the "Tlaloques" as a Judeo-Christian paradise:

They held it as a certainty that souls are immortal, and they were convinced that incorporeal souls inhabited one of three regions, to wit: heaven, hell, and earthly paradise. They said that those who fell in war have conquered the sky, where the sun presided, as have those who were taken prisoner in battle and were sacrificed on the altars of the gods, whatever form of death might have befallen them. . . . They believed that heaven was a flat and wooded place ruled by the sun, and thus, on leaving, one was greeted with loud voices. . . . They said that this place consisted of beautiful woods filled with different kinds of trees, domesticated animals, and the songs of a multitude of the most beautiful birds. . . . It is also said that among those who were received into the earthly paradise were those who had been shipwrecked, and those who died after being struck by lightning, those who died of leprosy, mange, and rash and the Indian disease which the natives call *nanahuatl* (which infected the entire globe) and those who died of dropsy. This earthly paradise bore all sorts of fruits and earthly delights. There were never any problems in this place of eternal spring, where the climate was most beautiful. In this place the earth yielded up squashes, corn, chili, and all kinds of blite, orach, vegetables, and fruits. It was also said that those who lived in these regions were the gods who brought the rains and were commonly called *tlaloques* in the native tongue.[20]

But, to return to Ximénez at Huaxtepec, we might remember that he said that he had received the Recchi manuscript of Hernández "by extraordinary means," suggesting underhand activity. Ximénez received this document while at Huaxtepec and, as is well known, undertook a Spanish translation that paradoxically contributed to Hernández's misfortune as an author. Ximénez published his work in 1615 as *Quatro libros,* which would become, without his knowing it, one of the principal vectors of the globalization of Hernández, ironically the opposite of Ximénez's purpose.[21] He meant to produce a local handbook based on observation and experimentation, to be used where there are neither physicians nor pharmacies. We should also remember that Marcgraf, de Laet, and Piso compared Brazil's "book of nature" with that of Recchi and Valles, that is, with Hernández.[22] Quite different from Ximénez's enterprise, Nieremberg enjoyed the privilege of copying "drafts in the author's hand" and copying original drawings from the Hernández papers at the Imperial College in Madrid.[23] Ximénez not only translated Hernández's materia medica, which had passed through the readings, selections, and annotations of two previous readers, but also added personal information based on his own observations at that great laboratory, the hospital at Huaxtépec.[24]

Hernández concluded his stay in New Spain at the Royal Indian Hospital (Real Hospital de los Naturales). In his monk's cell at the hospital he created a small type of cabinet of curiosities, which included herbaria, and he kept live animals such as the axolotl, as well as birds, minerals, plants, drawings, maps, and manuscripts. While he was at the hospital, he and López de Hinojosos carried out the first autopsies in the New World, in 1576, dissecting the bodies of people who had died as a result of the *cocoliztli* epidemic.

In 1587 the *protomédico* died in Madrid, without ever having received full compensation for his efforts.[25] In his will (1578) he names as executor Juan de Herrera, who was then in charge of teaching at Europe's first scientific academy.[26] Two years after Hernández's death, Recchi returned to his native Italy with his manuscript selection of Hernández under his arm. Like Hernández, Recchi, who died in 1595, never saw his work published. In spite of Hernández's anger at what Recchi did to his work, it was Recchi's selection that became the principal vector of globalization, whether by means of Ximénez's translation in America or through the noble efforts of Prince Federico Cesi, Duke of Aquasparta.[27] As we know, in Rome in 1603 the young prince founded the Accademia dei Lincei, the second such scientific society, whose purpose was to carry out the new science based on observation and experiment with natural phenomena. The prince's mentor was the "universal man" Giambattista della Porta, who initiated him in the practice and study of natural magic and co-wrote the new academy's statutes known as *Lynceographum.*[28]

In this invisible college the members of the Lincei, first funded by Cesi, took three decades to prepare the elegant, costly, and monumental edition based on Recchi's selection.[29] Cesi had bought the Recchi manuscript from Marco Petilio. According to Casanova and Bellingeri, this treasury of the materia medica of New Spain is a "Baroque attempt to reconstruct the world," an example of building a monadic "theater of the world," as Cesi liked to call it.[30] The Mexican natural history exemplifies the Lincei's dream of recapturing the secret order of the universe. This view of the book of nature of the Americas, while it lacked one section, would still allow an understanding of the New World, in which microcosm and macrocosm come together in a nutshell, in whose kernel man was the unifying umbilical cord, the point of convergence of the natural and the supernatural.[31] This doctrine was most certainly at the center of Hernández's beliefs.

Cesi read Hernández and studied the plants with the help of a microscope that Galileo had given him, and thanks to della Porta's influence he could study Hernández's descriptions of plants phytosophically. Cesi's twenty phytosophical tables, or "Mirror of Reason," were to be the introduction to the Lincei's edition. These tables outlined a complicated system that dealt with groups of living organisms, with every individual known plant described exactly according to its diverse varieties, uses, and virtues. The ultimate purpose was to establish possible interrelations between planetary and sublunar bodies. Cesi's "tables," much like Lull's *Ars magna (ars combinatoria)* (Lyon, 1517), applied the doctrine of signatures so dear to Paracelsus, and that he had surely learned from della Porta, to the reconstruction of the secret correlations that God had established between the structure of medicine and the natural and moral uses of plants. Again there was an attempt to discern the intimate relationships between the "Garden of Health" and spiritual paradise.[32]

This eclecticism was much more common than is generally thought during the century of scientific revolution. The combination of, on the one hand, classical humoral theory and hermetic/cabbalistic pan-vitalism with, on the other, mechanistic experimentalism and propagandistic and discursive practices during the times of religious wars was typical of the "invisible colleges" of the eighteenth century.[33]

Prince Cesi with all his intellectual baggage not only set out to edit the most important natural history of the times—a stature accorded Hernández's text by Ray's numerous citations, for instance—but also introduced the concept of "family" in botanical studies.[34] However, Hernández's work had to wait until the last third of the eighteenth century before it could be published for the first time in Spain, and then it was as part of another imperial enterprise, much the same as the way it was originally envisaged. During the

reign of the Bourbon Charles III, and in the atmosphere of the enlightened reforms of eighteenth-century Spain, Casimiro Gómez Ortega, the director of the Royal Botanical Garden in Madrid, published three volumes of the Hernández corpus in 1790. The publication of this work was undertaken for "the glory and honor" of the Spanish nation.[35] But before this, about 1780, Juan Bautista Muñoz, the cosmographer of the Indies, had found in the Imperial College a copy of almost all of the Hernández manuscripts, which had belonged to the Jesuits. As I have indicated already, Nieremberg had copied many passages and images from these same manuscripts and had included them in his own natural history. It is necessary to ascribe both of these events—Muñoz's "discovery" ("by divine design") at the time he was researching and looking for materials to be used in his apologetic *Historia del Nuevo Mundo*, as well as Gómez Ortega's publishing of Hernández—to a reforming impulse among Charles III's enlightened ministers, which led to an attempt to recover control of colonial lands as well as to appropriate them scientifically.[36]

About 1762, the Spanish minister Campománes indicated that one of the main reasons that the "laws of the Indies" were not being observed was that the practice of "writing about natural history, geography, and the customs of the Americas, so that the state might know which products are produced," had fallen into total neglect.[37] It is no coincidence that in that same year the Spanish physician José Quer, after a European journey during which he met some of the most notable naturalists of the time, published his *Flora española*. The prologue to this book reprints the "Isagoge" of Tournefort's *Institutiones rei herbariae* (Paris, 1700), which Quer himself had translated into Spanish and to which he added praise of Hernández. But, as I suggested above, Quer's praise of Hernández was recycled Sigüenza. Thus Hernández's work continued to circulate in Spain, but at the hands of the anti-Linnean Quer.

Hernández's natural history entered the century of the Enlightenment within the rhetoric of contemporary Spanish polemics. In my view, while I recognize the risk of being overschematic, there are three series of polemics in which Hernández thus makes an appearance in the second half of the eighteenth century. All three are intimately related to one another and overlap, and all of them indicate an ideological position with respect to natural history, outside Europe, in Spain, and in the Americas. The first is the polemic of the New World; the second, the polemic of science in Spain; and the third, the polemic of the New Botany in New Spain. I shall deal with each in turn, albeit briefly.

If we are to look for a scientific work that cites Hernández as an important authority during the 1700s, we will surely find it in the *Storia antica del Messico* [*The Ancient History of Mexico*] (1780), published in Italy by the Mexican Jesuit Francisco Javier Clavijero. It is noticeable that Hernández is used as an authority alongside Montesquieu, Sloane, and Valmont de Bomare and against Cornelis de Pauw in the context of natural and moral history. He is cited with more respect than Buffon, and at times with more authority than William Robertson, the Scottish historian and well-known leader of the La Condamine scientific expedition to Peru.

In the second half of the eighteenth century, two important events coincide that underscore perhaps one of the most important polemics of the Enlightenment. On the one hand was the "degenerist" view of American nature espoused by one of the major figures of the Enlightenment, which Antonello Gerbi has studied in detail for many years; on the other, the reunification and exile of the Jesuits in Italy after their expulsion from Spain and Spanish America in 1767.[38] These Jesuits came to Italy from all parts of the globe, bringing with them as their only consolation the possibility of intellectual exchange, which was without a doubt one of the best *aggorniamenti* of the Catholic Enlightenment.

It is within this context that we must situate Clavijero's *History* and the importance of his reading of Hernández's work. In the face of Buffon's "degenerative" views, the "miasmatic" ideas of de Pauw, and Robertson's natural law, with its concepts of individualism and balance of power—the three had important implications and consequences for the Americas—Clavijero constructed his history with the help of a complex tradition. Clavijero appropriated elements from the writers of chronicles from the sixteenth century to the baroque period, among them Athanasius Kircher, Sigüenza, Juan de Palafox (sometime viceroy in Mexico), René Descartes, and Benito Jerónimo Feijoo (a great educational

reformer), and he constructed a history of pre-Columbian Mexico in which he not only challenges and refutes the theories of Buffon, de Pauw, and Robertson but also establishes the cultural foundation for what would later become the basis of political nationalism espoused by Francisco Miranda, Simón Bolívar, Fr. Servando, Miguel Hidalgo, and others in Peru, Mexico, Venezuela, and Colombia at the beginning of the nineteenth century.[39]

But in which particular version of Hernández's thought did Clavijero support his beliefs? Was it in the views of the noted Swiss physiologist Albert Haller or in the views of lesser greats such as Marcgraf or even John Ray? Or was it, as we might suspect, in the views of the Lincei from Rome and in the ideas of the Jesuit Nieremberg?[40] In issues concerning questions of nature (plants and animals) he sided with the Lincei; in terms of moral questions (religion and the construction of temples), with Nieremberg. Take, for example, the lengthy and complex argument of *Dissertation No. 4* on Mexican animals, in the section on quadrupeds. Here Clavijero refutes Buffon and de Pauw's idea that American animals are timid because of the softness of the air and other issues of climatic determinism:

> These writers, De Pauw and Buffon, do not have any specific knowledge of American fauna. The truth of the matter is that the *miztli* or Mexican lion is in no way comparable to the lions of Africa. Either the latter species never came to the New World or it was brought to extinction by man. But in no way are the wild beasts of the Americas weaker than any other species such as the lions with no mane of the Old World, as Hernández has said, since he was familiar with both species. The Mexican tiger, whether or not it belongs to the same species of the true tiger of Africa [*sic*], it makes no difference, has great power, and exhibits extraordinary ferocity. If some authors whose work we might respect were to enumerate only small evidence of the prowess of the Mexican tiger, their authority would be debunked as if they were speakers of ridiculous fables. . . . [Clavijero adds as proof that] one need only be aware of what Mr. de la Condamine has written about American tigers, in spite of the fact that Condamine is held in high repute as a mathematician.[41]

If he was able to marshal such a defense for American fauna, what sort of arguments would he advance for the defense of Mexican Indians? In his arguments in defense of the native inhabitants of the New World, Clavijero demonstrates that there was a high degree of rationality and knowledge among pre-Colombian cultures and civilization. His study of the Aztec calendar allows him to show the native people's capacity for abstract thought as well as their vast knowledge of astronomy. The Spanish Jesuit Lorenzo Hervás and the Italian Salvatore Gilij were both interested in updating and carrying out Leibniz's project of classifying cultures according to their languages and in so doing constructing a universal comparative dictionary. Following this method, Clavijero, Hervás, and Gilij set out to study the origin of the Aztec people and their language.[42] In his treatment of the Aztec religion and in his description of Aztec temples, Clavijero bases his information on Hernández, citing the work of fellow Jesuit Nieremberg.

However, Clavijero's eclectic thought is best seen in his treatment of the origin of native populations, in America and Mexico in particular. After observing the Creole Mexican Catholic invention that Quetzalcoatl was the apostle Saint Thomas, and positing this as a probable hypothesis, Clavijero goes on to review, always in a scholarly fashion, all the known intellectual positions on the origin of humans in the Americas, from Acosta to Buffon.[43] After considering these, he goes on to choose the most convincing theories and attempts to accommodate them with the Scriptures. Having no other option, he adheres to Hernández's arguments as stated in the *Antiquities,* in which the protomédico attempted to demonstrate the Hebraic origin of the ancient Mexicans. Clavijero agrees with him on two other points: the necessity of establishing a unity in human lineage, and the argument that humans were transported to the New World after the Flood.[44]

Accordingly, Clavijero's *Ancient History* takes its place alongside Juan Ignacio Molina's great work on Chile, Sánchez Labrador's on Paraguay, and Guille's *Orinoco.* All these works are based on one tradition of natural history in which, if it were structured as a fugue, Hernández would play the basso continuo. All written by Jesuits during their Italian exile, they created an enlightened countercurrent. These works are characterized not by Kantism or individual pietism but rather by a polemic based on eclectic, ecumenical, and syncretic reasoning.[45]

But let us return to Spain during the government of Charles III and his minister José Moñino y Redondo, Count Floridablanca, and the polemics that arose concerning the monarchy and Spanish science. The so-called polemics of Spanish science began in 1782 with the writings of the Frenchman Masson de Morvilliers, who attacked the very notion of Spanish science. The Spaniard Juan Pablo Forner was enjoined to defend Spanish science against the Frenchman's attacks.[46]

In 1788 José Gálvez, general minister of the Indies, charged Nicolás Azara, royal Spanish emissary to Rome, with the task of searching for original manuscripts or documents pertaining to Francisco Hernández and his work, all so that Gómez Ortega might carry out his task of publishing the most nearly complete edition yet of Hernández's work. In a similar manner, the minister asked the viceroy, Bernardo de Gálvez, and Martin Sessé, director of the Royal Botanical Garden of New Spain, and his assistant, Vicente Cervantes, to seek the aid of Creole scientists Alzate, Bartolache, and García Jone in searching for Hernández materials, especially drawings, because Gómez Ortega believed that Hernández's work without illustrations (whether drawings or printed images) would be monstrous, "a body without eyes." None of them was successful in the attempt to recover any Hernández materials.

Nicolás Azara (1730–1804), according to Jean Sarrailh "one of the most intelligent, cultured, and ingenious men of the eighteenth century," recounted his failures to Minister Gálvez in a long letter of July 20, 1785. This letter is in reality a small anthology of the polemic of Spanish science, in which Azara, in a most scholarly way, demonstrates his historiographic knowledge of Hernández's work and his strong negative beliefs about Floridablanca's efforts and underscores the importance of Spanish science:

> It would happen that in wanting to give credit to our country, we might remove credit and produce things which do not belong to the genius of [the eighteenth] century. Natural sciences are not like the speculative sciences, nor are they like history, poetry, or the study of

rhetoric. Those disciplines become perfect with time and experience, so that anyone who wants to speak of them as they were two centuries ago finds no help from contemporaries. Take for example Juan de Valverde, one of the most important masters of anatomy of the sixteenth century, whose work was published and translated into Italian and Latin with great success. However, if one wanted to honor Spain (and Spanish science) by publishing his work, all of Europe would laugh at him as they would at the mathematics and astronomy of Pedro Ceruelo and at the studies on navigation by Spanish scientists from the same era. In a similar manner they would laugh at the works of da Orta, Christopher Acosta, Monardes, Oviedo and others who were engaged in the task of writing works of natural history. Based on what little I have to judge, Hernández was a unique case. His work at that time was most useful and the development of natural science owes a great deal to him because he was the first to make known, using a scientific method, the natural products of New Spain. However the only method he had at his disposal was that of Dioscorides, which is merely empirical. His work does not have the honor of standing next to such modern scientists as Tournefort or Linnaeus, who have changed the face of botany and have developed that discipline to the state of the art in which we find it today. However, I do not know what the judgment of the scholars of our day would be with respect to an author who seriously wrote about the discovery in Mexico of human skeletons which had two heads (like Janus), two noses, two mouths, four eyes, and so on. The only part of Hernández's work whose utility we might emphasize is his illustrations of plants and animals, because they were executed under his direction and because they demonstrate the characteristics and description of a work of art.[47]

It is in this polemical manner, which is recorded in the history of science and colored with the bias of modernity, that Francisco Hernández was read in eighteenth-century Spain and edited by some of the most enlightened thinkers of the day. Hernández's scientific expedition, according to Azara, is the "hidden foundation" of "a great man" on whose shoulders rests a new expedition of the eighteenth century, much like a Lilliputian (inverting Swift's image) reorganizing the foreign lands of the kingdom.[48] His name, more of a hero than an author, is engraved on both coasts of the

Atlantic, with gold letters on the frontispiece of the New Republic of Letters so that it might provide its citizens with a rhetorical device—to some, like the Jesuits and the Creoles, as a tool for regionalizing culture and to others the tools to refertilize the antique laurels of the ancient empire. The recently born American motherland, the emerging spirit of Creolism, used this rhetorical device as a geographical, physiological, and descriptive paradigm, which would legitimate the native tradition against the Linnean thought of such Spanish scientists as Mutis, Sessé, and Cervantes.[49] However, in the hands of men such as Bartolache, the work of Hernández was put to political use as a pretext for disobedience, and for men such as Alzate it was used as an argument against Spanish systems of taxonomy. Finally, for the followers of Mociño and Mutis it was used as a symbol of hegemonic prestige and a monument to those who had found royal funding for their scientific endeavors.

NOTES

1. Ludwig Binswanger, *Drei Formen missglükten Daseins: Verstiegenheit, Verschrobenheit, Manieriertheit* (Tübingen: Niemeyer, 1956); José María Valverde, *El Barroco, una visión de conjunto* (Barcelona: Montesinos, 1980), 9; José Gaos was one of the first to detect the sense of modernity in the traveler who, in the time of Hernández, sailed around the world in search of a Utopia that had been foreseen even before the European discovery of the New World (*Historia de nuestra idea del mundo* [Mexico City: Colegio de México and FCE, 1973], 133–41).

2. Lucien Febvre, *Le Problème de l'incroyanse au XVIe Siècle, la religion de Rabelais;* English edition, translated by Beatrice Gottlieb, 1942, as *The Problem of Unbelief in the Sixteenth Century* (Cambridge: Harvard University Press, 1982); and Leszek Kolakowski, *Cristianos sin iglesia en el siglo XVII* (Madrid, 1982).

3. *La Celestina* is a long prose drama in twenty-one acts, with a tangled bibliographical history. See the parallel text edition by Dorothy Sherman Severin (Warminster: Aris & Phillips, 1987), which uses James Mabbe's English translation of 1631.

4. See *Mexican Treasury,* especially the two introductory essays.

5. One of the first of these contributions to this concept of globalization, although not precisely coinciding with our understanding of this idea, can be found in the work of Xavier Polanco in "Une science-monde: La mondialisation de la science européenne et la création de traditions scientifiques locales," in *Naissance et développement de la science-monde,* ed. Xavier Polanco (Paris: Editions La Découverte, 1990), 10–51; also, a conversation with Antonio Lafuente and María Luisa Ortega, "Modelos de mundialización de la ciencia," *Arbor* 142, nos. 558–60 (1992): 93–117.

6. See Jesús Bustamante, "The *Natural History of New Spain,*" in *Mexican Treasury.*

7. Bustamante emphasizes the important point that "all the Hernández manuscripts used by Casimiro Gómez Ortega for his

edition, which were believed to have been lost, have now reappeared" ("De la naturaleza y los naturales americanos en el siglo XVI: Algunas cuestiones críticas sobre la obra de Francisco Hernández," *Revista de Indias* 52, nos. 195–96 [1992]: 297–328).

8. In this essay I use the underpinnings of the theory of reception from Wolfgang Iser, *The Act of Reading* (Baltimore: Johns Hopkins University Press, 1978), the subject of recent commentary by the Spanish philosopher Emilio Lledó in *El Silencio de la escritura*, 2d ed. (Madrid: Centro de Estudios Constitucionales, 1990).

9. José de Sigüenza, *Historia de la Orden de San Gerónimo* (Madrid: Imprenta Real, 1600), especially pt. 3, bk. 4, discourse 11, fol. 778, column 1a: "This enterprise was ordered by the King, and Dr. Francisco Hernández, a learned and diligent man from Toledo as the preface states, spent a little more than four years in the Indies. There he organized all his work, leaving no part of his charge unfulfilled. With the power granted him by the King, he carried out the writing of fifteen books of folio size. In each book he placed illustrations in color of the plants and animals he had described to the best of his abilities. Where he could not provide drawings or paintings he provided a description of the virtues and names of the plants and animals, according to the knowledge and experience of natives and Spaniards alike. He was able to make sense of this information but at times he could only conjecture the names, virtues, and uses of the plants and animals based on the information supplied by his informants, who had tested the usefulness of the natural products that he was studying. This vast enterprise could well compete with what Alexander had done with Aristotle. However, Hernández's work is not as complete as it could have been. It is but a beginnning for those who might wish to carry out this endeavor. It is not a task for one man alone." Sigüenza's history was widely disseminated not only during his own time but also during the eighteenth century, when José Quer copied Sigüenza's text in its entirety in his *Flora española* (1762), 1.37, without acknowledgment. See Antonio Hernández Morejón, *Historia bibliográfica de la medicina española*, 4 vols. (Madrid, 1842–45; reprint, New York: Johnson, 1967), 3:398–400.

10. It is no coincidence that Arias Montano dealt with "the medicine of salvation" in his *Humanae salutis monumenta*, written in Latin hexameters and published in Antwerp by Christophe Plantin, with illustrations, in 1571. See Benito Arias Montano, *Monumentos de la salud del hombre: Desde la caída de Adán hasta el Juicio Final*, translation into Spanish by Benito Feliú de San Pedro (Madrid: Swan, 1984).

11. It is interesting to note that in the *Book of Stoic Questions*, chap. 1, Hernández deals with the origin of the world and refers explicitly to the "science of the Cabala" in order to demonstrate the basic similarity between Plato and Aristotle on the preexistence of Chaos ("common mother" or "basic substance") before the Creation. In cabalistic thought the preexisting Chaos, or "Tohu," is one of the principal myths. Despite these interesting points of coincidence in the thought of Hernández, Sigüenza, and Arias Montano, it was fray Luis de León who was accused of being a cabalist and was called to Rome to answer charges of heresy for his biblical commentary, *De arcano sermone*, which greatly influenced his censored *Nombres de Cristo*. Hernández, Sigüenza, and Arias Montano were involved in the same thaumaturgy or theurgy, which in the sixteenth century was connected to the medical humanism of Marsilio Ficino and Pico della Mirandola. Writings representing this hermetic and cabalistic current of thought were carefully collected by Ambrosio Morales y Montano in the library of the Escorial. The tradition is also visible in the frescoes on the vaulted ceiling of the choir by Luca Cambiaso and those in the library by Pelegrino Tibaldi. See René Taylor, "Architecture and Magic: Some Considerations on the *Idea* of the Escorial," in *Essays in the History of Architecture Presented to Rudolf Wittkower*, ed. Douglas Fraser,

Howard Hibbard, and Milton J. Lewine (London: Phaidon, 1967), 81–109. See also B. Rekers, *Arias Montano (1527–1598)* (London: Warburg Institute, University of London, 1972; Leiden: E. J. Brill, 1972), 105–30.

12. For the significance of the theme of the Hesperides in America and the myths it generated at the time of the discovery, see Juan Gil, *Mitos y utopías del descubrimiento* (Madrid: Alianza, 1989) 1:73–77.

13. See Francisco Losa, *Tratado del apocalipsis y vida del siervo de Dios Gregorio López (1536–1624)* (Madrid, 1727), 297. Despite the implication of this title, López lived from 1542 to 1596.

14. See *Mexican Treasury*, Letter 3: [November/December 1571], in which Hernández compares himself to Aristotle and his protector to Alexander.

15. [Apparently typhus, according to the implication of Francisco Bravo, *Opera medicinalia* (Mexico City, 1570), fols. 1–5.—Ed.]

16. See Francisco Guerra, *El "Tesoro de Medicinas" de Gregorio López, 1542–1596* (Madrid: Cultura Hispánica del Instituto de Cooperación Iberoamericana, 1982). I have compared this work of López (c. 1589) with other medical texts of the period and noticed his philosophical ideas based on the Apocalypse ("Medicina novohispana del siglo XVI y la materia médica indígena: Hacia una caracterización de su ideología," *Quipu* 5, no. 1 [1988]: 19–48). See also Carlos Zolla, "La obra de Gregorio López en el Hospital de Guastepec," in *Gregorio López y su Tesoro de Medicinas para todas las enfermedades,* ed. Antonio Zedillo (Mexico City, 1983), xv–xxviii.

17. On the codices, see *La historia tolteca-chichimeca: Anales de Quauhtinchan,* ed. Heinrich Berlin and Silvia Rendón (Mexico City: Porrua, 1947), which includes the story of a lost paradise and the source of many ancient Mexican lineages according to the interpretation offered by Serge Gruzinski, *Painting the Conquest: The Mexican Indians and the European Renaissance,* trans. Deke Dusinberre (Paris: Flammarion, 1992), 103–14. In particular, see the section on the murals of Tepantitla, Teotihuacán, where the Tlalocan is represented. For the chronicles, see Alvarado Tezozomoc, *Crónica mexicana* (Mexico City: UNAM, 1944), with notes by Manuel Orozco y Berra; also Bernal Díaz del Castillo, *The Discovery and Conquest of Mexico*, trans. Irving A. Leonard (New York: Farrar, Straus and Cudahy, 1956).

On the *Relaciones* of Huaxtepec, see Gutiérrez de Liévana (1580), especially the "Description of Huastepec," in an appendix to E. J. Palacios, *Huastepec y sus reliquias arqueológicas* (Mexico City: SEP, n.d.), and René Acuña, ed., *Relaciones geográficas del siglo XVI* (Mexico City: UNAM, 1984), 206. For a study of the "geographical descriptions" and their connections with medicine, see Raquel Alvarez, *La conquista de la naturaleza Americana* (Madrid: CSIC, 1993). Finally, on the concept of "Tlalocan" and its place in the Náhuatl worldview and afterlife, see Francisco del Paso y Troncoso, *La botánica entre los Nahuas y otros estudios* (Mexico City: SEP, 1988), esp. 39–73; Alfredo López Austin, *The Human Body and Ideology: Concepts of the Ancient Nahuas,* trans. Thelma Ortiz de Montellano and Bernard Ortiz de Montellano (Salt Lake City: University of Utah Press, 1988), 1:331–43; Bernard Ortiz de Montellano, *Aztec Medicine, Health, and Nutrition* (New Brunswick: Rutgers University Press, 1990), 37–55.

18. Jeanette F. Peterson, "La flora y la fauna en los frescos de Malinalco: Paraíso convergente," in *Iconología y sociedad: Arte colonial hispanoamericano, XLIV Congreso Internacional de Americanistas* (Mexico City: UNAM, 1987), 23–42, and her full-length study, *The Paradise Garden Murals of Malinalco: Utopia and Empire in Sixteenth-Century Mexico* (Austin: University of Texas Press, 1993). The quotations cited by Peterson are compelling evidence of the "convergence" of metaphors that she finds in the cloisters of Malinalco.

With considerable critical acumen she identifies and disentangles many of the plants represented in the complex mural. She identifies such plants as the *huacalxochitl, ololiuhqui, cacaoxochitl,* and the *zapote* tree, whose fruit is similar to the "apple from the Garden of Eden." She also describes an image of a snake hypnotizing a bird. All these are also described by Cruz and Badianus, by Sahagún in the *Florentine Codex,* and by Hernández. The paintings of plants and animals carried out by native artists or "tlacuilos" served to educate European friars and physicians in the hospitals of New Spain and brought about "inculturization" during the sixteenth century. See Ignacio Chávez, *México en la cultura médica* (Mexico City, 1947), 51–68, and Jaime Vilchis and José Salá, *Pensamiento utópico y profético hispano-americano* (Toluca, Mexico: Universidad Autonoma del Estado de México, 1990). For a comparison of these three works and their relation with natural history in general, see Debra Hassig, "Transplanted Medicine: Colonial Mexican Herbals of the Sixteenth Century," *Res* 17–18 (1989): 31–53, esp. 48–53. Also, Jacqueline Durand-Forest, "Aperçu de l'histoire naturelle de la Nouvelle-Espagne d'après Hernández, les informateurs indigènes de Sahagún et les auteurs du codex Badianus," in *Nouveau monde et renouveau de l'histoire naturelle,* ed. M. C. Bénassy-Berling (Paris: Université de la Sorbonne, 1986), 3–28. On the different types of pre-Hispanic gardens according to their use of space and their ideological function, see Alain Musset, "Les jardins préhispaniques," *Trace* 10 (1986): 59–73.

19. Somolinos, "Vida y obra," 1:198 ff., and Rafael Chabrán and Simon Varey, "Entr'acte," above.

20. See Hernández's *Antiquities,* 1.15, in *Mexican Treasury.* In the *OC* 6:73–74 n. 61, Miguel León-Portilla notes that bk. 1, chap. 15, is based on Sahagún (and see Eduardo Seler's edition [Mexico City: Robredo, 1938], 1:283–88), bk. 3, chaps. 1–3. It is interesting to note that in this comparison Hernández tries to "semitize" the concept of "tlalocan," which, as León-Portilla indicates, omits Sahagún's concept of limbo. No less interesting is chapter 11, which deals with "the origin of the people of New Spain" and combines the legend of Chicomoztoc, or "the place of the seven caves," with the conjecture that they form part of the Lost Tribes of Israel dispersed by Salmanasar, king of the Assyrians.

21. See *QL.* In the *Epistle to Arias Montano* Hernández complains of the mistreatment of his text by a foreign hand (that is, Recchi). I think that one reason that Philip II might have ordered Recchi to make his selection from Hernández's work was to control the protomédico's encyclopedic ambition (which Hernández himself admitted in the preface to the *Antiquities*). I believe that Hernández's desire to write an encyclopedic natural history would have had the effect of making publication of his work more difficult as well as inducing the king's displeasure.

22. For the Dutch diffusion of Hernández, see Rafael Chabrán and Simon Varey, "The Hernández Texts," in *Mexican Treasury* and their "Hernández in the Netherlands and England," above. Also, José M. López Piñero, "Los primeros estudios científicos sobre la materia médica americana: La historia medicinal de Nicolás Monardes y la Expedición de Francisco Hernández a Nueva España," in *Viejo y nuevo continente: La medicina en el encuentro de dos mundos* (Madrid: Saned, 1992), 221–79.

23. Nieremberg is important not least because his work contains copies of five original illustrations of plants as well as those from the *Antiquities* made by native artists in New Spain. Nieremberg's illustrator was Christopher Jegher, a student of Rubens's. Recently, López Piñero has demonstrated that the *Codex Pomar* (c. 1590) includes some thirty copies in color and watercolor of paintings and copies of illustrations from the Hernández expedition. See *Códice Pomar* and López Piñero, "The Pomar Codex (ca. 1590): Plants and Animals of the Old World and from the Hernadez [sic]

Expedition to America," *Nuncius* 7, no. 1 (1992): 35–52. The issue of cosmography is central in evaluating the work of Hernández in Mexico. The value of the iconographic works was noticed long ago: for example, Enrique Alvarez, "El Dr. Francisco Hernández y sus comentarios a Plinio," *Revista de Indias* 3, no. 8 (1942): 251–90. Alvarez speaks of Hernández's work in terms of an "encyclopedic naturalism" with a new vision of the world. Along these lines, see Somolinos, "Sobre la iconografía botánica original de las obras de Hernández y su sustitución en las ediciones europeas," *Revista de la Sociedad Mexicana de Historia Natural* 15, nos. 1–4 (1954): 73–86.

24. Guillermo Gándara carefully compared Ximénez's translation and Hernández's manuscript, in "La obra de fray Francisco Ximénez comparada con la del doctor Francisco Hernández, recompuesta por el Dr. Nardo Antonio Recco," *Memorias y Revista de la Sociedad Científica "Antonio Alzate"* 39 (1921): 99–120. Although there is little space here, I would like to cite one example of the type of commentary that Ximénez added to Hernández's work. In speaking of the *ololiuhqui,* he agrees with Hernández in terms of the plant's description, basic nature, medicinal virtues, and various mixtures. When Hernández comes to describe the plant's use by native priests, he recounts how it is used to communicate with the gods, to induce delirium and invoke spirits and demons, but Ximénez modifies the text, and, at the point where Hernández says that the Indian priests "wanted to make believe that they were talking to the gods," Ximénez omits the section altogether, perhaps because he did not want to emphasize what was happening and wanted to attack Amerindian shamanism. This is what David Goodman believes (see the chapter "The King's Control of Medical Practice," in *Power and Penury* [Cambridge: Cambridge University Press, 1988]). Similarly, although Hernández indicates where one can find the plant, Ximénez decides that "it would be a great mistake to say where it grows, because it is not important, even if the Spanish do not know about this plant"(*QL* bk. 2, sec. 1, chap. 14).

When considering the notion of sixteenth-century hospitals in New Spain as "social laboratories of transculturation," one should remember that the "pueblo-hospital" communities founded by Quiroga in Michoacán were established in imitation of the statutes of the lay brotherhoods, written and promulgated by fray Alonso de Molina for Franciscan hospitals. We must underscore three characteristics of these hospitals: (1) their utopian function; (2) their "intercultural" function; and (3) their experimental and pharmacological mission. See Guenter B. Risse, "Shelter and Care," above.

25. Upon his return to the court of the Escorial, sick and infirm, with little energy left to continue living, Hernández gave himself over to obtaining indulgences in order to "die well." The obstacles he had encountered during the expedition were eventually overshadowed by his remarkable and diverse writing projects. The disparity between what he was sent to do and the amount that he wrote certainly provoked the envy of the "palace rats" as well as the king's displeasure that he had overstepped the bounds and scope of his mission. Having lost the support of Juan de Ovando, the head of the Council of the Indies, Hernández registered his bitter complaint in his poem to Arias Montano. The complaint reads like the cry of a dying swan in the opinion of the noted nineteenth-century Spanish natural historian Marcos Jiménez de la Espada. Another reason for Hernández's fall from favor was his heterodox thought, to which he himself alluded in his poem. Although his heterodoxy is easy to explain, it should be seen in terms of its double meaning: Erasmianism (which Elias Trabulse has postulated) is not enough to explain heterodox thought, especially in light of the recently discovered translation of Pseudo-Dionysus, which in turn leads to revaluation of Hernández's *Christian Doctrine.* Second, B. Rekers includes the thought of Arias Montano in the context of the

Flemish "Family of Love," which was closely tied to the Hebraic thought of fray Luis de León and which caused the latter so many problems with the Inquisition. Only after considering these factors can we have a sketch of the possible heterodox nature of Hernández's thought. See Elías Trabulse, "El erasmismo de un científico: Supervivencias del humanismo cristiano en la Nueva España de la contrareforma," *Historia Mexicana* 28, no. 2 (1978): 224–96, and Rekers, *Arias Montano*, 70–104.

26. The project for the creation of the Academy of Mathematics was carried out by Herrera during the first decade of the 1570s when he held the post of chamberlain at the Escorial. But it was not until December 1582 that the academy began to function with the express purpose of bringing together experts in cosmography and nautical sciences, in order to standardize the routes to the Indies according to established nautical charts.

27. Nardo Antonio Recchi was born in Montecorvino in what is now the province of Salerno. He received his medical degree in 1564 from Salerno's medical school. In 1589 he returned to Naples with his copy and selection of Hernández's work as well as with copies of the original illustrations. In Naples he worked as so-called chief physician. On his death he bequeathed his Hernández manuscript to his nephew Petilio along with all his other writings.

28. G. B. Marini Bettòlo, *Una guida alla lettura del tesoro Messicano: Rerum medicarum Novae Hispaniae thesaurus* (Rome: Accademia Nazionale dei Lincei, 1992), 11–67. It was in this academy that Galileo, a member of the Lincei since 1611, disseminated his ideas on Copernican heliocentrism and applied experimental rigor to the new Baconian sciences. Among those who collaborated in the foundation of the Lincei were Prince Cesi along with his young cousin Anastasio de Filles, the Dutch physician Johan Heck, and the Galilean scientist Francesco Stelluti, who was the driving force and guiding spirit of the academy. Stelluti was responsible for summarizing the work of his teacher Giambattista della Porta's work *Della fisonomia* (Rome, 1637) as well as preparing the indexes for the Rome edition (but cf. José M. López Piñero and José Pardo Tomás, "Contribution of Hernández," above), and was in charge of publishing the last seven "phytosophical tables," which Cesi had left incomplete. See Julio Caro Baroja, *Historia de la fisiognómica* (Madrid: Istmo, 1988), 107–34.

29. The following is a chronology of the publication of the Rome edition by the Lincei:

1618   Johannes Terrentius goes to Madrid to consult the Hernández originals.

1625–28 Johannes Faber finishes the treatise on animals.

1626–28 Fabio Colonna writes his annotations on the work on plants.

1626   Cassiano dal Pozzo goes to Madrid and obtains a copy of Hernández that was not included in Recchi's manuscript.

1628   Cesi completes the first thirteen "phytosophical tables" and finishes the Lincei edition of Hernández up to page 936 as it would eventually be printed, with the "first" title page by Mattias Greuter.

1630   The death of Cesi and the printing of the "second" title page by Greuter.

1648   Printing of the "third" title page by J. F. Greuter.

1649–51 Olimpia Cesi gives Alfonso Turrienus all the material from the *Thesaurus* prepared in 1630. Vitale Mascardi uses this material, placing the title page successively on the respective editions, 1648–49 and 1651.

1649   The printing of the "fourth" title page by J. F. Greuter and pages 937–50 (the tables and later materials). Publication of volume 2 (pp. 1–95) based on Hernández's descriptions of Mexican animals, taken from the copy Dal Pozzo had brought to Rome.

1651   Printing of the "fifth" title page by G. Greuter and a new title page requested by Turrienus. Printing of the index.

30. Rosa Casanova and Marco Bellingeri, *Alimentos, remedios, vicios y placeres: Breve historia de los productos mexicanos en Italia* (Mexico City: INAH-OEA, 1988), 63–83.

31. The Renaissance idea of man as microcosm was first developed in Spain by Raimundo de Sabunde. Hernández writes on this concept in two paragraphs of his *Book of Stoic Questions*. In the first paragraph ("On the Community of Love") he connects the Renaissance notion of man as microcosm with Giordano Bruno's doctrine of Neoplatonic pantheism, and in the second ("Whether the Light of the Sun Is a Corporal Quality or an Accident, and on the Eyes and Vision") he relates the same idea of the microcosm to Pico della Mirandola's "Spiritual Heliocentrism." See Eugenio Garin, "The Philosopher and the Magus," in Garin et al., *Renaissance Characters,* trans. Lydia G. Cochrane (Chicago: University of Chicago Press, 1991), 123–53, and José Antonio Maraval, "Sobre naturaleza e historia en el humanismo español," *Arbor* 64 (1951). However, Hernández gives the doctrine of man as microcosm, especially in terms of its relation to Pythagorean music of the spheres, an unusual turn with respect to heliocentrism. He accepts that the earth does not move because it does not have the same "sound" (or music) as the other spheres, and on the other hand he invites readers not to be surprised if it seems that the doctrine of free will is questioned. In summary, Nature takes part in our moral decisions to do good or evil.

32. In 1657 the English botanist William Coles took the doctrine of signatures to an extreme in *Adam in Eden,* but the most famous and heterodox thinker to apply this alchemical doctrine to botany was Theophrastus Bombast von Hohenheim, known as Paracelsus (1493–1541). According to him the three principal substances—not elements—of all living bodies were sulfur, salt, and mercury. These substances determine the particular virtues of each plant according to the combination in which they are found in that plant. The Neapolitan della Porta combined the doctrine of signatures with that of physiognomy in *Phytognomonica* (1588), in which he explains how the virtues and curing powers of plants can be seen in their external appearance. See Agnes Arber, *Herbals: Their Origins and Evolution* (Cambridge: Cambridge University Press, 1938), 247–70.

In table 14 (Rome edition, 939) Cesi offers a classification for the sciences and the arts based on the various sections of his phytosophia and the followers of this discipline.

33. Francis Yates has demonstrated this to be true of the Royal Society and for the Rosicrucians of Bohemia, as has Akerman for Queen Christina's Academy in Sweden. Vicenzo Ferrone has said much the same of Italian scientific societies. Without a doubt the Lincei's *Thesaurus* was meant to be a propaganda effort on behalf of the Catholic reform supported by Cardinal Barberini from Rome. See Yates, *The Rosicrucian Enlightenment* (London: Routledge & Kegan Paul, 1972); S. Akerman, "The Forms of Queen Christina's Academies," in *Shapes of Knowledge from the Renaissance to the Enlightenment,* ed. D. Kelly and Richard H. Popkin (Dordrecht, the Netherlands: Kluwer, 1991), 165–88; and Vicenzo Ferrone, *The Intellectual Roots of the Italian Enlightenment: Newtonian Science, Religion, and Politics in the Early Eighteenth Century,* trans. Sue Brotherton (Atlantic Highlands, N.J.: Humanities Press, 1995).

34. Yet it is possible that Ray might have further developed the concept of species for plants after Cesi. What is certain is that the concept of "family" based on affinities of species on an empirical basis in botany appears again in a meaningful manner in the work of Michel Adanson (1727–1806) and A. P. de Candolle (1776–1837)

as an alternative to Linnaean functionalism. See Antonello La Vergata, "La specie: Il problema della sua fissita en l'evoluzione biologica: Da Linneo a Darwin, 1735–1871," in *Storia della scienza,* ed. Paolo Rossi (Turin, UTET, 1979), 95–133.

35. For the Madrid edition, see text vol., intro. See Javier Puerto, *Ciencia de Cámara: Casimiro Gómez Ortega (1741–1818) el científico cortesano* (Madrid: CSIC, 1992), 242–47, and Leoncio López-Ocón, "Circulation of the Work of Hernández," below.

36. Antonio Lafuente, "Las expediciones científicas del setecientos y la nueva relación del científico con el Estado," *Revista de Indias* 47, no. 180 (1987): 373–79.

37. P. Rodríguez Campománes, *Reflexiones sobre el comercio español a Indias,* ed. Rosa Llompart (Madrid: Instituto de Estudios Fiscales, 1988), 247.

38. On the "degenerist" view, see Antonello Gerbi, *The Dispute of the New World: The History of a Polemic, 1750–1900,* rev. ed. trans. Jeremy Moyle (Pittsburgh: University of Pittsburgh Press, 1973). Edmundo O'Gorman notes that the Hegelian thesis that the Americas were inferior had actually originated with de Pauw and Buffon (Gerbi, pref., n.p.). [The polemical battle is, in some respects, still being fought: see Elsa Malvido, "Illness, Epidemics," above.—Ed.] Recently Jorge Cañizares has returned to this topic, emphasizing the moral history viewed from the Americas: "Entre Maquiavelo y la jurisprudencia natural: William Robertson y la disputa del Nuevo Mundo," *Quipu* 8, no. 3 (1991): 279–91.

39. Francisco Javier Clavijero, *Storia antica del Messico Cavata da' migliori storici spagnuoli, e da' manoscritti, e dalle pinture antiche degl'indiani,* 4 vols. (Cesena, Italy, 1780–81). I have used Joaquín de Mora's Spanish translation (Jalapa, 1868).

Among the most accessible titles in the extensive bibliography on Clavijero are Charles Ronan, *Francisco Javier Clavijero, S.J. (1731–1787), Figure of the Mexican Enlightenment: His Life and Work* (Rome: Institutum Historicum, S.I., 1977; Chicago: Loyola University Press, 1977); Giovanni Marcheti, *Cultura indígena e integración nacional: La Historia Antigua de México de F. J. Clavijero* (Jalapa: University of Veracruz, 1986); A. Martínez Rosales, ed., *Francisco Xavier Clavijero* (Mexico City: Colegio de México, 1988); and Anthony Pagden, *Spanish Imperialism and the Political Imagination* (New Haven: Yale University Press, 1990).

40. In speaking of the incomparable beauty of the flower known as "Viper's head"(*cabeza de víbora* or *coatzontecoxochitl*), Clavijero is clear that his source is the Rome edition of Hernández of 1651, noting how the Lincei adopted this flower as an emblem (*Historia antigua,* 23 n. 1). In addition to listing useful plants, the Mexican Jesuit discusses another plant (34) that Hernández had described for the first time, one believed to cure kidney problems: the *tlapalezpatli* (or *ezpatli,* meaning "scarlet medicine") or *lignum nephriticum* (meaning "kidney wood") (see *Mexican Treasury,* "Seven English Authors" [Petiver]). Clavijero tested this famous plant on himself. Kircher and Grimaldi knew of the fluorescent qualities of this plant and experimented with the diffraction of colors when its stems are submerged. In the *Optics,* bk. 2, pt. 3, sec. 5, Newton speaks of how it reflects rays of one color but transmits another.

41. *Historia antigua,* 217. Clavijero was aware of what the Lincei believed, but he was also critical of this view of Mexican wolves: "Johannes Faber, a member of the Academy of the Lincei, published in Rome a long and erudite dissertation in which he tried to prove that the xoloitzcuintli is the same animal as the wolf from Mexico. However, he let himself be fooled by the picture of the quadruped which, among other illustrations, Dr. Hernández sent [*sic*] to Rome. However, if he had read the description given by this learned naturalist in his book "On the Quadrupeds of Mexico," he would have saved himself the trouble of writing that work and spared the cost of its printing. Buffon accepted Faber's error" (40 n. 4). This work by Hernández was carefully read and studied by the eighteenth-century military natural historian Félix de Azara. After taking part in an expedition to the borders of Paraguay, Azara wrote about the quadrupeds of that region in his *Natural History.* According to Enrique Alvarez, this is not only the place in which one can read about a theory that would ultimately influence Darwin but also a place where Azara could respond to Buffon and de Pauw concerning their views of and polemics on the New World. Azara was without a doubt the first Spaniard to carry out this type of work (Alvarez, "Félix de Azara, precursor de Darwin," *Revista de Occidente* 12, no. 128 [1934]: 146–66).

42. In Italy, Clavijero certainly enjoyed the sparkling intellectual ambience produced by the convergence of the similarly exiled Hervás and Gilij—and, of course, he brought with him a rich Spanish linguistic tradition—and between 1767 and 1787 he compiled the *Reglas de la lengua mexicana con un vocabulario.* Filipo Salvatore Gilij, *Saggio di storia americana* (Rome, 1784), vol. 3, is a treatise on linguistics that was translated into German and used by Humboldt; Lorenzo Hervás, *Idea dell'universo* (Cesena, Italy, 1778). See Jesús Bustamante, "Asimilación europea de las lenguas indígenas americanas," in *Ciencia colonial en América,* ed. Antonio Lafuente and José Sala (Madrid: CSIC, 1992), 45–77.

The encyclopedic mentality of Hervás and Panduro encompassed the Mexican calendar and led to a polemical public debate with Clavijero on the accuracy or otherwise of the *Ciclografía mexicana* of the baroque scientist Sigüenza y Góngora and of the great Italian traveler and collector Boturini. See Clavijero, *Historia antigua,* 324–41.

43. On the Mexican temple, Clavijero, *Historia antigua,* 190 n. 1, and for the relation between Saint Thomas and Quetzalcoatl, 182.

44. The discussion on the origin of the human race in the Americas is in Clavijero, *Historia antigua,* dissertation 1, 148–67. For the tradition of the idea of the unity of the human race, see E. Sauras, "La unidad del linaje humano según Francisco de Vitoria," *Anuario de la Asociación Francisco de Vitoria* 10 (1972).

45. Three important themes converged, in my view, in the understanding of the Jesuit missionary project in the Americas: (1) *Galicanismo,* which assumes the autonomy of local churches as agreed by the Synod of Pistoya; see Mario Góngora, "Estudios sobre el Galicanismo y la ilustración católica en la América española," *Revista chilena de historia y geografía* 125 (1980): 96–151; (2) agrarian republicanism, which recovered the Visigothic concept of *cortes* and councils, and then Lascasiano's of "sovereignty over sovereigns"; see Victor Frankl, "La idea del imperio español y el problema jurídico-lógico de los estados-misiones en el Paraguay," *Instituto Panamericano de Geografía e Historia* (1948); and (3) *la pedagogía visualizadora.*

46. See Enrique García Camarero and Ernesto García Camarero, *La polémica de la ciencia española* (Madrid: Alianza, 1970). It is very interesting to note that Forner, like a good traditionalist, resisted the utilitarianism of the new sciences as if they were seeds of disbelief and social disorder. And holding to Tomaso Campanella's traditional concept of universal Spanish monarchy, he, too, recommended cultivating the political, theological, and military sciences, to which Spain owed its military might.

47. Archivo Histórico Nacional, Diversos 490, 30 folios. See Enrique Beltrán, "Una polémica sobre Francisco Hernández y su obra en 1785," in *Anales de la Sociedad Mexicana de Historia de la Ciencia y de la Tecnología* 5 (1979): 59–73.

48. There was a reason that his name was officially yoked to the royal decree that established the Botanical Garden in Mexico City, with which, in turn, Sessé's scientific expedition was inaugurated. See Enrique Alvarez López, "Noticias y papeles de la expedición

científica mejicana dirigida por Sessé," *Anales del Jardín Botánico de Madrid* 10, no. 2 (1955): 5–79. Fermín del Pino has critiqued the causal relation that, on the basis of these documents, had been established between the "discovery" of the Hernández manuscripts and the expeditionary program of Charles III ("América y el desarrollo de la ciencia española en el siglo XVIII: Tradición, innovación y representaciones a propósito de Francisco Hernández," in *La América española en la epoca de las Luces: Tradición, innovación y representaciones* (Madrid: Ediciones de Cultura Hispánica, 1986), 121–43.

49. Vicente Cervantes, *Exercicios publicos de botánica* (Mexico City, 1793), 1–9; Rogers McVaugh, *Botanical Results of the Sessé and Mociño Expedition (1787–1803)* (Ann Arbor: University of Michigan Press, 1987), 155–71; José Luis Peset, "Las polémicas de la nueva botánica," in *La Real Expedición Botánica a Nueva España, 1783–1803,* ed. Belen Sánchez, Miguel Angel Puig-Samper, and José de la Sota (Madrid: CSIC, 1987), 95–116; Gracielo Zamudio, "El Jardín Botánico de la Nueva España y la institucionalización de la botánica en México," in "Los orígenes de la ciencia nacional," ed. Juan José Saldaña, *Cuadernos de Quipu* 4 (1992): 55–98. It is interesting to note the coincidence in the anti-Linnaeanism in America and Spain alike of the value attached to the work of the Swiss Albert von Haller. Apart from representing descriptive physiology, which rejected the concept of the constancy of species and the definition of binary botanical nomenclature, in his *Bibliotheca botánica* (1771), he also included a short biographical sketch and a favorable assessment of Hernández. See Erich Hinzsche's entry on Haller in *Dictionary of Scientific Biography* 6:61–67 and see Somolinos "Vida y obra," 321.

THE CIRCULATION OF THE WORK OF HERNÁNDEZ IN NINETEENTH-CENTURY SPAIN

LEONCIO LÓPEZ-OCÓN

In 1790, when Casimiro Gómez Ortega, director of the Royal Botanical Garden in Madrid, published some of the Hernández manuscripts that had been rediscovered late in the eighteenth century by the historian Juan Bautista Muñoz, his edition created a watershed in the circulation, assimilation, and diffusion of the legacy of Francisco Hernández in both the Americas and Europe. Several studies have improved our sense of the cultural ambience in which the legacy of Hernández was revived at the end of the eighteenth century, and we now know more about the personality of Gómez Ortega.[1] Furthermore, we are now beginning to recognize that Gómez Ortega's editorial labors were the culmination of a long process in which the knowledge recorded by Hernández had traveled back and forth across the Atlantic in different Euro-American scientific circles throughout the early modern era.[2]

The "rediscovery" of Hernández's work at the end of the eighteenth century led, in the nineteenth, to a sustained interest in the man and his work among various Euro-American scientific communities. My main purpose here is to describe how and why the work of Hernández circulated in Spain in the nineteenth century. My thesis is that Hernán-dez came to occupy a special place in the Spanish scientific heritage for a variety of representatives of the few scientific communities that emerged in Spanish society in the nineteenth century.[3] These scientists, immersed in the double polemic of Spanish science and colonial activity in the Americas, which are two sides of the same coin—the export of Spanish culture—promoted throughout the century the task of recovering and reevaluating Spanish scientific activity in the Americas in the early modern period. As this work of recovery took place, the accomplishments of Hernández naturally turned up time and again and came to be considered a paradigm of the most civilized work carried out in the Indies by the Spanish nation.

During the nineteenth century, naturalists, doctors, and writers on a wide variety of subjects were attracted to Hernández within the framework of a cultural movement related to the double polemic, which drew in Spanish scientists of the Enlightenment, romanticism, and positivism. Hernández and his work came to be seen as an exemplum that could be used to justify Spanish colonial activity in the Americas and as a founding moment in a scientific heritage that modern Spain was constructing in close relation to the colonial American experience. As I shall show, this vision of the Hernández project as occupying a special place in the scientific heritage of Spain, inasmuch as it was seen as the origin of continuous scientific effort, would come to be maintained by several generations of Spanish scientists, principally naturalists. This interpretation of the original Hernández project can be seen developing quite clearly in three distinct periods, each one roughly corresponding to one-third of the nineteenth century.

The Recovery of a National Scientific Tradition

The first phase coincides with existing interest in Hernández in the early years of the nineteenth century, especially in the core of the publication of the *Anales de historia natural,* published from 1799 to 1804.[4] In the pages of this periodical, the first Hispanic journal to specialize in the natural sciences, the dialogue with the legacy of Hernández was continuous, though problematic, as can be appreciated in various contributions undertaken by the main force behind the journal, Antonio José de Cavanilles (1745–1804).[5]

Cavanilles, the new mandarin of Spanish botany during the reign of Charles IV, usurped Gómez Ortega and dislodged him from his positions of power in something like a palace coup. Cavanilles used some of his works to settle scores with his rival and to criticize his effort to recover the legacy of Hernández, using "modernist" criteria, antitraditional and Linnaean.[6] Thus in a work published in June 1800, a decade after the appearance of the Madrid edition, Cavanilles dismissed Gómez Ortega's editorial work on the botanical writings of Hernández, on the grounds that the resulting edition of Hernández, "like the writings of his age, contains no scientific descriptions, nor any identifying features of the plants; these defects would have been less important if the original illustrations had not been lost." And he added that if the "learned" Hernández, along with other travelers of his time, contributed to an increased knowledge of the number of plants by virtue of his iconographic efforts, nonetheless all these prints were "imperfect because they did not depict the fruits; an understandable defect for the time, but reprehensible in this day and age when the science has reached such a stage of advancement."[7]

Yet at the same time the Aragonese illustrator Ignacio de Asso was showing some interest in reconstructing the scientific tradition of the Spanish naturalists, insisting that the impact of Hernández's work on the evolution of botanical science in Europe was important. To demonstrate his point he used a dualistic approach. On the one hand he translated the Swedish work on natural history in Spain and the Americas by Linnaeus's pupil Peter Löfling, to demonstrate just how important the legacy of Hernández was among the most influential naturalists in Europe in the mid-eighteenth century, including these two eminent Scandinavians.[8] On the other hand his keen but cautious sense of history impelled him to "consult the monuments of the past." One of those monuments was precisely what resulted from Hernández's commission in New Spain. It was exactly because of the monumental character of this work and its role in spreading knowledge of America—owing to which discovery "there was a sharp increase in the study of natural history by the Spanish, in view of the treasures they could observe in a region previously unknown to them"—that Ignacio de Asso outlined a genealogy of Spanish naturalists, among whom Hernández occupied a place of honor. Asso's text generated topics, such as the professional jealousy and envy that Hernández's work provoked—and it generated biographical errors, too, for example, that Hernández came from Seville—that remained rooted for decades.

For showing the paths that Asso followed in his effort to follow Hernández's footsteps, his text is worth quoting at length:

> The city of Seville . . . brought Dr. Hernández into the world. He is famous in Spanish literary history of the sixteenth century, and can reasonably take his place alongside Teofilo Spicelio among unfortunate writers, if we consider the jealousy and copying prompted by his botanical travels, and the meager recompense he obtained for his toil and travail, as attested by Livino de Suca and Ferrante Imperato, his contemporaries, in a number of manuscript letters that I have seen at the public library in Leiden. The former says in a letter to Charles de l'Ecluse in 1592 that he knew about Hernández in Naples, and that he marveled at the manuscript containing descriptions of plants and animals, along with illustrations, and that it would be most desirable if this

treasure remained hidden from public view no longer, from which one may infer that it did remain unpublished throughout the reign of Philip II. In another letter to Clusius, dated 7 January 1598, Ferrante Imperato mentions the testimony of Doctor Montecorvino, that some Spanish physicians blocked the publication of Hernández's work, putting obstacles in its way to prevent approval in the Royal Council: this was without a doubt exactly what happened in Naples, where it was being proposed that his work should be printed, but this still had the desired effect, though quite why nobody knows. What is certain is that Nardo Antonio Recho remained charged with organizing and publishing the works of Hernández, as his dedication to Philip II makes manifest, a document I have seen among the letters of Vicente Pinelo.[9]

It may have been Asso's emphasis on the importance that European botanists attached to Hernández's work that persuaded Cavanilles to reconsider his verdict on the legacy of Hernández and to revise his assessment of Gómez Ortega's historiographical work. Thus in 1804, in a lecture given at the Royal Botanical Garden, he presented some biographical data about Hernández, such as the fact that in 1555 he had botanized with the learned Juan Fragoso of Toledo in the kingdom of Seville. He gave a full account, laden with praise, of these scientific activities and accorded Hernández a prominent place in the pantheon of illustrious Spanish botanists, because he had the good fortune "to go to the New World in the reign of Philip II to cover himself with glory, immortalize the nation, and stimulate his successors." And he withdrew his earlier strictures on Gómez Ortega, justifying the deficiencies of Hernández's work:

Unfortunately the monuments of Francisco Hernández's expedition perished in the Escorial fire, and all vestiges of them would have been destroyed had it not been for the happy discovery by Juan Bautista Muñoz, who found five volumes in the library of the Imperial College, now published in part by . . . Ortega. It cannot be denied that the descriptions are almost always so compressed that, today, it is difficult if not impossible to be certain to which plant they correspond. As Mr. Cervantes has noted [in a letter from Mexico City, August 28, 1803], proper identification depends on knowing that in one place there were several plants, in Hernández's time given the same name, even those with considerable differences. But let us

remember to excuse our genius for what he frequently repeated: convinced as he was of the accuracy of his illustrations, "plantarum formas ex imaginibus cognosces" (you recognize the forms of plants from images). For this reason, no doubt, he limited himself to the virtues and uses of each one, only indicated the place in which it grows, without describing in detail the plant's dimensions, or the shape of its flowers, leaves and other vital parts.[10]

Cavanilles proposed to explain how all this work of constructing a scientific tradition based on a cultivation of memory and the establishment of a kind of cult of ancestors was projected into the present and the future, to establish a connection between the recovery of the work of Hernández and the organization of the botanical expedition to New Spain in the 1780s: "To recover what was lost in the fire, to communicate to scholars the natural riches of the Mexican Empire, His Majesty ordered a scientific expedition, which was entrusted to Martín de Sessé, and which was brought to a successful conclusion. The members of the expedition finally found themselves at Court with descriptions and illustrations of insects, fish, birds, quadrupeds and plants, all done with such truth and precision, that to some extent we should be happy about the earlier loss that prompted this expedition, which restored the collection of Hernández to us with interest."[11]

The explorers who came back from New Spain—armed with twenty-five hundred plants unknown in Europe, among them about two hundred new genera, and five hundred birds described and drawn, one-third of which were completely unknown—activated new interest in the work of Hernández in scientific and political circles in Madrid. At the end of 1805 one Madrid periodical gave an account of the rediscovery by Martín de Sessé of the paintings from the Hernández expedition:

Of all the discoveries turned up by this expedition, none has caused its director [Sessé] so much rejoicing as the recent finding of the most valuable paintings, which our celebrated Dr. Francisco Hernández, doctor to Philip II had had made in New Spain in the 1570s not very long after the conquest: that is, when none of the nations that now accuse us of backwardness in the study of natural sciences even thought of leaving their homes to study

Nature, and copying it at first hand the way Dr. Hernández did.

This valuable monument to the generosity of our monarchs and to Spanish illustration in those times was thought to have been destroyed in the terrible fire at the Escorial. But as luck would have it, providence kept it in a basement room under that monastery, until it came into the hands of Sessé, the very man whose principal task it was to illustrate the work of the learned Spaniard.

This discovery was much appreciated by His Excellency José Antonio Caballero, Minister of Peace and Justice, who at once accompanied Sessé to the room in the basement where these precious works had been found, and ordered that they be collected and placed in the Library with the old manuscripts, warning the Prior that they were to be looked after with the greatest of care, so that Sessé could rectify and compare his discoveries with those of Dr. Hernández and preserve this testimony of so much honor to the Spanish nation.

It is not easy to estimate when the public will have the pleasure of seeing such an interesting and valuable work; because although its arrangement is quite far advanced, the number of plates that have turned up is very large, and the illumination of these prints is very costly.[12]

This desire to publish the discovery never came to anything, because among other reasons, after Napoleon's invasion of the Iberian Peninsula in 1808, the scientific system constructed in the eighteenth century was dismantled, and Spanish science entered its own dark age. All the same, in the most difficult of these dark times, which lasted roughly from 1808 to 1840, interest in Hernández's legacy was kept alive, as two facts will attest.

After the counterrevolutionary movement of 1823, the exiled Spanish liberals who fled to London took with them the legacy of Hernández and did their utmost to disseminate it. Thus in one of their publications, entitled *Ocios de españoles emigrados* [Leisure of Spanish émigrés], produced in London from 1825 and to which one of Cavanilles's disciples was a prominent contributor—the botanist Mariano La Gasca—there appeared a "Notice of the discovery and printing of the manuscripts on the natural history of New Spain by Doctor Francisco Hernández."[13] Much of this text was adopted en bloc from *Mercurio peruano de historia, literatura, y noticias públicas* (March 10, 1793), which itself

reprinted portions of Gómez Ortega's preface to his Madrid edition of Hernández. In this text (see appendix 1 below), American and European readers received an account of the scientific importance of Hernández's American expedition, under the generous patronage of Philip II, and of the context in which the discovery of the Hernández manuscripts occurred in the time of Charles III, and whose contents are mentioned. Ironically, Gómez Ortega and his editorial efforts received not a word.

The impact of this article is unknown to us today. But we do know that when one of the exiled liberals, the bibliophile Bartolomé José Gallardo (1776–1852), returned to Spain with an obsessive eagerness to rearrange the written record of Spanish culture, he spent many hours of research and labor confronting the problem of the Hernández legacy. Prior to the 1830s, shortly after the exile's return, he spent some time working in the library of the Escorial and there made a discovery of which two contradictory accounts have come down to us in his posthumous "Essay on a Spanish Library of Rare and Curious Books," published by the scholars Zarco del Valle and Sancho Rayón between 1863 and 1889. There, after describing the article on Sessé's discovery in the *Variedades,* mentioned a few lines above, Gallardo said: "This passage, which I copied from the *Variedades,* gave me a taste of what it must have been like to have been the one who discovered this treasure, so I went back to the upper library of the Escorial in the year 1835, and there I found thirteen very learned and exhaustive volumes in large folio. But they had nothing to do with herbs." And in another note he added: "In November 1836, living with the monks at the Escorial, and spending all the daylight hours shut up in the upper library, I found among the banned books, where this had finished up, 13 volumes (at least I remember 13) in large fol[io], of botanical works by Dr. Hernández, with the corresponding examples of the plants. I communicated this affair to Dr. Lagasca."[14]

This relative interest in the work of Hernández in certain circles of Spanish society in the early nineteenth century prompted an increase in the number of known manuscripts of Francisco Hernández. At a given moment in this period, in an act of *evergetismo* typical of the scientific culture of liberal patriotism, a certain Blas Hernández, deputy inspector of the National Militia in Toledo, presented to the Cortes a valuable autograph manuscript. Gallardo described it tersely: "Autograph manuscript in large folio, 233 leaves paginated, leather-covered boards, edges gilt, with the royal arms stamped in gold on the covers," and he listed the contents of the most important work contained in this manuscript: the three books of *Antiquities of New Spain*. This manuscript contained three other works by Hernández: *The Conquest of New Spain, Stoic Questions,* and *Stoic Problems*.[15] Gallardo likewise compiled an index of manuscripts at the Biblioteca Nacional, noting that this repository of the national heritage held two manuscripts by Hernández in its collections: the first contained a translation of Pliny's *Natural History,* up to book 35 (thus lacking the last two books), and the second, the compendium of five books of ethics by Aristotle, the compendium of the book on the soul, and the compendium of the physics.[16]

The Cultivation of a Heritage

Attention to the legacy of Hernández gathered momentum in the mid-nineteenth century, from 1840 to 1870. In this period, coinciding more or less with the reign of Isabella II, when liberalism had become established and Spanish science was rebuilt following its destruction during the ancien régime, interest in conservation was revived along with increased interest in the national heritage, and various scientific groups did all they could to strengthen their individual scientific traditions.

Thus in 1842 three members of the Academy of History, Martín Fernández Navarette, Miguel Salvá, and Pedro Sainz de Baranda, resolved to publish a collection of unpublished documents on the history of Spain. The first volume of this great historical project contained an important sequence of Hernández documents preserved in the Archivo de Indias in Seville, originating from the Archivo of Simancas, including six letters sent by Hernández to Philip II from Mexico between 1572 and 1576, on the natural history he was writing at the king's behest, one letter to Ovando on the same subject, and one written at the end of 1581 to the king from Francisco Domínguez, the cosmographer who originally accompanied Hernández to New Spain.[17]

The editors of this historical material added a footnote on Hernández and his expedition in which they supplied new information, taken from the work of Dr. Porreño, *Los dichos y hechos del rey Felipe II,* published in Brussels in 1666, as follows:

[Philip II] sent Dr. Francisco Hernández, native of Toledo, to the west Indies to write a history of all the animals and plants of those remote regions: he proved himself to be a learned and diligent man in little more than four years, writing fifteen large folio books which I have seen at the Escorial, with accompanying colored images of the plants and animals, each part of the tree or herb painted appropriately: the root, trunk, branches, leaves, flowers, fruits; the cayman, spider, snake, serpent, rabbit, dog and the fish with its scales; the most beautiful plumage of a wide range of birds, . . . and even the heights, colors, and clothing of people, and the costumes they wear for galas and fiestas, and the manner of their songs, dances, and sacrifices, something that is a special delight and a wonder to behold. In some of these books he put down the face, shape, and color of the animal and plant, working as best he could, for the rest referring to the numbers he had written in the margins in his history. For each thing, the qualities, properties, and names of all conformed to what could be gathered from this barbarous people and from the Spanish who were born and raised there and who lived there. In addition to these fifteen books there are two others, one an index of the plants, and a comparison of them with ours; the other is on the costumes, laws and rites of the Indians, with descriptions of specific sites in the provinces, lands, and places in those regions and new world, arranged by climate. His Majesty paid the expenses of all this with an open hand, and arranged for the volumes to be handsomely bound in blue leather, with gold tooling, clasps, corner-protectors, and bosses of very thick silver, all evidence of excellent workmanship.[18]

Doctors, too, paid attention to Hernández during these years. In fact, in the 1840s, two of the great histories of Spanish medicine, by Anastasio Chinchilla and Antonio Hernández Morejón, referred extensively to Hernández.[19] But the work that expresses the deepest and most systematic interest in Hernández in the middle third of the nineteenth century in Spain was that of Miguel Colmeiro: *La botánica y los botánicos de la peninsula hispano-lusitana* (1858). The author, who was already a distinguished botanist at the Museum of Natural Sciences, Central University of Madrid, had written about the history of botany from its beginnings to the 1840s.[20] But it was at the end of the 1850s, at a time when the most influential circles in Spanish society revealed a distinct desire to be linked with enlightened science, that the work acquired more consistency. Colmeiro's work, a prizewinner in a public competition run by the Biblioteca Nacional and printed at government expense, became an important repository of collective heritage for Iberian botanists. Nationalist zeal and scientific interests were the driving forces behind a historiographical project in which the botanist would be the most influential in the later nineteenth century, becoming like a patron to this small group of naturalists: "The nation's honor and interest in science demand that our scientific writers, living or dead, start to be better known, because there are many more of them, and they are much more important than is commonly believed."[21]

Colmeiro conceived this book as a comprehensive bibliographical survey of Iberian botany, arranged chronologically to demonstrate the progress of botanical studies and including a table of authors to provide some orientation in this ocean of hundreds of books and titles. Hernández figures in the book in the following way. The first section of this re-creation of Iberian scientific heritage is devoted to interpretation, extracts, commentaries, and Spanish and Portuguese editions of the Greek and Roman authors who had some connection with botany. Hernández appears in this section as the commentator and translator of Pliny's *Natural History*. Section 5, dedicated to "Spanish works describing exotic plants, or containing some information about them, and almost all pertaining to the West and East Indies," includes three long and accurate references to the legacy of Hernández. In the first of these he is mentioned for the way his work was the cornerstone of the *Quatro libros*. The second concerns the publication of the Rome edition of 1651, acknowledging Recchi's role in selecting extracts from the Hernández manuscripts, and the third, Gómez Ortega's Madrid edition of 1790. In each of these four references Colmeiro undertook the long job of describing both the published and unpublished works of Hernández, according to the principles of nineteenth-century bibliography, with its exhaustive detail.

Colmeiro completed his account of Hernández in two ways: he indicated how the memory of Hernández had been preserved and how he had been enshrined as a scientific hero, one who had had a genus named after him (*Hernandia* Plum.), and he offered a full biographical sketch of "one of the most learned and industrious naturalists of the sixteenth century."[22] Colmeiro's biographical sketch mentions topics already established previously, such as that "emulation and envy prevented the important fruits of his voyage from becoming known," while other points were designed to prove that the doctor was from Toledo, "though some say from Seville," and he organized all the information that was collected in his bibliographical files, adding some new material, albeit rather confused, about how some scholars had followed in the footsteps of Hernández in the first half of the nineteenth century, in a fruitless manner, Colmeiro thought: "When Tournefort crossed the peninsula in 1688 he was shown an herbarium in several volumes, thought to be that of Hernández; but this experienced botanist declared it to be European, and that it could be the same one that was acquired by Philip II from the library of Diego de Mendoza in 1576, as a signature attests, and is preserved today in the library at the Escorial. These could have been the fourteen volumes which a modern bibliographer claims to have seen in 1836."[23]

Revival of a Legacy

The work of Colmeiro seems to be a decisive turning point in the evolution of Hernández's place in the historiography of science in nineteenth-century Spain. It is a turning point insofar as Colmeiro meant to organize the botanical bibliography of previous generations and list the formal characteristics of the whole known Hernández corpus, published or unpublished. This task of organizing the historical material was prompted by a learned bibliophilic movement in the middle third of the nineteenth century in Spain and was dominated by the desire to establish a scientific tradition. Colmeiro's study was also a point of departure because, by giving prominence to the legacy of Hernández, he called attention once again to the importance of Hernández's achievement and piqued curiosity about the man and his work among various historians, scholars, and Spanish naturalists during the last third of the nineteenth century.

In fact, one of the most important historical works on the history of the Americas to come out of "Restoration" Spain, the *Cartas de Indias* published by the Ministry of Economic Development, Public Education, and Culture in 1877, took as its rationale the publication of the letter of the viceroy count Coruña to Philip II, signed in Mexico, October 15, 1581, in which Dr. Juan de Vides was recommended by the *protomedicato* of New Spain for the mission of continuing the history that Hernández had begun, on the virtues and properties of the plants of New Spain. A full biographical account of Hernández in the *Cartas* presented him as a scientific hero, with an intelligent bibliographical survey and a synthesis of his project.[24] The author insisted on such diverse facts as the major contribution of Hernández's son to the project and Hernández's personal interest in creating a trilingual work (in Latin, Spanish, and Náhuatl) with the goal of making the diffusion of the work as widespread as possible—not just in Europe but among the native Mexican population as well (see appendix 2 below).

This biographical account has been attributed to Justo Zaragoza, one of the five editors of the *Cartas de Indias,* but in my view the author was Marcos Jiménez de la Espada, another of the editors responsible for this collection.[25] There are two kinds of evidence in support of this attribution to Jiménez de la Espada, who traveled across American territories between 1862 and 1865 as a member of the Scientific Commission of the Pacific and who, on his return to Europe, became one of the late nineteenth century's leading authorities on American antiquities and on the history of the colonization of the Americas.[26]

On the one hand one may point out that among the papers of Espada's private archive, which survive today in Madrid, several documents prove his interest in following in Hernández's footsteps.[27] Four years after the edition of the *Cartas de Indias,* in 1881, Espada published the first volume of one of his most ambitious historical projects—his edition of the geographical account of Peru—in whose introduction was a defense of the pioneering and modern spirit

of the Hernández expedition, based on the royal instructions of 1570, a copy of which he had found preserved in Madrid's Archivo Histórico Nacional and which was published in the *Colección de documentos inéditos de Indias*.[28]

Espada said in the introductory study:

I will record, with all due attention to its importance, the travels of Dr. Francisco Hernández to the Indies in 1570. It was the first scientific expedition of its kind, and was designed—though by no means exclusively, as has been thought—to study of the animals, vegetables and minerals of New Spain, but also those of Peru, not to mention the geography and history of both regions. The expedition is memorable not just for the scope of this concept, but also for being prepared and organized in such a way that although expeditions today might be more numerous and more narrowly focused on natural resources, when it comes down to the kind of people, the purpose of the assignment, and the method of carrying it out, there are in the end very few differences. Hernández directed the expedition and took with him a geographer, Francisco Domínguez, a draftsman and one "who gathered plants." [Here follows a summary of the royal instructions.]

Hernández successfully completed this vast and difficult task, including the material on the geography, history, and antiquities, as witnessed by the originals, which he sent shortly before his return to Spain; nonetheless he did not come up to expectations, and perhaps the end of his mission coincided with the death of his protector, Ovando. A footnote added: "A letter from Hernández to Ovando (published in volume one of the Salvá collection) informs him about the project, and encloses with it a statement of the necessary reasons for his return and his abandonment of the journey to Peru: his age (sixty years), his weakness of body and weariness of mind, and his desire to supervise the printing of his work in Spain. I do not know if the president of the Council of the Indies ever read this letter."[29] And on the other hand, the paragraph of the biographical sketch that appeared in the *Cartas de Indias,* in which there is an allusion to the obstacles that he had to overcome to accomplish his task, seems to refer as much to Hernández's difficulties as to those of Espada himself. Espada was another Spanish naturalist who was displaced to the Americas, who ran into financial difficulties, bureaucratic obstructions, and professional jealousy. That is, in describing the Hernández expedition, the author of the biography seems to speak of his own experience, and who better than Espada, of the five editors of the *Cartas,* to know the problems confronting Spanish naturalists sent to the Americas? In composing this biographical essay, Espada certainly saw Hernández as his alter ego.

The attention that Espada devoted to Hernández was to be continued in the twentieth century by fray Agustín Barreiro, the first scholar of the Scientific Commission of the Pacific and heir in great measure of Espada's historical projects.[30] It is certainly a possibility that the historical works of Barreiro, who was the chief force behind a retrospective project of the Spanish Natural History Society in the 1920s and 1930s, helped to prompt Somolinos, who also suffered the experience of exile, to undertake his great project of an edition of the complete works of Hernández.

These are some of the facts that may affect our image of the reception and circulation of Hernández within the Spanish scientific community. The received opinion is that between the Madrid edition of 1790 and the *Obras completas* that began to appear in 1960 there was no interest in the accomplishments of Hernández, but my evidence shows that, on the contrary, one generation after another never lost sight of the work of Hernández and continued a dialogue about it. In so doing, the scientists and scholars of the period generated a long series of links in the continuous process of understanding the life and work of Francisco Hernández.

APPENDIX 1

Ocios de españoles emigrados, no. 21 (December 1825), 4.473–75

Notice

On the discovery and printing of the manuscripts on the natural history of New Spain by Dr. Francisco Hernández

Recognizing the importance of examining the precious natural resources of his American dominions, King Philip II

entrusted this charge to his distinguished protomédico, Dr. Francisco Hernández, who to his vast knowledge of medicine added no common learning in natural history, geography, mathematics, and humane letters. The king spent 60,000 ducats (a considerable sum when we think of the value of money in those days) on the Hernández expedition. In the seven years he spent in New Spain, Hernández fully discharged his duty, filling seventeen large volumes with dried plants, depictions, and descriptions of the structure, uses, and virtues; he did the same for animals and minerals, as well as the antiquities and topography of that realm. The death of the author, and other occurrences, prevented publication of a work containing discoveries of consummate benefit to medicine, the arts and sciences, and commerce, until the appearance of an abridgment, which was printed in Rome in one folio volume in 1651, with notes by the academicians of the Lincei, who graced this work with the grand title, *Treasury of the Medical Things of New Spain,* even though it was incomplete and diminished, because its principal editor or compiler, Nardo Antonio Reccho, had considered all the natural history useless, as is usual in the medical profession.

In the fire at the Escorial in 1671, the flames consumed, among many of the library's treasures, the original work of Hernández which had been deposited there. Consequently all hope was lost of ever seeing these valuable manuscripts published, to the great disappointment of men of letters, as is shown by several eminent writers, such as Tournefort, Linnaeus, and others. This was the state of affairs, at a time when expectations were low, when five folio volumes of manuscripts were discovered in the library of the Imperial College in Madrid. These manuscripts were known to have served as the first draft of the works of Dr. Hernández, who had polished them with additions and interlinear corrections in his own hand.

Apprised of this discovery by the Minister for the Indies, Charles III resolved at once to bring these Latin originals to light for the public good, and to make up for the loss of the original designs by having a new botanical expedition replace them. He ordered such an expedition to New Spain to take place at this time, at his expense, with the task of gathering, describing, drawing, and illuminating all the natural resources of that territory, especially those noted by Hernández.

The whole work consisted of five volumes, as outlined in the preface: the first three covering the history of Mexican plants in 24 books, and in the last one, three indexes were to be added for clarification: in the first, Mexican names of plants; in the second, the places where they grow; in the third, the most notable things.

Volume 4, besides containing an essay by the editor on the life and writings of Dr. Hernández, contains a natural history of quadrupeds, birds, reptiles, insects, fish, and minerals from New Spain, with an unpublished dedication addressed by the author to Philip II, followed by descriptions of plants from the east Indies and the Philippines, which Hernández also examined. The first book and part of the second consisted of the history of Mexican plants, translated by the author into Spanish, to which were added four books on the nature and virtues of the plants and animals which are used in medicine in New Spain, written by fray Francisco Ximénez, which came to form an epitome of the works of Hernández printed in Mexico in quarto in 1615, and which is extremely rare.

The fifth volume is all unpublished short works, such as the treatise on the Great Mexican Temple; which Hernández had managed to see, and whose seventy-eight parts, the number of priests, their ceremonies, hymns, and circumstances of the women dedicated to worship and service, he described in detail. One book on the province of China. The description of a certain illness peculiar to New Spain, which broke out in 1576. The explanation of the Christian doctrine in hexameters, with notes by the archbishop of Mexico, and a personal friend of the author, Pedro Moya de Contreras. A book of Stoic questions with the prologue to Philip II, and other philosophical works which testify to the varied and profound erudition of Dr. Hernández.

The first volume is prefaced by an elegant epistle in Latin verse, addressed by the author to the famous Beito [sic] Arias Montano, in which he tells of his return to Spain, his works and his past efforts, and the condition and nature of his writings, and he complains about the injustice of his detractors, to whom the censorship and coordination of his works had been entrusted.

APPENDIX 2

Biographical Sketch of Francisco Hernández from *Cartas de Indias* (Madrid, 1877), 3.773

HERNÁNDEZ (Francisco).—Born in the city of Toledo about 1514, studied medicine, graduated doctor in the University of Salamanca and became royal physician to Philip II. Charged by this monarch to write the natural, ancient, and political history of New Spain and the topography of the land, accompanied by the noted cosmographer Francisco Domínguez, to whom this last part of the work fell, he traveled in 1570 to this province with the title of protomédico, and stayed there until 1576, one year beyond the projected terminal date for this enormous work. The obstacles he had to overcome in carrying out his commission are those that Spanish naturalists sent to the Indies always encounter: inadequate funding, lukewarm support as well as the ridiculous demands of the governor and the local authorities, and the envy of those in office. But Hernández, upon whom fortune had bestowed intelligence, wisdom, patience, and a firm character, proceeded to overcome them all, and with only his son, who was sent with him, to help him, he finished the work by September 1575, which brought to an end his permitted time. He prepared his work to see the light of day in sixteen folio volumes, six of text, with the descriptions of the animals, plants, and minerals of New Spain, and ten of illustrations, including those of the antiquities; four books which he judged necessary for the perfection of his natural history, entitled: Método de conocer las plantas a ámbos orbes (Method of identifying the plants of both hemispheres), Tabla de los males y remedios de esta tierra (Table of the illnesses and cures of this land), Las plantas de ese orbe que crecen en éste y los provechos que tienen entre los naturales (The plants of this hemisphere that grow here and their usefulness to the natives), and Experiencias y antidotario del nuevo orbe (New World experiences and antidotes); the topography of New Spain; one book on the conquest and another on its antiquities; translation and commentary on the thirty-six books by Pliny, and two other books, one of questions, the other of problems, of Stoic philosophy.

Doctor Hernández wrote his original treatises in Latin; but at some date he had finished or nearly finished a Spanish version of the history of animals, plants, and minerals, with another just on the plants, in Náhuatl, which was done under his supervision by a native of the country. Further, on his return to Spain, he left there three or four copies of all his manuscripts and drawings of the images, and he did not leave Mexico without testing for himself the virtues of the simples that his work described, curing and attending at the hospitals gratis, trusting the experience of other doctors. Besides all this, he brought back millions of seeds and a number of the most useful trees and shrubs of that land, alive and grown quite sizable, so that they would better survive the journey and could later be transplanted to His Majesty's gardens.

Despite his having declined to complete his commission by continuing his work in the kingdoms of Peru and other parts of the Indies, with the object of returning early to Spain and occupying himself with editing his work before infirmity and age could prevent him, our eminent naturalist died (we do not know in which year) without having the pleasure of seeing even a small part of his most important works published. However, we have seen a sample of the printing of the illustrations in color which he projected for his natural history, with an estimate of the cost, and to judge from that, the edition would have been magnificent, and perhaps the best of all of them in that era.

NOTES

1. For the studies, see, for example, Enrique Beltrán, "Una polémica sobre Francisco Hernández y su obra en 1785," *Anales de la Sociedad Mexicana de Historia de la Ciencia y de la Tecnología* 5 (1979): 49–73, and Fermín del Pino, "América y el desarrollo de la ciencia española en el siglo XVIII: Tradición, innovación y representaciones a propósito de Francisco Hernández," *La América española en la epoca de las Luces: Tradición, innovación y representaciones* (Madrid: Ediciones de Cultura Hispánica, 1986), 121–43. On Gómez Ortega, see Francisco Javier Puerto Sarmiento, *Ciencia de cámara: Casimiro Gómez Ortega (1741–1818): El scientífico cortesano* (Madrid: CSIC, 1992).

2. See Jaime Vilchis, "Globalizing the *Natural History*," above.

3. On the notion of a place in the cultural heritage, see Pierre Nora, "Entre mémoire et histoire: La problématique des lieux," in *Les lieux de la mémoire,* ed. P. Nora (Paris: Gallimard, 1984–93), 1:xv–xlii, and "Le passé recomposé," interview with Mona Ozouf by Jean-François Chanet, *Magazine littéraire,* no. 307 (February 1993): 22–25.

4. This journal has been meticulously edited by Joaquín Fernández Peréz: see *Anales de historia natural, 1799–1804: Estudio preliminar y edición,* 3 vols. (Aranjuez: Doce Calles and Secretaría General del Plan Nacional de I+D-Comisión Interministerial de Ciencia y Tecnología, 1993). Fernández Peréz studies the characteristics of this journal in vol. 1, pp. 15–130.

5. For a recent account of the life and work of this noted naturalist, see the articles collected in *Asclepio* 47, no. 1 (1995): 135–260.

6. For the rivalry, see Diana Soto Arango, "Cavanilles y Zea: Una amistad político-científica," *Asclepio* 47, no. 1 (1995): 169–96, esp. 177–81.

7. Antonio José de Cavanilles, "Materiales para la historia de la botánica," *Anales de historia natural* 2, no. 4 (June 1800): 5.

8. "Observaciones de Historia Natural hechas en España y América por Pedro Loefling, traducidas del sueco por D. Ignacio de Asso," *Anales de ciencias naturales,* nos. 9, 11, 12, 13, and 15 (1801–2). Ignacio de Asso cited references to Hernández in Löfling's letters to his teacher, from Aranjuez, June 24, 1753 (no. 13, 99–100), from Madrid, October 15, 1753 (p. 316), from Puerto de Santa María, December 18, 1753 (p. 326), and from Cumaná, April 18, 1754 (p. 337).

9. Ignacio de Asso, "Discurso sobre los naturalistas españoles," *Anales de ciencias naturales* 3, no. 8 (February 1801): 170–79.

10. Ignacio de Asso, "Discurso sobre algunos botánicos españoles del siglo XVI," *Anales de historia natural* 7, no. 20 (April 1804): 99–140, esp. 111 on the relation between Fragoso and Hernández. Other references to Hernández at 112, 124–26.

11. Ibid., 126 and n.

12. *Variedades de ciencias, literatura y artes* 2, no. 24 (December 15, 1805): 357, col. 4a.

13. *Ocios de españoles emigrados* 4, no. 21 (December 1825): 473–75.

14. Gallardo, "Essay," 3:177.

15. Ibid., 3:177–79. [Our thanks to Cynthia Buffington and David Szewczyk for giving us the correct English equivalents of the Spanish bibliographical terms, here and again below.—Ed.]

16. Ibid., vol. 2, appendix, p. 73.

17. *Colección de documentos inéditos para la historia de España* 1 (Madrid: Academia de la Historia, 1842; reprint, Vaduz, Liechtenstein: Kraus Reprint, 1964), 362, 376, 379.

18. Ibid., 362–63.

19. Anastasio Chinchilla, *Historia de la medicina española,* 4 vols. (Valencia: López y Mateu, 1841–46); Antonio Hernández Morejón, *Historia bibliografía de la medicina española,* 7 vols. (Madrid: Widow of Jordan, 1842–52). Both works were reissued in 1967 by Johnson Reprint, New York: Chinchilla as *Anales históricos de la medicina en general y biográficos-bibliográficos de la española en particular,* intro. by Francisco Guerra.

20. Miguel Colmeiro, *Ensayo histórico sobre los progresos de la botánica desde su origen hasta el día considerados más especialmente con relación a España* (Barcelona: A. Brusi, 1842).

21. Miguel Colmeiro, *La botánica y los botánicos de la península hispano-lusitana* (Madrid, 1858), viii.

22. See Colmeiro's "Lista alfabética de los géneros de plantas dedicados a españoles y portugueses por los botánicos de la Península y fuera de ella, e índice para hallar en el escrito que precede las noticias biográficas correspondientes a cada uno de los españoles y portugueses que en el mismo se contienen" (ibid., 211).

23. Ibid., 154.

24. *Cartas de Indias* (1877; reprint, Madrid: Atlas, 1974), 1:346–47 for recommendation of Dr. Juan de Vides, 3:773 (appendix) for biographical account of Hernández.

25. On Zaragoza as author, see Somolinos, "Vida y obra," 361. The other three editors were Vicente Barrantes, Francisco González de Vera, and José María Escudero de la Peña.

26. See Leoncio López-Ocón, *De viajero naturalista a historiador: Las actividades americanistas del científico español Marcos Jiménez de la Espada (1831–1898)*, Colección Tesis Doctorales no. 162/91, 2 vols. (Madrid: Editorial de la Universidad Complutense, 1991).

27. These documents are deposited in the library of Patronato Menéndez Pelayo in Madrid (their call numbers are temporary): Caja 11/4/17 doc. 17 contains a bibliographical essay on the works of Hernández; Caja 11/4/23: an account of documents acquired by the Archivo Histórico Nacional for the purpose of inclusion in the *Cartas de Indias;* Caja 14/3 doc. 37, essay and notes on the letters of Hernández and Francisco Domínguez, the description of New Spain, which are in the *Colección de documentos inéditos,* vol. 1.

28. *Colección de documentos inéditos de . . . ultramar,* ed. Joaquín Francisco Pacheco, Francisco de Cárdenas y Espejo, and Luis Torres de Mendoza, 2d ser., 15:280ff.

29. In *Relaciones geográficas del virreinato del Perú* (Madrid: Atlas, 1965) 1:46–47. See also *Marcos Jiménez de la Espada: Tras la senda de un explorador,* ed. Leoncio López-Ocón and Carmen María Pérez-Montes (Madrid: CSIC, in press)

30. See Leoncio López-Ocón, "Las relaciones científicas entre España y la América Latina en la segunda mitad del siglo XIX: Un balance historiográfico," *Revista de Indias* 50, no. 188 (1990): 305–33. Barreiro edited Hernández's will in "El testamento del doctor Francisco Hernández," *Boletín de la Real Academia de la Historia* 94 (1929): 475–97, and see *Mexican Treasury.* Jiménez de Espada's archive is currently being put online, as a result of two projects with financial support from the city of Madrid and Spain's Ministry of Education. See <www.csic.es/BGH/espada/pagina.htm> and <www.pacifico.csic.es>.

PART IV   POSTSCRIPT: CONTINUING TRADITIONS OF MEXICAN MEDICINE

LATINO CATHOLIC CIVILIZATION
PATTERNS OF HEALTH AND DEMOGRAPHY

DAVID HAYES-BAUTISTA

Historians have begun to view epidemics as causative agents in historical developments and as mirrors of society.

—Gert Brieger (1994)

Nearly four hundred years after Francisco Hernández's epic study of life, society, health, and death in post-conquest Mexico, the descendants of that meeting of two worlds have burst into general public awareness in North American society. Although California's missions and pueblos were well established in the 1760s by Mexican missionaries, settlers, and soldiers—sprinkling the state with villages that would shortly spring to worldwide prominence with names such as Los Angeles, San Francisco, and San Diego—the massive in-migration of Anglo population (spurred by the discovery of gold at Sutter's Mill in 1848) swamped the California population, and from 1850 through 1910, Latinos accounted for barely 1 percent of California's total population.

Once no more than a colorful footnote in the state's history, the Latino population in the twentieth century has grown to nearly one-third of California's total today.[1] There are about ten million Latinos in California and nearly thirty million in the United States; most projections predict that by the year 2020, close to one out of every two Californians will be Latino. This apparently sudden growth has prompted many reactions from the non-Latino population, ranging from the desire for corporate investment to outright political hostility. The present and future role of a large and growing Latino population in California and the United States is fiercely debated in many venues, yet what is often lost to sight is the fact that the current size and growth of the Latino population, and its particular patterns of social behavior, are the direct result of the fateful "encounter" that occurred more than five centuries ago.

Since the civil rights movement of the 1960s, minority groups have been popularly assumed to be "dysfunctional." Minority group status is usually linked to poverty and low levels of education, two variables that are assumed to generate social ills: high unemployment, high labor force desertion, high levels of welfare dependency, rapid disintegration of the family, short life expectancies, high levels of illness and disease, and high levels of health-harming behavior such as smoking, drinking, and drug use. Contrary to the common assumption, Latino patterns of behavior do not on the whole sustain the thesis of a dysfunctional minority.

The Latino Epidemiological Paradox

Sudden epidemics aside, health indicators change very slowly for a population. These stable patterns reflect, to a large extent, the stable ways of life of a given population. The Latino population, at least in California, exhibits stable patterns of health behavior that surprise those expecting a "minority" population pattern of behavior, but they will not surprise anyone who has read Hernández's descriptions of Mexican medical traditions.

Long life expectancy

In 1990, the Office of Minority Health released a chart book that bluntly stated that "blacks and minorities have a shorter life expectancy than whites."[2] It is commonly said that a young man in Bangladesh has a greater chance of reaching age 65 than a young man in inner-city America.[3] Driven by these and similar statements, the image of "minority" life expectancy is that it is substantially shorter than "mainstream" American society. However, this is not the case with Latinos. In California, an average newborn has a life expectancy of 76.9 years, a newborn Latino 80.2 years. The comparable figures for Texas are 76.3 and 77.5 years, respectively.[4]

Low death rates

A death rate is a figure for the number of deaths per 100,000 persons of a given population. The crude death rate is simply a measure of how many persons will die in a year, irrespective of any age bias. The 1993 crude death rate in California was 943.0 per 100,000 Anglo-Americans, yet only 288.3 among Latinos.[5] The Anglo population in California has a median age of 34 years, the Latino 23. The age-adjusted rate for Anglos in California in 1993 was 471.3 per 100,000 of the Anglo population.[6] The corresponding rate for Latinos was 363.7. Thus even when the effects of age are factored out, the Latino death rate is still substantially lower than the Anglo. This pattern of lower Latino death rates (both crude and age-adjusted) holds for Latino populations in Arizona and Texas as well.

Heart disease, cancer, and stroke are the top three causes of death in California, Arizona, Texas, and the United States as a whole, among Latinos as well as Anglos, but the age-adjusted rates at which these deaths occur are much lower for Latinos.[7] Of the top fifteen causes of death, Latinos also have lower death rates for chronic obstructive pulmonary diseases, pneumonia and influenza, AIDS, suicide, and hereditary and degenerative diseases.[8] These patterns of health behavior and health outcome are very stable, being observed in the sizable Latino populations of Arizona and Texas as well as in California. They are also unexpected, as a result of which they are called "the Latino epidemiological paradox": the health indicators of this group are expected to be substantially worse than the Anglo yet turn out to be substantially better.[9] The health paradox is repeated in various stable, long-term patterns of sociodemographic indicators, such as high male labor force participation, lower rates of dependence on welfare, and strong family formation.

In a recent editorial in the *American Journal of Public Health* pondering the existence of the Latino epidemiological paradox, Scribner came to the conclusion that "a group level effect for cultural orientation is far more important in determining the risk of chronic disease among Mexican-Americans, than genetic, biologic or socioeconomic factors operating at the individual level."[10] This phenomenon we could call "culture." From the health data, it is clear that there is a relation between this indefinable thing called Latino culture and the paradoxical outcomes. Even in the sociodemographic data, we find evidence pointing to the daily effects of Latino culture. Whence came this culture, and what is its likely future?

Population, Civilization, and Culture

During the Quincentenary observance of 1992, some commentators depicted the encounter as the start of five hundred years of unmitigated catastrophe: blood, death, rapine, subjugation, plunder, and enslavement. Others took the polar opposite view that the encounter was an offering of a civilization, religion, tongue, knowledge, and its own children, from Spain to the New World. Almost lost amid the fiery debates was the simple fact that the encounter did occur and that, because of it, the Western Hemisphere would never be the same. As we can appreciate in the life and works of Dr. Francisco Hernández—as the essays in this volume demonstrate in different ways—the Old World, too, would never be the same.

It is nearly impossible to imagine what life would be like today in the Americas if there had been no "encounter." Certainly, the major features that describe social life in Mexico and Latin America—a mestizo, Spanish-speaking population descended from the Iberian Catholic experience—would not apply. And yet, the civilizations of Mexico, the Caribbean, and Latin America were not simply and only an extension, a transplantation, of the Iberian world. Hernández showed that he knew this when he compiled his *Antiquities* and his *Natural History*. Over the past five hundred years, the sequelae of the encounter have continued to stew and sediment into the now recognizable patterns of behavior and thought that are considered to be so "typical" of the Americas but that need to be seen not as simply traditional and oriented to the past but as "behavior in process of formation," still evolving, changing, and emerging before our eyes. Instead of thinking of the nearly thirty million Latinos in the United States as a quaint, ethnic minority group "clinging to its cultural heritage," we would do better to see Latinos in the United States as the hemisphere's third-largest Spanish-speaking "country" (after Mexico and Colombia), stemming from the same larger civilization shared with nearly 500 million other residents of the New World.

The Clash of Civilizations

S. P. Huntington recently offered a novel way of conceptualizing the major geocultural regions of the world. For him, the operant, underlying, impelling force that defines these regions is religious, rather than merely linguistic, ideological, or ethnic.[11] Huntington defines some of the major civilizations of the world: the Western Christian, Eastern

Orthodox, the Muslim world, the Confucian/Buddhist, and the Hindu. In passing, he alludes to Latin America, but without elaborating on the region in much detail. I would like to take the liberty of picking up where he ends and, through the vehicle of this Hernández project, to illustrate the primary dynamics and features of what I shall call "Latino Catholic civilization." As we shall see, Latinos in the United States are part and parcel of a much larger civilizational shell.

The Latino Catholic Civilization

The meeting of two worlds set in motion dynamics—demographic, linguistic, religious, economic, political—that are still at work today. Their evolution over the past five centuries has formed a recognizable civilization that is much greater than a single culture: indeed, this larger shell of civilization is so large and transcendent that it can give birth to smaller, more localized cultures yet stamp them indelibly with its larger characteristics such that the smaller cultures resemble one another to an amazing degree. Although it has been customary to speak of Latin American "culture," any traveler to the region recognizes two seemingly contradictory aspects of daily life: uniformity and diversity.

It matters little if one is in Mexico City, Caracas, Santiago, Havana, San Juan, or Buenos Aires, because much of the language, architecture, modes of social behavior, and ideas discussed by intellectuals during their *tertulias* will be instantly recognizable. Yet, even though the larger sociocultural envelope is so readily recognizable, there are myriad smaller, local variations. Foods, vocabulary, genetic composition of the residents, and regnant political ideologies can differ radically from one area to another, yet the differences are not so great as to be unintelligible: the differences seem to be contained in a larger envelope, which I call the Latino Catholic civilization.

I use this term advisedly, and not with just a little trepidation. The term may seem grandiose, raising the ideas, values, and behaviors of an area to an undeservedly high level of abstraction, yet I will argue for the use of *civilization* rather than *culture*. One feature of Huntington's definition of *civilization* is that it transcends language, providing a "mentality" that is greater than any number of languages contained within it. Unlike the world's other great civilizations, the Latino Catholic world functions with only two, very closely related languages—Spanish and Portuguese, in which, it is safe to estimate, more than 90 percent of the population of Latin America can communicate. And, with just a little patience, a Spanish speaker can communicate with a Portuguese speaker on just about any topic: imagine a German speaker attempting to communicate with an Italian with only a little patience as a guide! Although linguistic unity was not a requirement for Huntington's definition of *civilization,* the Latino Catholic civilization is the most linguistically unified of them all.

Because Catholicism is a fundamental of Huntington's Western Christian civilization, one might be inclined to consider the Latino Catholic civilization as merely another variant on the Judeo-Christian Western tradition. If Mexico and Latin America were simply a transplant of Iberian culture, one could agree with this, but Iberia was not merely transplanted across the ocean, as the writings of Hernández illustrate in vivid detail. Iberia met with a number of then living societies that absorbed it into their own life patterns and whose descendants shaped, and continue to shape, the sequelae of the meeting of two worlds.

The Iberian Overlay

For non-Latinos, perhaps the most recognizable and familiar elements of Latino Catholic civilization are the Iberian ones. The Iberian Peninsula was, and is, a central part of the Western Christian civilization. Itself an amalgamation of various peoples and religions, Iberia presented a mosaic of languages, cultures, genetics, and politics, all tucked by 1492—sometimes none too tidily—under the covering tent of militarily triumphant Catholicism. Yet this diversity was artificially reduced to an imposed homogeneity when brought to the New World. Officially, Castilian was imposed as the official language of territories controlled by Spain. This artificial linguistic uniformity has resulted, five hundred years later, in relative linguistic unity. It is worthwhile to remember in this context that, simply by translating his

Latin manuscripts into Náhuatl as well as Spanish, Hernández was registering his heterodoxy.

A key element of the Latino Catholic civilization was, obviously, Catholicism. Under the authority granted the Spanish Crown by the pope, the civil authority was able to select (and, at times, deselect) the religious who traveled to the New World and the ecclesiastical authorities who managed them. Yet this unity of religion was tempered by the nature of Catholicism: it is by its nature a religion of diversity, encompassing a wide variety of opinions manifested in the multiple orders—Franciscans, Dominicans, Jesuits—that were given authority for specific regions for specific periods of time for specific purposes. As others in this volume have shown, unity of religion still allowed for the possibility of a *converso* doctor's writings to be published in the Protestant north of Europe.

Administrative authority was imposed, through the massive bureaucratic structure of the Spanish Crown. Viceregal authority responded to a highly centralized command structure. Yet, when the centralized orders were patently unworkable in a local situation, the elaborate bureaucratic structure was sidestepped, through the reasoning of "Obedezco, pero no cumplo" (I will obey the order, but I will not fulfill it). This was the context of Hernández's inability to do much in his capacity as *protomédico.* So, the Iberian society was artificially reduced, and the diversity of the peninsula hopefully (and futilely) averted, as the homogeneous reflection was overlaid on the indigenous societies of the New World.

The Indigenous Substrate

The population of New Spain when Columbus arrived is variously estimated to have ranged from 18 million to 30 million.[12] These millions of people were already organized into urban complexes of millions of residents, rural villages of thousands, and nomadic tribes of a few hundred or mere dozens. The fact of hundreds of different indigenous societies interacting, over the centuries, with the artificially homogeneous Spanish overlay brought the texture of diversity back to the Iberian overlay, but with a diversity completely different from that known in the peninsula.

Although the Crown imposed a linguistic unity, the tongue of Castile encountered hundreds of indigenous languages and dialects. In a process lasting centuries, indigenous populations adopted Spanish grammar, and Europeans learned the indigenous terms for native plants, animals, foods, and social behaviors. Hernández, of course, made a major contribution to this interplay by undertaking the massive task of naming new realities and organizing them in the indigenous way.[13] In an even more diverse fashion, the Catholicism of diversity met with the diverse religious beliefs of the different indigenous societies. As the *Antiquities* of Hernández demonstrates, key Catholic beliefs resonated with indigenous beliefs—finding salvation in community, the importance of ritual, the sacramentality of life's events—to reveal critical areas of nearly immediate convergence, such as the appearance of the Virgin of Guadalupe at the site of the former area of worship to the Aztec earth-mother goddess, Tonantzin.

The extent to which indigenous societies should or should not be influenced by the Europeans was a subject of continuous debate. Some argued (and acted) in favor of incorporating the indigenous as a source of labor and commerce, expecting that they should adopt Iberian ways of life. Others—for example, the first generation of evangelizers—argued that Iberian influence was corrupting and should be held at bay by the continued use of American languages and the formation of American utopias, where the Spanish would not be allowed to intrude.

To some extent, there was the possibility of two societies living cheek by jowl, the numerically small Iberian society held accountable to Spanish law, and the numerically much larger American society regulated by the Law of the Indies. The history of Mexico under the Spanish Crown might have been similar to that of India under the British two centuries later—a thin layer of law and custom familiar only to a small elite group at the top, but remote, foreign, and inaccessible to the large masses of people at the bottom, who live in India today much as they did 250 years ago before the British set foot on the subcontinent. This possibility was rendered unlikely because of the simple fact elaborated on earlier in this volume: the epidemiology of the conquest.

The Mestizo

When Hernández lamented that the *cocoliztli* took the lives of so many people in New Spain in 1576, he added that with those people went their specialized knowledge. The ravages of cocoliztli took an estimated 95 percent toll on the indigenous population and so created a demographic vacuum that was slowly filled in Mexico by a new population, the mestizo. Ultimately, the various waves of cocoliztli created the population dynamics of California in the 1900s. The "depopulation" of New Spain in the 1570s was not a new experience for the Spanish Crown: it had already witnessed the virtual disappearance of the Caribbean indigenous populations (Carib, Arawak, Siboney) within a few years of the first landings. In the Caribbean, the lost indigenous population was replaced by another brought from Africa. In New Spain, slavery was not as important a factor relative to the surviving population. Instead, New Spain was slowly repopulated by the mestizo, the offspring of Spanish and American, with pockets of African and Asian.

The emerging mestizo society was more than simply a bridge or mediator society between the Spanish and American. It was a fusion between the two, more than simply an Iberian transplant, yet very different from the indigenous. Mestizo society was developed largely in the Castilian tongue, but with a great appreciation for Náhuatl terminology for the emotive, everyday things of hearth, home, table, and kin. Thus, while the grammar was Castilian, the words for items such as turkey and child were, in everyday mestizo language, *guajolote* and *escuintle*.

It was in the spiritual realm that the mestizo paid particular reverence to both Iberian and indigenous. Whereas the recently converted American might be suspected in the worst of cases of hiding pre-Columbian gods underneath a supposedly incomplete conversion to Christianity, the mestizo was rarely so suspected. Life for the mestizo was filled with sacrament, the presence of the sacred and a joyful release into ritual. The complementarity between the indigenous and the Catholic found full, unquestioning expression in the religious beliefs and practices of mestizo society.

The content of meaning in mestizo society—the values, beliefs, and behaviors—was created and sustained by two sources: the formal, institutional church, and the popular Catholicism that lived independent of, but linked to, that church. The institutional church of papal announcements and royal appointments provided a link, albeit at times tenuous, to the world of Protestant reformation and Catholic baroque Counter-Reformation. The edicts and papers related to that lengthy conversation, however, played a relatively small part in the daily life of meaning constructed by emergent mestizo society.

More important, on a daily basis, was popular Catholicism, the unconscious welding of pre-Columbian moral discourse with a pre-Tridentine Catholicism unaware of the search for individual perfectionism unleashed by Luther and Calvin. Mestizo popular religiosity built on the foundation of indigenous practices of ritual and the Iberian popular cults of saints. In this emerging worldview, a number of messages were distilled from both the indigenous and the Iberian and communicated from generation to generation. Definitions of the desirable and undesirable, the acceptable and the unacceptable, the beautiful and the ugly, the good and the bad, were the product of a sedimentation of social construction, reinforced by tales, jokes, and daily gossip. "¿El que dirán?" (What will people say?) became an important element, as did the claims of family and community on the individual. Only occasionally reinforced by the formal sacramental life of the institutional church, this mestizo worldview (or "mentality," to use the terminology of the Annalistes) was built up over centuries of commonplace, everyday life.

This, then, formed the moral matrix that would nourish thoughts and behaviors of numerous future generations of Latinos. Gradually Mexico, and the hemisphere, repopulated itself with an increasingly mestizo population. About 1930, the population of Mexico was once again about 25 million, approximately what it had been nearly four hundred years earlier. As Mexico began the process of industrial development, its population began the "demographic transition" from an agrarian, preindustrial society of high fertility balanced by high mortality to an urban, industrial one. With the development of basic urban infrastructure—sewage, clean water, adequate housing—mortality dropped quickly, while fertility remained high for decades, causing, during the middle part of the twentieth century, a rapid population growth due to an excess of births over deaths. In the space of a few decades, the population of Mexico exploded from 25 million in 1930 to more than 100 million by the dawn of the twenty-first century.

The demographic-cultural process of formation of mestizo society, illustrated here by the case of Mexico, was repeated up and down the mountainous spine of Latin America and across its wide, low plains. There were subtle textural variations, depending on the characteristics of the indigenous society (that is, language, social structure such as urban or nomadic, religious beliefs, and so on) and on varying genetic inputs (some parts of Latin America have a more indigenous genetic heritage, others a more European, still others a more African, and most with more than just a soupçon of Asian). There was much variation at the local level, yet the overarching presence of the Catholic religion—both the formal and the popular—with its mental and spiritual constructs of appropriate human behaviors, provided a basis of continuity from region to region.

Perhaps the closest similar and familiar demographic-cultural dynamic to the formation of mestizo America might be the outer provinces of the Roman Empire, but unlike the provinces of the Roman Empire that developed their own distinctive languages and cultures, the centrifugal tendencies of Latin America have been increasingly outweighed by the centripetal ones. True enough, Latin America has always had its sentiments of *patria chica*, local areas of intense pride, such that one is not simply Mexican, but is more proudly a "Poblano" from Puebla, a "Jarocho" from Veracruz, or a "Tapatio" from Guadalajara. These feelings of *patria chica* might have formed the nucleus for the development of increasingly different languages and cultures. But technological improvements in communication and travel reinforced by the Latino Catholic tradition provided a different history and future.

Travel by sea, although slow and sporadic, kept the Americas in contact with one another during the colonial and early independence periods, staving off a complete isolation as was seen in post-Roman Iberia, Gaul, and Germania. Gradually, during the late nineteenth century and early twentieth, railroad networks, then paved road connections, and finally jet age travel knit the regions of Latin America together for purposes of trade, travel, and education. Perhaps the most profound centripetal force has been the revolution in communications. Certainly, the printed word helps to slow the process of linguistic shift and change, and the Latino Catholic civilization benefited from the first printing press in the Americas.[14] However, the twentieth-century improvements in communication stitch the region together even more tightly. Thus the Latino Catholic civilization has remained flexibly intact, elastic, able to stretch and to accommodate new inputs, yet always keeping its threads whole.

If any region of the Latino Catholic civilization were to be lost to it, that would be the northern border with the present United States. Although settled as early as 1594, the area was thinly populated. Distant from the metropolitan centers such as Mexico City, Havana, or Lima, lacking universities or viceregal courts, it relied largely on popular religion and culture to provide a world of meaning for its people. After the American conquest and annexation, the early Latino population was suddenly swamped by an influx of peoples from the east (coast, that is). Four phenomena intervened to prevent a complete loss of this population to the Latino Catholic civilization.

First, the early Latino population lived somewhat in isolation, left alone or avoided by the Anglo in-migrant population. Second, a degree of segregation was imposed by the incoming order, relegating Latinos to live a separate life, whether that was desired or not. Third, unlike the fallen Roman Empire with its looted capital, the rest of the Latino Catholic civilization did not suffer other large-scale permanent invasions, and it remained alive and viable, only yards away from its overrun children. And fourth was the demographic recovery from the epidemiological consequences of the meeting of two worlds.

Current Demographic Effects of the Epidemiological Encounter

Mexico's population finally reached its pre-encounter levels just at the time when political and economic forces in both the United States and Mexico drew a portion of it back to its former territories. The political instability during the Mexican Revolution, from 1910 to 1917, caused the first trickles of population movement north of the border. Then, the economic boom years of the Roaring Twenties created a demand for an enlarged workforce. While cities on the Atlantic seaboard had relied on European immigrants for their labor force earlier, both the proximity to Mexico and the stoppage of European immigration created a situation mutually advantageous to U.S. employers in the Southwest and Mexican immigrants. As California's economy boomed in the years after World War II, it required ever greater numbers of workers in certain segments of the economy. At precisely the time California required such a growing population, Mexico had finally shaken off the last of the epidemiological effects of the encounter and was able to supply the needed workforce. California's Latino population grew from 1 million in 1960 to about 10 million by the late 1990s. The Latino population of the state now finds itself woven back into the Latino Catholic civilization, owing to demographics, technology, and proximity.

It is tempting, albeit pragmatically useless, to imagine an alternative history of California had the epidemics of cocoliztli not occurred, or had they occurred with European levels of mortality. Had either of these been the case, there might be no United States as we know it, stretching from sea to sea. Had the estimated 25 million inhabitants of Mexico in 1519, rather than suffering a 95 percent mortality, increased instead, even at preindustrial levels of growth, by the time the pilgrims left Plymouth in 1620, the population of Mexico might well have been close to 35 million. Such a population base would have created population pressures to establish large urban centers in Albuquerque, San Antonio, San Diego, and Los Angeles. By the time of the American Revolution in 1776, the population of Mexico could have been around 50 million, with, no doubt, large metropolitan centers with cathedrals, universities, and viceregal courts, anchoring the cities of a densely populated northern border region. Probably Mexican miners would have discovered the mother lode of gold in California and the Comstock silver lode of Nevada, and part of the riches would have been used to finance the construction of mining cities that would have looked like Guanajuato or Taxco but located in California, Nevada, Arizona, or Colorado.

Had any of this happened, the 5 million Anglo-Americans in the newly independent United States would have faced a deeply rooted Latino Catholic population around ten times its size. Westward expansion would have been difficult, if not impossible, and the United States would have been likely limited to a narrow band of land between the territories of Mexico and the British territories of Canada. The United States as we know it would not have existed.

However, wave after wave of cocoliztli did sweep the hemisphere, the population was ravaged, and in that window of time between the sixteenth and nineteenth centuries, Mexico could not anchor its northern borders sufficiently to withstand the in-movement of new and different peoples, and this gives us our current demographic situation: the Latino population is nearly one-third of California's population and is growing, while the Anglo population is slightly less than half and will experience very little growth throughout the twenty-first century.

Latino culture will change in the twenty-first century. It is a dynamic culture, accustomed to change, indeed springing from the momentous changes wrought by the meeting of cultures five hundred years ago. But its rate and direction of change are now dictated by the internal dynamics of the culture, rather than being imposed by external forces. These internal dynamics that are now the motor force for the construction of meaning in California have their origins in the topic of this volume, the encounter of two worlds.

NOTES

1. *Latino* covers a vast array of people from North, Central, and South America and the Caribbean.

2. *Health Status of the Disadvantaged* (Washington, D.C.: Health Resources and Services Administration, U.S. Public Health Service, 1990).

3. For example, C. McCord and H. Freeman, "Excess Mortality in Harlem," *New England Journal of Medicine* 322 (1990): 173–79.

4. David E. Hayes-Bautista, "Work Force Options and Issues in the Border States," paper presented to the Clinical Directors Network, 1996.

5. Although the crude death rate provides one picture of the health status of different populations, it can be biased by a population that is disproportionately old or young: deaths are more common among an older population than a younger one.

6. The age-adjusted death rate removes the effects of differential age structure, by artificially making all populations identical in age structure.

7. For death from heart disease: Anglos 127.0, Latinos 90.9; cancer, Anglos 126.5, Latinos 75.7; stroke, Anglos 24.3, Latinos 21.1.

8. There are some causes of death for which Latinos have higher age-adjusted death rates than Anglos, but these causes are much less frequent than heart disease, cancer, or stroke, and the rates are around one-tenth that for heart disease: unintentional injuries, diabetes, homicide, and cirrhosis. Latinos have a lower rate of infant mortality and a lower likelihood of smoking, drinking, and drug use among females (see K. H. Acree, D. G. Bal, D. O. Lyman, and K. W. Kizer, *Behavioral Risk Factor Surveillance in California* [Sacramento: Department of Health Services, 1990]; H. Amaro, R. Whitaker, G. Coffman, and T. Heeren, "Acculturation and Marijuana and Cocaine Use: Findings from the HHANES, 1982–1984," *American Journal of Public Health* 80, supplement [1990]: 54–60).

9. K. S. Markides and J. Coreil, "The Health of Hispanics in the Southwestern United States: An Epidemiological Paradox," *Public Health Reports* 101 (1986): 253–65.

10. Richard Scribner, "Paradox as Paradigm: The Health Outcomes of Mexican Americans," *American Journal of Public Health* 86 (1996): 304.

11. Samuel P. Huntington, "The Clash of Civilizations?" *Foreign Affairs* (Summer 1993): 22–50.

12. W. Borah and S. F. Cook, *Essays in Population History: Mexico and the Caribbean* (Berkeley: University of California Press, 1971), 1:115, and see N. Sánchez-Albornoz, *The Population of Latin America: A History* (Berkeley: University of California Press, 1974).

13. See Carmen Benito-Vessels, "Hernández in New Spain," and José M. López Piñero and José Pardo Tomás, "Contribution of Hernández," above.

14. Printing began in Mexico possibly in 1535, definitely by 1539 (the date of the earliest surviving imprint). Spain acquired its first printing press in the decade of the 1540s. See the basic summary information in Douglas C. McMurtrie, *The Book: The Story of Printing and Bookmaking* (New York, 1989), 390–400, and Lucien Febvre and Henri Jean Martin, *The Coming of the Book: The Impact of Printing 1450–1800,* trans. David Gerard, ed. Geoffrey Nowell-Smith and David Wootton (London: Verso, 1984), 208–9; and of course Joaquín García Icazbalceta, *Bibliografía mexicana del siglo XVI* (Mexico City: Fondo de Cultura Económica, 1954).

THE POPULAR LEGACY OF FRANCISCO HERNÁNDEZ

SIMON VAREY

RAFAEL CHABRÁN

At the Real Jardín Botánico in Madrid, near the graceful neoclassical main gate, is a small gift shop in which books, potted plants and seeds are displayed for sale to visitors. Just outside the door of the shop is a wooden stand on which some of the merchandise is displayed. Pinned to that stand one torrid day in June 1995 was a handwritten list of the names of perhaps twenty plants, together with an indication of the diseases, disorders, or discomforts that they cure. The tradition of Pliny, Dioscorides, and Hernández was visible in that modest scrap of paper. Five thousand miles away, across the Atlantic Ocean, the traditions recorded by Hernández are visible in equally tangible ways, but they are far more widespread.

Five of the contributors to this volume attended a conference in November 1992 that was brought to a triumphant close with a day spent at the Botanical Garden in Cuernavaca. Historically arranged so that plants imported into Mexico at various times since 1492 will not be confused with natives, the garden itself preserves the tradition of botany as a medicinal source. Dr. Margarita Aviles graciously gave a guided tour of the garden to a large crowd of academics, as well as to two less academic visitors who turned

out to be healers with an obvious interest in the medicinal applications of the plants and who repeatedly asked specific questions, especially about dosages, and with intense concentration wrote down the answers in their notebooks. This is only anecdotal evidence, true, but as one UCLA researcher discovered in a study of folkloric tradition among Latinos in Los Angeles, the traditional medicine practiced by healers is still thriving.[1] So too are the *herbolarios* that dot the landscape wherever Mexican culture has asserted itself, practically unchanged since the time of Hernández.

The streets of downtown Los Angeles near the Grand Central Market bear witness to the continuing popular tradition of botanical, or herbal, medicine. In East Los Angeles, with its predominantly Latino population, there are even more such shops dispensing herbal remedies, dried roots for making infusions, and so on.[2] Some of these shops have a tendency to combine medicine for the body with medicine for the soul: hence many of them have names such as Botanica Cristo Rey (translated roughly as Christ the Lord Herb Shop) and offer a wide range of "religious articles" as well as spiritual advice, in addition to boxes and packets of dried herbs. This is perhaps not so much evidence of "our blessed Saviour as the glorious Physician of Souls" as it is a sign that body and soul are not so easy to separate.[3]

One of these retail businesses, named Herbs of Mexico: Herb Emporium, sells about eight hundred different herbs and spices from all over the world, perhaps 10 to 15 percent of them Mexican, most of those listed by their Náhuatl names. Another, Jardines Botánicos de Oaxaca, which declares itself "guardian of your health," issues a leaflet that reads almost like the *Index medicamentorum* of Hernández. Virtually every box of dried leaves or powders is supposed to cure six or seven different conditions. For example, a product named simply Aromatico, which contains such familiar plants as guayabo and mint, is recommended for "diarrhea, vomiting, dysentery, constipation, colic, lethargy, colitis, stomach ache, and stomach upsets (intestinal illness)." Hernández probably would not be surprised to learn that *tlanchalagua* helps fat people to lose weight, because its two principal ingredients are *cocolmeca[tl]* and *tejocotl*. It is not that Hernández is directly necessary for the survival of enterprises such as these, but as the essays in this volume should attest, his words have constituted the principal written scientific authority on Mexican herbal medicine for more than four centuries, not only where Latinos live but, as we have seen, in the Puritan north of Europe, too. In the Americas the received knowledge of the medicinal properties of so many Mexican plants has been passed on orally, within families, especially rural families, and to some degree limited by region, so that the plants of the Yucatán are not necessarily familiar to the inhabitants of Michoacán. With complex patterns of migration and cultural change, especially northward to California, that body of knowledge has come to depend not for its survival but for its coherence on Hernández, because it was he who organized it, urbanized it, and ultimately controlled it.

Now and then Hernández turns up by name, as an authority, in other relatively unexpected places. A popular history of herbs and spices mentions his role in "identifying" allspice; a brief article in *Herb Quarterly* at least alludes to him, quite properly, as "the foremost Spanish naturalist of his day" and "the first European authority on" vanilla.[4] Scattered allusions such as these clearly do not amount to much. The real key to Hernández's authority today is perhaps Mex-

ico's most popular book on the subject of herbal medicine: Maximino Martínez's *Las plantas medicinales de México* (Mexico City: Botas, 1933). There are, of course, many published books in circulation today that describe Mexican medicinal plants, many of them, like this one, in a practical paperback format. As far as we know, Martínez is the only author of such books who bases many of his descriptions of the plants and, particularly, their applications on the authority of Hernández, quoting from the *Quatro libros* and the Rome edition throughout the book. And surely this one must be unique among such publications in that it not only reproduces the title pages of the Rome edition, the *Quatro libros,* the Madrid edition, and Cardenas but is even dedicated to the memory of Hernández, "the immortal protomédico of the Indies in the era of Philip II."

In his time a distinguished professor of natural sciences and head of Mexico's national herbarium and of the botanical division of the Museum of Natural History, Martínez is a valuable indicator of the legacy of the native Mexican medical tradition with which Hernández is associated. Part of the usefulness of *Las plantas* is that it gives the scientific as well as native names of the plants. It is also organized helpfully, in four parts: plants that have a known botanical classification and have been the subject of scientific study; those that have the classification but have not been studied; unidentified plants that are popularly called remedies; and plants from Yucatán.[5] The description of each plant is organized, tersely, under some permutation of headings: its other names; places where it grows; popular uses; written sources and references; parts of the plant that are used in medicine; characteristics; chemical composition; and dosages.

In his prologue, Martínez points out that some plants are commonly dismissed as medicinally ineffective only because they have been identified incorrectly. He recognizes that some plants have different effects according to differences between organisms, he is aware of the vagaries and dangers of oral tradition, and he knows that healers wish to keep their knowledge secret. All these signs of the author's judiciousness are reinforced by his selection: he does not dwell on plants that are no longer in use, such as guaiacum as a cure for syphilis (even though it is still considered good for purifying the blood), and so demonstrates

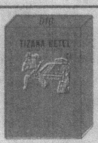
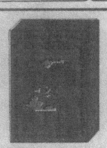
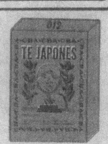
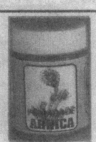
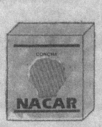
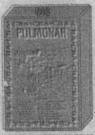

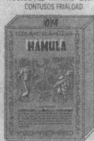
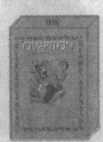
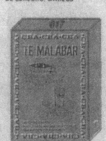
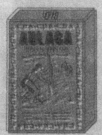
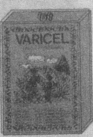
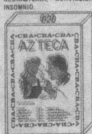
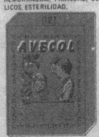
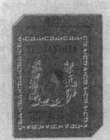
A modern advertising leaflet, showing Mexican herbal medicines.

that his interest is not in any sense antiquarian. His emphasis on modern practice and scientific taxonomy really strengthens his respect for Hernández, whom Martínez quotes as his authority on seventy-one plants.

Martínez is a perfect example of a scholar who was able to write for a popular market. Scholarly attention to Hernández has never really abated in either Mexico or Spain; Italian scholars have paid careful attention to the Rome edition and to occasional Italian publications that adopted and quoted him, but in England and the Netherlands, where Hernández should have figured in botanical and medical history, he has been largely absent.[6] Yet the kind of work that Hernández undertook in the field in Mexico in the 1570s continues to be done in various parts of the region, and the Mexican traditions of indigenous medicine that he described continue to thrive. In Mexico particularly, researchers have found again and again that the traditions enshrined in the work of Hernández change very little as they are passed down from generation to generation, as Martínez's manual testifies. Once populations move, especially from rural to urban cultures or from Mexico to the United States, their medicinal traditions undergo transformations, perhaps retaining a core of traditional knowledge and practice.

Expeditions in the spirit, and in the footsteps, of Hernández took place in the first four centuries after his death, and they continue to do so in the fifth. As the Renaissance shaded into the Enlightenment, botanists and physicians, cosmographers and engineers painstakingly pieced together their knowledge of the Americas. From the era of de Laet, Piso, and Marcgraf to that of Sloane, then Humboldt, Muñoz, and Sessé, practical men went to those regions of the world that Hernández had sought to describe systematically. They went with ideological agendas, as others in this volume have shown, but surely the most important point is that they went at all.

From the 1980s to the present there have been many more, very extensive investigations and publications of the uses, physiology, and pharmacology of Mexican folk plants. The most recent investigator in a long and distinguished line that includes Howard and Mary Cline, Arthur Rubel, Xavier Lozoya, Robert Bye, Edelmira Linares, Carole Browner, and

Michael Heinrich, Dr. Mark Plotkin has received due plaudits for his field research in Costa Rica and Ecuador, where he has patiently sought out the necessary information about medicinal plants. In addition to the publication of his remarkable book, *Tales of a Shaman's Apprentice,* articles describing his work have appeared in places that demonstrate the popular (as well as scholarly) appeal of botanical medicine.[7] If Plotkin and his immediate predecessors are in a sense following the lead of a botanist/explorer such as Hernández, the pharmaceutical manufacturing industry could be said to be following Philip II. It would probably be stretching the evidence too far if we were to claim that the welcome that is accorded to "alternative" medicines in the Netherlands has any connection at all with the Mexican traditions described by Hernández, even if we now know that many Mexican plants found their way there. Nonetheless, it is widely recognized in the scholarly world as well as the drug industry that medicinal plants are potential and actual sources of new therapeutics, and, not surprisingly, the worldwide market for medicinal plants has grown steadily in recent years.[8] To their credit, Plotkin and some of the drug companies have sought to protect the resources and people of those countries from possible ravages at the hands of Western governments, businesses, and unprincipled profit motives, by arranging for financial compensation payable to the country where the plants are found that are used for the drugs.[9] However, we have not found any evidence of a modern effort to transplant medicinally useful plants as Hernández endeavored to do. Not yet.

NOTES

1. Beatrice A. Roeder, *Chicano Folk Medicine from Los Angeles, California,* California Publications in Folklore and Mythology Studies, vol. 34 (Berkeley: University of California Press, 1988), esp. 28–38.

2. Many of the plants that were considered medicinal still appear frequently as foods, whether or not they are still used as medicines today. The most obvious ones, such as corn, tomatoes, and chili, are universal now, but Mexican restaurants in the United States as well as Mexico can be found today serving dishes that include *cempoalxochitl* flowers, or *huitlacoche* (corn smut, as American farmers disgustedly call it, but "in Mexico we consider it our truffle," according to Zarela Martínez, *Food from My Heart* [New York: Macmillan, 1992], 9). Scholarly and popular research on the implications and consequences of 1492 has led to a plethora of explorations of "The Great Food Migration," as John Schwartz called it in a special issue of *Newsweek* in 1992. For the best account, prob-

ably, see Raymond Sokolov, *Why We Eat What We Eat* (New York: Summit Books, 1991). The intricate cultural connections between foods and drugs have been addressed by Timothy Johns, *The Origins of Human Diet and Medicine* (Tucson: University of Arizona Press, 1996).

3. The phrase is Cotton Mather's: it was the subject of his first sermon, in 1680, and reflects Mather's dual interests: the church and medicine (Samuel Mather, *The Life of the Very Reverend and Learned Cotton Mather* [Boston, 1729], 27).

4. J. O. Swahn, *The Lore of Spices: Their History and Uses around the World* (New York: Crescent Books, 1991), 172. Raymond Schuessler, "Vanilla—from Orchids to Extract," *Herb Quarterly* 68 (Winter 1995): 42.

5. The Yucatán section is, rather surprisingly, a slightly revised version of an herbal known as *El libro del Judío*, written probably at some time before 1770 and first published in 1834.

6. The Rome edition is discussed, and a small selection from Hernández appears briefly, but as cited by Giuseppe Donzelli, *Teatro farmaceutico* (Venice, 1686), in Rosa Casanova and Marco Bellingeri, *Alimentos, remedios, vicios y placeres: Breve historia de los productos mexicanos en Italia* (Mexico City: INAH and Organization of American States, 1988). There is no comparable work that shows the transfer of Mexican *realia* to northern Europe, probably because northern Europe's collective cultural memory no longer recognizes that there ever was much traffic from Mexico, as we have attempted to show above.

7. For example, Karen Allen, "Mark Plotkin: 1994 Conservation Medalist," *Zoonooz* 58, no. 1 (January 1995): 16–21. This journal is a publication of the Zoological Society of San Diego, which, on October 7, 1994, made the award to which the title of the article alludes. One caption describes Plotkin as "a leading rain forest ethnobotanist and modern medicine man" (20).

8. See Paul Hersch-Martínez, "Commercialization of Wild Medicinal Plants from Southwest Puebla, Mexico," *Economic Botany* 49, no. 2 (1995): 197–206, and Walter H. Lewis and Memory P. Elvin-Lewis, "Medicinal Plants as Sources of New Therapeutics," *Annals of the Missouri Botanical Garden* 82 (1995): 16–24, with a judicious bibliography, 23–24. There is, of course, a growing interest in herbs and medicinal plants generally, witnessed by the publication of popular magazines addressed to herbalists, gardeners, and others. There is even an international herb symposium, held for the third time in June 1996.

9. See Marjorie Shaffer, "Going Back to Basics," *Financial Times*, September 29, 1992.

GLOSSARY

Although we translate virtually everything into English, there are inevitably some terms that either (1) have specialized meanings in Spanish that resist exact translation into English; (2) are used by our contributors in a specialized sense; or (3) are unfamiliar to Anglophone readers in any form. In a few cases (*protomédico*, for example) we use the Spanish term and its English translation indifferently. With our "rules" strictly defined by pragmatism, we list all the relevant terms here.

America, American The Americas, particularly Spanish America; not the United States.

Audiencia Strictly speaking, an appellate court, but commonly used to indicate a local governing body in the colonial administrative structure.

Don The honorific title that in certain circumstances means "esquire" or "sir" but otherwise cannot be translated directly into normal English ("el rey don Felipe" would be King Sir Philip) and is therefore omitted silently.

Imperial College The Jesuit seminary in Madrid. This venerable teaching institution, founded in 1346, has been through many incarnations with corresponding changes of name. Today it is the Instituto Nacional de Enseñanza Media de San Isidro. At the end of Hernández's life it was known as the College of the Society of Jesus, and for the whole of the seventeenth century and most of the eighteenth, its official name was the Imperial College of the Society of Jesus (Colegio Imperial de la Compañía de Jesús).

Mexico/New Spain From the early sixteenth century, the Spanish referred to New Spain to indicate territories that came under the jurisdiction of the *audiencia* of Mexico, territories that correspond, more or less, to the modern country of Mexico. When referring to the territories, we use "New Spain" in appropriate historical contexts, and "Mexico" otherwise. Until independence (1821), when "Mexico" was adopted as the name of the whole country, Mexico was just one part of the viceroyalty of New Spain. Hernández speaks of "Mexicans" without always being careful to specify exactly whom he meant.

Náhuatl Náhuatl is the language spoken by a large group of peoples who, in Hernández's time, inhabited the central Valley of Mexico and points southeast, as far as Guatemala. It is an Uto-Aztecan language, whose speakers included the Azteca.

Names of plants We give the Náhuatl names of plants, not necessarily as Hernández spelled them, but as they are most commonly spelled today. Wherever identification has been established, we provide a scientific name as well and an English equivalent if there is one.

Personal names and place names   These are given in whatever form is most familiar to Anglophone readers: thus, Columbus (not Colón), Philip II (not Felipe II), Carolus Clusius (not Charles de l'Ecluse). With such obvious exceptions, most names are left in the vernacular. For Mexican place names that have variant spellings we usually follow the recommendations of Ricardo J. Salvador (and others, possibly) found in <http://www.public .iastate.edu/~rjsalvad/scmfaq/PLACENAM>.

Protomedicato   An official board of overseers of the medical profession in general. The regulatory concept was taken from Spain to the Americas but not put into practice according to the Spanish model until 1646.

Protomédico   Chief medical officer. Generally used in this volume to refer to the *protomédico general de las Indias,* or chief medical officer in the Spanish colonies—the position that Hernández held throughout his time in New Spain.

Pueblo   A village or a small town, especially a country town.

Units of currency and units of weight   It is virtually impossible to gloss or translate units of currency such as the ducat, maravedis, peso, and real. Units of currency and weight are explained in our text volume, where they are used extensively.

INDEX

scalding oil. *See* remedies and treatments

Schreck, Johannes. *See* Terrentius

science, 4, 5, 8, 11, 12, 15, 18 n. 2, 33; Hernández's place in the history of, 9; versus humoral and pan-vitalistic theory, 174; and Philip II, 16–17

Scientific Commission of the Pacific, 189, 190

scientific revolution: 15, 16; and eclecticism, 174

Scribner, 198

scurvy. *See* diseases and symptoms

Sebastian, Dom, 17

Sechium. See botanical taxonomies

Second Epistle to the Corinthians, 94

"second version," of Hernández's *Natural History* (1626), 122, 123. *See also* Escorial, fire; Madrid edition; Recchi, Nardo Antonio; Reyes; Rome edition

seeds. *See* plants and plant products

Segal, Sam, 158, 164, 166

Segha, Philippo (Bishop of Piacenza), 127

Seghers, Daniel, 164

semaneros, 72. *See* charity; nurses

Seneca, 31 n. 43

senna. *See* remedies and treatments

Sephardim, 33, 39 n. 1. *See* Jews

serpents. *See* remedies and treatments

Serra, Dr. Jacinto de la, 96

Servando, Fr., 175

Sessé, Martin de, 134, 137 n. 59, 176, 177, 181 n. 48, 185, 186, 208; wants to continue in Hernández's footsteps, 135. *See also* Asso, Ignacio de; Jiménez de la Espada, Marcos; Spanish botanical expeditions

Seville (kingdom), 185

Seville, 16, 29, 35, 111, 112, 115, 117, 152, 163, 170, 184, 188. *See* botanical gardens

Sherard, William, 146. *See* Ray, John

shipbuilding, 17

shortness of breath. *See* diseases and symptoms

Siam, 146

Siboney, 201

Sicana. See botanical taxonomies

side aches. *See* diseases and symptoms

Sigüenza y Góngora, fray José de, 34, 48, 171, 172, 174, 175, 178 nn. 9,11, 181 n. 42

"simples," 5, 123, 128

sin. *See* disease

Sixtus IV, Pope, 51 n. 34

skin and bone diseases. *See* diseases and symptoms

skin lesions. *See* diseases and symptoms

slavery, 84

Sloane, Sir Hans, 141, 142, 143, 144, 145, 146, 147, 148, n. 29, 149 nn. 28,29,30,44, 175, 208. *See* Ray, John; Uvedale, Robert

smallpox. *See* diseases and symptoms

Smilax. See botanical taxonomies

social diseases, 83–85

Society of Apothecaries, and catalog of medicinal ingredients, 146–47

Society of Jesus, 3

Solanaceae or "species of solano." *See* botanical taxonomies

Solanum mexicanum flore magno C.B. *See* plants and plant products

Solanum. See botanical taxonomies

Somolinos d'Ardois, Germán, 23, 29, 34, 35, 42, 47, 128, 130, 171, 190

Soto, Nicolás de, 45

souchet d'Amerique or *cyperus americanus* (*Cyperus articulatus* L.). *See* plants and plant products

soup kitchens, 73. *See also* hospitals; poor / poor relief

Spaniards, 66, 67, 69, 74, 76, 79 n. 28, 86, 87, 89, 89 n. 23, 98; and hospital care, 66, 74

Spanish baroque paintings: and reach of Hernández's work, 151–69; and representation of American plants, 151–66

Spanish baroque paintings and artists (individual works): *Christ in Martha's House / Cristo en casa de Marta* (Velázquez), 153; *Food of the Angels / Cocina de los angeles* (Murillo) 153, 155; *Frutero con dulces* (Hamen y León), 155; *Holy Family* (Murillo), 158; *Holy Family* (Zurbarán), 158, 160; *Mystic Wedding of Saint Catherine / Desposorios místicos de Santa Catalina* (Sánchez Cotán), 156; *Old Woman Frying Eggs / Vieja friendo huevos* (Velázquez), 153; *Still Life with Flowers / Florero* (Hiepes), 159, 162; *Still Life with Flowers, Birds, and Fruit / Florero con pájaros y frutas* (Arellano), 166; *Still Life with Fruit Basket and Bunches of Grapes / Bodegón con frutero y racimos de uva* (Hamen y León), 158; *Still Life with Game / Bodegón con piezas de caza* (Sánchez Cotán), 155; *Tribute to Flora / Ofrenda a Flora* (Hamen y León), 165; *Two Trinities (Las dos Trinidades)* (Murillo), 156, 157; *Vase of Flowers / Jarrón de flores* (Belvedere), 161; *Vertummus and Pomona* (Hamen y León), 153, 155. *See also* plant illustrations

Spanish America, 59, 69, 78, 70, 175

Spanish botanical expeditions: and inspiration of Hernández's work, 134; and melding of Hernández's native names of plants with binomial Linnaean terms, 135; and missions to complete Hernández's work, 135, 184, 189; to New Spain, 7, 133–35. *See also* Asso, Ignacio de; classification techniques; Jiménez de la Espada, Marcos; Sessé, Martin de

Spanish chroniclers, 106

Spanish colonists, native perceptions of, 108 n. 2

Spanish Crown, 71, 78

Spanish empire, 12–14, 35, 100; in the Caribbean, 141. *See also* Philip II

Spanish Indies, 55, 62

Spanish medicine, 30 n. 15, 33, 35, 36

Spanish monarchy, 12

Spanish plants, 148 n. 13

Spanish Renaissance, 4, 33

Spicelio, Teofilo, 184

squashes (Cucurbitae). *See* plants and plant products

starvation. *See* remedies and treatments

Stelluti, Francesco, 128, 180 n. 28

Stevens, Philip, 140

Still Life with Flowers / Florero (Hiepes) (painting), 159, 162

Still Life with Flowers, Birds, and Fruit / Florero con pájaros y frutas (Arellano) (painting), 166

Still Life with Fruit Basket and Bunches of Grapes / Bodegón con frutero y racimos de uva (Hamen y León) (painting), 158

Still Life with Game / Bodegón con piezas de caza (Sánchez Cotán) (painting), 155

stimulants. *See* remedies and treatments

stomach ache. *See* diseases and symptoms

stomach upsets (intestinal illnesses). *See* diseases and symptoms

Storia antica del Messico (*The Ancient History of Mexico*) (Clavijero), 175–76

stramonium (*Datura stramonium* L.). *See* botanical taxonomies; plants and plant products

Stubbe, Henry, 142, 143, 149 nn. 29,30

Stubbers (Essex). *See* botanical gardens

studia humanitatis, 25

sugar. *See* plants and plant products

Suma y recopilación de cirugía (López de Hinojosos), 76

Sumach. See remedies and treatments

Sumario de la natural y general ystoria de las Indias (Fernández de Oviedo), 164

sunflower. *See* plants and plant products

surgeons, 57, 59, 62, 66, 72. *See also* physicians

surgery, 27, 29

Sutter's Mill, 197

swallow wings, pulverized. *See* remedies and treatments

sweat houses, 70

sweat pad, of mule. *See* remedies and treatments

sweating. *See* remedies and treatments

Swedish Academy of Science. *See* Handilgar

sweet potatoes. *See* plants and plant products

Swift, Jonathan, 177

swine lard. *See* remedies and treatments

symptomatology, 74–75

syphilis: European mortality rates, 77; therapeutic regime, 77. *See also* diseases and symptoms

tabardete (*cocoliztli*). *See* diseases and symptoms

Table of Illnesses and Remedies of this Land. See Hernández's work

Tagetes. See botanical taxonomies

tagetes patula or *damasquina. See* plants and plant products

Taino, 124

Talavera, fray Gabriel de, 46

Talavera, Hernando de (Archbishop of Granada), 45

Tales of a Shaman's Apprentice (Plotkin), 208

tamarinds. *See* plants and plant products

tapir hoof. *See* remedies and treatments